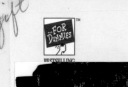

Allergies & Asthma For Dummies

D0599218

Major Myths about Allergies and/or Asthma

The following ideas are myths and misinformation that you may often hear about allergies and asthma. This isn't a true or false test — all of these statements are incorrect! Refer to the chapters in parentheses for the real story about these topics.

- Moving to Arizona will cure my allergies and asthma (Chapter 5).
- A cat or dog with short hair is safer for my allergies and asthma than a long-haired pet (Chapter 6).
- Allergies and asthma are contagious (Chapter 1).
- I can't exercise because I have asthma (See Chapter 11).
- I just have a recurring chest cold. I don't need to check for allergies or asthma (Chapters 4 and 10).
- My children don't need to be evaluated or treated for allergies or asthma because they'll outgrow them anyway (Chapter 14).
- My friends and family say that my allergies or asthma are all in my head (Chapter 1).
- The only medication I'll ever need for my asthma is a quick-relief rescue inhaler such as albuterol, Proventil, or Ventolin (Chapter 12).
- I get stomach cramps and diarrhea every time I drink milk, so I must be allergic to it (Chapter 19).
- Allergic rhinitis (hay fever) is just a minor annoyance and won't cause any serious problems (Chapter 9).
- I can take as many over-the-counter (OTC) medications as I want, because if I don't need a prescription for them, these products probably don't cause any side effects. Besides, because my doctor didn't prescribe them, it's none of his or her business if I'm taking them (Chapters 7 and 12).
- I'm breaking out in hives mainly due to stress, and if I would just calm down they would go away (Chapter 18).
- I should stop taking all my allergy and asthma medication while I'm pregnant (Chapter 15).
- I'll try to drop by my doctor's office for allergy shots when it's convenient for me. I don't need to stick to a regular schedule for immunotherapy (Chapter 8).
- I don't need to check with my doctor. I can just give my child half an adult dose of my asthma or allergy medication (Chapter 14).
- What's the big deal? They're just bunch of annoying little bugs, and no one ever died from an insect sting (Chapter 21).
- Nothing's going to happen during the flight, so why bother packing my asthma and allergy medications in my carry-on bag (Chapter 22)?
- Why waste money on a MedicAlert bracelet just because I had a life-threatening reaction to penicillin? I can just tell the doctor about my allergy if it happens again (Chapter 20).
- I'll figure out how to use an epinephrine kit (AnaKit or EpiPen) when I need it (Chapter 1).
- Not much can be done to improve my asthma, so I'll have to settle for less and just live with my condition (Chapter 23).

AUG   2005

Allergies & Asthma For Dummies®

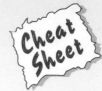
Cheat Sheet

Organs That Allergies and Asthma Affect

Allergies and asthma can affect several organs in the following ways:

- **Eyes:** Allergic conjunctivitis (Chapter 4).
- **Ears:** Otitis media, which is an inflammation of the middle ear, often leading to an ear infection — a frequent complication of allergic rhinitis (Chapter 9).
- **Nose:** Allergic rhinitis, which is the medical term for hay fever (Chapter 4).
- **Sinus:** Sinusitis — inflammation of the sinuses, a frequent complication of allergic rhinitis (Chapter 9).
- **Throat:** Allergic rhinitis and/or pharyngitis (a complication of postnasal drip associated with allergic rhinitis — Chapter 4), generalized reactions to insect stings (Chapter 21), food hypersensitivities (Chapter 19), and drug hypersensitivities (Chapter 20).
- **Airways of lungs:** Asthma (Chapter 10) primarily. Other allergic conditions that can also affect the airways of your lungs include food hypersensitivities (Chapter 19), generalized reactions to insect stings (Chapter 21), drug hypersensitivities (Chapter 20), and anaphylaxis (a widespread, potentially life-threatening reaction that affects many organs simultaneously; Chapter 1).
- **Gastrointestinal tract:** Food hypersensitivities (Chapter 19), generalized reactions to insect stings (Chapter 21), drug hypersensitivities (Chapter 20), and anaphylaxis (Chapter 1).
- **Skin:** Atopic dermatitis (eczema — Chapter 16), allergic contact dermatitis (Chapter 17), urticaria (hives) and angioedema (deep swellings — Chapter 18), and insect sting reactions (Chapter 21).

Dr. Berger's Top Ten List of Allergy Triggers

1. Dust mites (Chapter 5)
2. Pollens from certain grasses, weeds, and trees (Chapter 5)
3. Molds (Chapter 5)
4. Animal danders — especially from cats and dogs (Chapters 6 and 11)
5. Foods — especially peanuts and shellfish (Chapter 19)
6. Insect stings from yellow jackets, honeybees, wasps, hornets, and fire ants (Chapter 21)
7. Drugs — especially penicillin and aspirin and related NSAIDs (Chapter 20)
8. Latex — especially in rubber gloves (Chapters 10 and 17)
9. Nickel — especially in jewelry (Chapter 17)
10. Poison ivy, poison oak, and poison sumac (Chapter 17)

Hungry Minds™

Copyright © 2000 Hungry Minds, Inc.
All rights reserved.

Cheat Sheet $2.95 value. Item 5218-X.

For more information about Hungry Minds,
call 1-800-762-2974.

For Dummies: Bestselling Book Series for Beginners

Praise for Allergies & Asthma For Dummies

"Every person with asthma or allergies should own this book!"

> — Nancy Sander, president, Allergy and Asthma Network•Mothers of Asthmatics, Inc.

"I wish there had been a handbook like this when I was suffering from allergies, going from doctor to doctor, searching for relief. If you constantly suffer from a runny nose, itchy eyes, or a scratchy throat, you might have allergies. If left untreated, these symptoms can lead to more serious health problems. Dr. Berger's book will help you pinpoint your problem and find a solution."

> — Joan Lunden, New York

"Understanding what allergies and asthma are all about can be tricky for anyone, including doctors. But leave it up to Dr. Bill Berger to put everything in its place. He takes complicated subjects and breaks them into pieces that each of us can relate to, without talking down to anyone. This is a book that not only belongs in every home, but in every doctor's office as well."

> — Nancy L. Snyderman, M.D., F.A.C.S., associate professor of otolaryngology, medical correspondent for ABC News

"*Allergies and Asthma For Dummies* empowers the asthmatic patients and their families to understand allergy and asthma treatment in simple and concise terms. Dr. Berger is a nationally recognized allergist who distills tons of information into very readable chapters. It is a wonderful book for patient education."

> — Jean A. Chapman, M.D., M.A.C.P., past president, American College of Allergy, Asthma, and Immunology

"Dr. Bill Berger has a wonderful way of making complicated problems easy to solve. What's great about this book is that it can be read on several different levels — from browsing for a quick answer, to in-depth research that can make the difference in managing a really tough problem. I have it on my bookshelf — and not just for patients either. I've been known to sneak a peek now and then myself! It's a well thought out, entertaining work with great references and resources I use in developing TV spots for my syndicated *60 Second Housecall*."

> — Bob Lanier, M.D., creator and host, *60 Second Housecall*

"Take it from someone who knows what it's like to carry a handful of inhalers . . . THIS IS A BOOK TO BREATHE BY!"

> — Congressman Patrick J. Kennedy (D-RI)

"In *Allergies and Asthma For Dummies*, Dr. Berger takes some of the most difficult medical mechanisms and makes them clear and understandable for the ordinary person. This book answers your most common questions about allergies and asthma in witty, informative prose."

> — Linda B. Ford, M.D., past president, American Lung Association

"Asthma is complex. Anyone with this disease — and their family and friends — needs to understand it and work with it, for a full, active life. This book makes understanding asthma and allergies a whole lot easier. Read it, and you'll see.

> — Mary E. Worstell, M.P.H., executive director, Asthma and Allergy Foundation of America

"A must-read for all allergy sufferers. Dr. Berger has succeeded in simplifying the world of allergic disease while offering individuals who suffer from these disorders a clear and concise insight into their causes, as well as wonderful tips regarding their treatments. You will particularly love his BergerBits and Tips, which are tantalizingly scattered throughout the text. His chapter on food reactions is a classic which artfully deals with a controversial and much debated subject."

> — Phil Lieberman, M.D., past president, American Academy of Allergy, Asthma, and Immunology

"I know some great Olympic swimmers who have overcome their asthma and allergies to win the gold. This book will help keep you off the sidelines and in the race."

— Mark Spitz, winner of nine Olympic gold medals

"Millions of asthma and allergy sufferers now have a comprehensive, up-to-date, and medically correct compendium of self-help information. No patient with asthma or allergies should be without it."

— Rufus E. Lee, M.D., past president, American College of Allergy, Asthma, and Immunology

"Wow! Dr. Berger has captured the essence of what patients need to know. Those who read *Allergies and Asthma For Dummies* will be miles ahead of those who don't. Knowledge is power and that power is definitely here."

— Bruce M. Prenner, M.D., associate clinical professor of pediatrics, division of immunology and allergy, University of California-San Diego School of Medicine

"*Allergies and Asthma for Dummies* is an easy to understand, scientifically accurate tool, which will help patients improve their understanding and care of their allergic disease. The MythBusters sections are a must-read."

— Stanley Fineman, M.D., board of regents, American College of Allergy, Asthma, and Immunology

"*Allergies and Asthma for Dummies!* What a great idea! And Dr. Bill Berger is just the physician to make simple sense of asthma management. One of the nation's best asthma educators for decades, he brings an understanding of asthma that prompts his listeners to take action. You don't have to go to medical school to get your asthma under control. But it does take persistent, daily actions to prevent asthma and to live symptom-free. Then you can achieve anything."

— Nancy Hogshead, Olympic triple gold medallist, attorney and author, *Asthma and Exercise*

"Dr. Berger has a wonderful way of making the reader feel at ease with the tremendous amount of valuable information in this book. I will enthusiastically recommend it to my patients."

— Richard Nicklas, M.D., clinical professor of medicine, George Washington University Medical Center

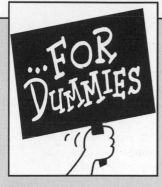
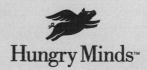

Allergies & Asthma

FOR

DUMMIES®

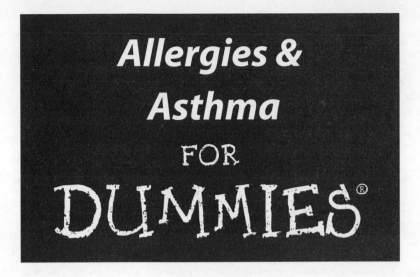

Allergies & Asthma
FOR
DUMMIES®

by William E. Berger, M.D.

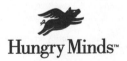

Hungry Minds™

Best-Selling Books • Digital Downloads • e-Books • Answer Networks • e-Newsletters • Branded Web Sites • e-Learning

New York, NY ◆ Cleveland, OH ◆ Indianapolis, IN

Allergies & Asthma For Dummies®

Published by
Hungry Minds, Inc.
909 Third Avenue
New York, NY 10022
www.hungryminds.com
www.dummies.com

Library of Congress Catalog Card No.: 99-69718

ISBN: 0-7654-5218-X

Printed in the United States of America

10 9 8 7 6 5 4 3 2

1O/QT/QU/QQ/IN

Distributed in the United States by Hungry Minds, Inc.

Distributed by CDG Books Canada Inc. for Canada; by Transworld Publishers Limited in the United Kingdom; by IDG Norge Books for Norway; by IDG Sweden Books for Sweden; by IDG Books Australia Publishing Corporation Pty. Ltd. for Australia and New Zealand; by TransQuest Publishers Pte Ltd. for Singapore, Malaysia, Thailand, Indonesia, and Hong Kong; by Gotop Information Inc. for Taiwan; by ICG Muse, Inc. for Japan; by Intersoft for South Africa; by Eyrolles for France; by International Thomson Publishing for Germany, Austria and Switzerland; by Distribuidora Cuspide for Argentina; by LR International for Brazil; by Galileo Libros for Chile; by Ediciones ZETA S.C.R. Ltda. for Peru; by WS Computer Publishing Corporation, Inc., for the Philippines; by Contemporanea de Ediciones for Venezuela; by Express Computer Distributors for the Caribbean and West Indies; by Micronesia Media Distributor, Inc. for Micronesia; by Chips Computadoras S.A. de C.V. for Mexico; by Editorial Norma de Panama S.A. for Panama; by American Bookshops for Finland.

For general information on Hungry Minds' products and services please contact our Customer Care Department within the U.S. at 800-762-2974, outside the U.S. at 317-572-3993 or fax 317-572-4002.

For sales inquiries and reseller information, including discounts, premium and bulk quantity sales, and foreign-language translations, please contact our Customer Care Department at 800-434-3422, fax 317-572-4002, or write to Hungry Minds, Inc., Attn: Customer Care Department, 10475 Crosspoint Boulevard, Indianapolis, IN 46256.

For information on licensing foreign or domestic rights, please contact our Sub-Rights Customer Care Department at 212-884-5000.

For information on using Hungry Minds' products and services in the classroom or for ordering examination copies, please contact our Educational Sales Department at 800-434-2086 or fax 317-572-4005.

Please contact our Public Relations Department at 212-884-5163 for press review copies or 212-884-5000 for author interviews and other publicity information or fax 212-884-5400.

For authorization to photocopy items for corporate, personal, or educational use, please contact Copyright Clearance Center, 222 Rosewood Drive, Danvers, MA 01923, or fax 978-750-4470.

About the Author

William E. Berger, M.D., M.B.A., is one of the nation's foremost experts on allergies and asthma. As a board-certified physician in two separate specialities (Pediatrics and Allergy and Immunology), Dr. Berger has had extensive clinical experience in diagnosing and treating patients with allergies and asthma for more than 20 years. He holds dual appointments at the University of California, Irvine, as Clinical Professor in the College of Medicine, Department of Pediatrics, Division of Allergy and Immunology, and as Adjunct Professor of Health Care Management in the Graduate School of Management. In addition, he has also served as Principal Investigator in numerous clinical research projects.

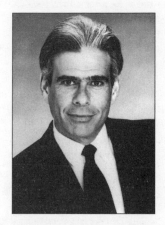

Dr. Berger is a member of the Joint Task Force on Practice Parameters that writes the national treatment guidelines for asthma and allergies. He has served as president of both the Orange County and California Societies of Allergy, Asthma, and Immunology. In recognition of his continued achievement in the specialty of treating allergic diseases, Dr. Berger was awarded the title *Distinguished Fellow* of the American College of Allergy, Asthma, and Immunology.

A former medical correspondent for the Orange County Newschannel, the Medical News Network, and ABC Television Network's *Mike and Maty Show*, Dr. Berger is also the author of many academic papers and lay press articles in the field of allergy, asthma, and immunology. He is a recognized international speaker in the field of allergy and asthma and is frequently invited to lecture at medical conferences and symposia held throughout the world. In addition, Dr. Berger has been the subject of medical reports on allergies and asthma that have appeared on Lifetime Medical Television, *NBC Dateline,* and Cable News Network (CNN). He has also been featured in medical articles published in *Time Magazine, The Wall Street Journal,* the *Los Angeles Times,* and *The Orange County Register.*

Dr. Berger founded the Allergy and Asthma Associates of Southern California Medical Group in 1981 in Mission Viejo, California, where he currently practices both adult and pediatric allergy medicine. In 1995, Dr. Berger established the Southern California Research Center, focusing on respiratory and allergy clinical research studies.

Dedication

This book is dedicated to my wife Charlette, my son Michael, and my daughter Johanna, for their loving encouragement and their inspiring confidence that I would actually get the writing done on time.

Author's Acknowledgments

I especially want to thank Acquisitions Editor Tami Booth, whose vision and foresight actually made this book possible. My project editor, Christy Beck, kept me on track throughout the writing process and insured that this book follows in the great line of the *For Dummies* tradition. I also greatly appreciate the artistry of Kathryn Born, our Medical Illustrator, whose drawings enhance the text.

I am also very grateful to the numerous other people who have made this book possible, most of all my indefatigable senior research editor, Carl Byron, who probably won't miss my midnight telephone calls to review the manuscript. Thanks also to Skye Herzog, agent extraodinaire, part-time psychologist, nurturer, and motivational expert. I am extremely grateful to Francene Lifson, Executive Director of the Southern California Chapter of the Asthma and Allergy Foundation of America, whose assistance was invaluable during the initial stages of this project.

A very special thanks to my friend, Olympic gold medalist Jackie Joyner-Kersee, the world's greatest female athlete, for writing the Foreword to this book and for her unceasing efforts in raising awareness of the importance of early diagnosis and effective treatment of asthma. Jackie has inspired asthmatics throughout the world by proving that having asthma shouldn't prevent you from achieving your goals — no matter what they might be.

I also want to express my deep-felt appreciation to Jean Chapman, M.D., who acted as technical editor for this book and who provided invaluable insights from his many years of experience in the field of allergy and immunology. In addition, thanks to Fred Beams, whose entomological expertise assisted in the editing of the chapter on insect sting hypersensitivity (Chapter 21).

Richard Nicklas, M.D., and Bob Lanier, M.D., also deserve my special thanks for taking time out from their busy schedules to review the manuscript and for providing excellent comments and suggestions.

Also, thanks to the following individuals who have been great friends, outstanding educators, and constant sources of inspiration due to their supreme dedication to providing excellent patient care: Brian Levine, M.D.; Eric Schenkel, M.D.; Joel Cristol, M.D.; Bob Lanier, M.D.; Stanley Galant, M.D.; Sherwin Gillman, M.D.; Charles Siegel, M.D.; Bruce Prenner, M.D.; Joseph Bellanti, M.D.; Phillip Lieberman, M.D.; Ira Finegold, M.D.; Don Mitchell, M.D.; John Zucker, M.D.; Tom Plaut, M.D.; and Mark Wohlgemuth, M.D.

Thanks to my fellow members of the Joint Task Force on Practice Parameters in Allergy, Asthma, and Immunology, including Stanley Fineman, M.D.; Richard Nicklas, M.D.; I. Leonard Bernstein, M.D.; Joann Blessing-Moore, M.D.; Mark S. Dykewicz, M. D.; Rufus Lee, M. D.; James Li, M.D., Ph.D.; Jay Portnoy, M.D.; Diane Schuller, M.D.; and Sheldon Spector, M.D., all of whose extraordinary commitment and hard work in developing and maintaining the highest quality parameters for the care of our patients inspired me to write this book.

I greatly appreciate the information provided by allergy historians Sheldon Cohen, M.D., and Guy Settipane, M.D., whose research helped in developing Chapter 23.

As always, I place special value on the support and understanding of my clinical and research staff, my associates in practice, Mark Sugar, M.D., Janis Davidson, R.N., C.P.N.P., and especially Ellen Schonfeld, R.N., C.P.N.P., who provided invaluable assistance in reviewing the manuscript and researching the illustrations for this book.

I am especially grateful to Georgia Beams and Jennifer Feaser, R.N., who helped me start Allergy and Asthma Associates of Southern California in Mission Viejo more than 20 years ago (we were all 12 years old at the time!) and who have always provided me with their generous support and advice in whatever professional goals and endeavors I have pursued (including this book).

Patient advocate and spokesperson, founder and president of Allergy and Asthma Network•Mothers of Asthmatics, Inc., Nancy Sander also deserves my gratitude for her friendship, insights, and especially for her dedication to raising awareness about asthma and allergies.

Most of all, I would like to thank all of my patients for allowing me the privilege of caring for them and their children. Over the years, I've learned a great deal from them and am a better person and physician for the experience. As Ralph Waldo Emerson once wrote: "To know that even one life has breathed easier because you have lived: That is to have succeeded!"

Publisher's Acknowledgments

We're proud of this book; please register your comments through our Online Registration Form located at www.dummies.com.

Some of the people who helped bring this book to market include the following:

Acquisitions, Editorial, and Media Development

Project Editor: Christine Meloy Beck

Executive Editor: Tammerly Booth

Acquisitions Coordinator: Karen S. Young

Acquisitions Assistant: Allison Solomon

Copy Editor: Billie A. Williams

Technical Editor: Jean A. Chapman, M.D., M.A.C.P.

Editorial Managers: Jennifer Ehrlich, Pamela Mourouzis

Editorial Assistant: Laura Jefferson

Production

Project Coordinator: Maridee V. Ennis

Layout and Graphics: Barry Offringa, Tracy K. Oliver, Jill Piscitelli, Brent Savage, Jacque Schneider, Brian Torwelle, Dan Whetstine, Erin Zeltner

Proofreaders: Laura Albert, Corey Bowen, Rachel Garvey, John Greenough, Marianne Santy

Indexer: Sherry Massey

Special Help

Amanda M. Foxworth, Beth Parlon, Susan Diane Smith, Linda S. Stark

---

Hungry Minds Consumer Reference Group

Business: Kathleen A. Welton, Vice President and Publisher; Kevin Thornton, Acquisitions Manager

Cooking/Gardening: Jennifer Feldman, Associate Vice President and Publisher

Education/Reference: Diane Graves Steele, Vice President and Publisher

Lifestyles/Pets: Kathleen Nebenhaus, Vice President and Publisher; Tracy Boggier, Managing Editor

Travel: Michael Spring, Vice President and Publisher; Suzanne Jannetta, Editorial Director; Brice Gosnell, Publishing Director

Hungry Minds Consumer Editorial Services: Kathleen Nebenhaus, Vice President and Publisher; Kristin A. Cocks, Editorial Director; Cindy Kitchel, Editorial Director

Hungry Minds Consumer Production: Debbie Stailey, Production Director

Contents at a Glance

Cartoons at a Glance

By Rich Tennant

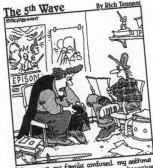

page 7

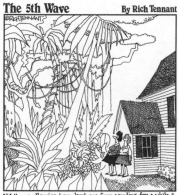

page 309

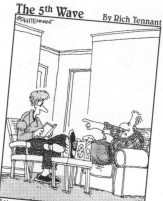

page 53

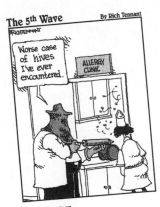

page 257

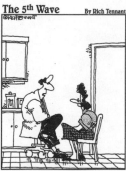

page 139

page 353

Fax: 978-546-7747

E-mail: richtennant@the5thwave.com

World Wide Web: www.the5thwave.com

Table of Contents

Foreword

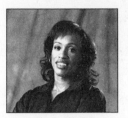

When I was first diagnosed with asthma back in college, I could have used a book like this. I really didn't know what asthma was all about or what I needed to do to manage it.

The truth is, I didn't take my asthma very seriously. I didn't want to think of myself – a serious athlete — as being sick. So I lived in denial. I took rescue medicine when my symptoms acted up, but mostly I tried to ignore it. I thought I could overcome it — that maybe it would go away on its own.

Finally, after one particularly scary attack, it hit me: Instead of controlling my asthma, I was letting my asthma control me.

Now, I work with my doctor and manage my asthma daily. It's made a big difference. My symptoms are much less frequent, and I can do the things I want to do without being limited by my asthma.

The more I talk to people with this disease, the more I realize that my story is a very common one. If symptoms and attacks are interfering with your life or if you limit your activities in order to avoid asthma symptoms, keep in mind that things don't have to be this way.

That's why this book is so useful. It tells you everything you need to know about how to keep your asthma under control, so you don't have to go through what I went through.

Read it carefully, and work with your doctor. Learn what you can do to help prevent symptoms from happening in the first place, and stick with it. Set your sights high, and never settle for less than your personal best.

It's not always easy, but you can do it. Take it from me: With the proper training and attitude, asthma doesn't have to slow you down.

Jackie J. Kersee

Jackie Joyner-Kersee

P. S. Through a program called Asthma All-Stars™ I'm helping others to learn more about asthma. To find out more, see the **FREE OFFER** card inside this book.

Introduction

● ●

"I feel like I'm breathing through a straw." "Oh, my aching sinuses." "I can't stop coughing." "My child keeps scratching his rash." If you've ever uttered words like these, you're not alone. These statements are some of the most frequent medical complaints that people in the United States and around the world report, and their complaints often describe allergy and asthma symptoms.

Allergies and asthma affect at least a quarter of the U.S. population and, when combined, represent the most common conditions seen in current medical practice. Allergies and asthma also prompt more doctors' office visits than any other medical problem. In fact, these ailments cause the greatest number of school and work days lost, affect the lives of millions of sufferers and their families, and cost billions of dollars annually in medical services and medications.

But enough about facts and figures. I want to talk about you: How are you feeling? Do you, or someone you know, think that having allergies or asthma means that feeling unwell is normal and that your condition can never improve? Unfortunately, many people answer yes to this question. However, as I explain throughout this book, the plain, simple, and accurate medical truth is this: Although no cures exist for allergies and asthma, when you receive effective, appropriate care from your doctor, combined with your motivated participation as a patient, you can lead a normal, active, and fulfilling life.

About This Book

I wrote this book to give you sound, up-to-date, practical advice, based on my over 20 years of experience with numerous patients, about dealing with your asthma and allergies effectively and appropriately. For that reason, I've structured this book so that you can jump to sections that most directly apply to your medical condition. You don't need to read this book from cover to cover, although I won't object if you do. (Be careful, though, because once you start reading, you may have a really hard time putting it down!)

This book can also serve as a reference and source for information about the many facets of diagnosing, treating, and managing allergy and asthma conditions. Although you may pick up this book for one form of allergy or asthma, you may realize later that other topics in here also apply to you or a loved one.

Don't worry about remembering where related subjects are in this book. I provide ample cross-references in every chapter that remind you where to look for the information you may need in other chapters or within other sections of the chapter that you're reading.

I intend the information in this book to empower you as a person with allergies and/or asthma, thus helping you to:

- Set goals for your treatment.
- Ensure that you receive the most appropriate and effective medical care for your allergy and asthma condition.
- Do your part as a patient by adhering to the treatment plan that you and your physician develop.

Foolish Assumptions

I don't think I'm being too foolish, but while writing this book, I assumed that you want substantive, scientifically accurate, relevant information about allergies and asthma, presented in everyday language, without a lot of medical mumbo-jumbo. In this book, you find straightforward explanations when I present important scientific aspects of allergies and asthma and when I use key medical terms. (You also get a chance to work on your Latin and Greek.)

If you've chosen to read my book, I know you're no dummy, so I'm willing to go out on a limb and make some further assumptions about you, dear reader:

- You or someone you care about suffers from some type of allergic condition and/or asthma.
- You want to educate yourself about allergies and asthma as part of improving your medical condition (in consultation with your doctor, of course).
- You want to feel better.
- You really like doctors named Bill.

How This Book Is Organized

I've structured this book in six parts, based on the major allergic ailments, to help you find the information you need as easily as possible.

Part I: Allergy and Asthma Basics

This part helps you determine what may affect you, explaining how allergies and asthma present themselves, the underlying immune system mechanisms involved in allergy and asthma ailments, and how you can — as well as why you should — get a proper diagnosis of your condition.

Part II: Taking Care of Your Nose

Part II discusses the triggers of allergic rhinitis (hay fever), the effects the ailment can have on many parts of your body, how those effects occur, the types of complications frequently associated with the condition, and what you and your doctor can do to effectively treat your problem.

You also discover ways of avoiding allergens and irritants, as well as appropriate medications that you can take to control and prevent your symptoms. Likewise, I explain why immunotherapy (allergy shots) may successfully manage your allergic rhinitis long-term.

Part III: Asthma: A Disease in Search of Good Management

In this part, you find an extensive discussion concerning the underlying inflammatory mechanism that characterizes asthma, what you need to know about how your doctor diagnoses your condition and avoiding triggers of this disease, the range of long-term and quick-relief medications that your doctor may prescribe for you, and essential information about developing an effective long-term asthma management plan. I also include chapters that focus on taking care of a child with asthma and on continuing your asthma treatment during pregnancy.

Part IV: Allergic Skin Conditions: Beauty Is Only Skin Deep

If you wonder why many people refer to atopic dermatitis (allergic eczema) as the "itch that scratches, or the scratch that itches," this part of the book is for you. In Chapter 16, I explain the atopic dermatitis condition, what can trigger it, how you can relieve the symptoms, and steps you can take to prevent your eczema from recurring.

The chapter on allergic contact dermatitis (17) explains the extensive range of substances in your everyday life (such as nickel and rubber) that can trigger skin (topical) reactions. I also provide vital tips for dealing with poison ivy, important preventive measures for avoiding exposures to other allergic contact dermatitis triggers, and advisable treatments for relieving symptoms if you experience them.

Chapter 18 deals with urticaria (hives) and angioedema (deep swellings). Urticaria and angioedema are two of the more perplexing problems known to allergists, primarily because most cases of these skin eruptions aren't due to allergic reactions.

Part V: Food, Drug, and Insect Reactions: A Really Bad Trip

Are your allergies what you eat? Mostly, no, as I explain in Chapter 19. However, identifying the type of food mishaps you experience, the specific foods that cause them, what you need to do about them, and how you can avoid those problems in the future is important. In fact, finding the answers to all these questions is especially important if you determine that you have a true food hypersensitivity (allergy), rather than a form of food intolerance.

I also deal with adverse drug reactions in Chapter 20. Understanding what may affect you is vital, because you can take steps to avoid potentially serious reactions, especially to medications such as penicillin or aspirin and related non-steroidal anti-inflammatory drugs (NSAIDs.)

In Chapter 21, I explain why having a sensitivity to the venom of *Hymenoptera* insects (honeybees, yellow jackets, wasps, hornets, and fire ants) is serious business. I also provide important and practical steps that you can take to avoid painful encounters with these creatures.

Part VI: The Part of Tens

All *Dummies* books contain one of these parts. The chapters in this part offer information that simply fits better in this more informal format, such as:

- ✔ What you need to take with you — and practical information and steps you should take into account — when traveling with allergies and asthma.
- ✔ Examples of significant people, from ancient times to today, who have excelled in many impressive ways in spite of their asthma.

Appendix

The appendix at the back of the book is a compendium of valuable allergy and asthma resources, information on numerous important allergy and asthma organizations, and suppliers and manufacturers of environmental control products that can greatly assist you in managing your condition. I've also included listings of other important books and information sources about allergies and asthma, and, of course, a survey of quality allergy and asthma Web sites.

Icons Used in This Book

Throughout the margins of the book, you'll see the following icons. They're intended to catch your attention and alert you to the type of information I present in particular paragraphs. Here's what they mean:

The Berger Bit icon represents me expressing my opinion on a topic.

A Caution icon advises you about potential problems, such as symptoms you shouldn't ignore or treatments that you may not want to undergo.

Spotting the Medicalese icon means that you are about to encounter medical and scientific terms. If it's all Greek to you, don't worry; I explain the technical terms that I use throughout the book.

Myths and misconceptions abound about allergies and asthma. (How about a little alliteration?) The Mythbuster icon indicates that I expose and correct mistaken beliefs that many people hold about allergies and asthma.

The Remember icon indicates things you shouldn't forget, because you may find the information useful in the future. (Now, where did I put my car keys?)

The See Your Doctor icon alerts you to matters that you should discuss with your physician.

To give you as full a picture as possible of allergy and asthma, I occasionally get into more complex details of medical science. The Technical Stuff icon lets you know that's what I'm doing so that you can delve into the topic further — or skip it. You don't have to read these paragraphs to understand the subject at hand. (However, reading the information with these icons may give you a better handle on managing your medical condition, as well as providing some great material for impressing your friends at your next party.)

You can find lots of helpful information and advice in paragraphs marked with the Tip icon.

Where to Go from Here

Although you can read this book from cover to cover if you want, I suggest turning to the table of contents (alright, check out Rich Tennant's cartoons first) and finding the sections that apply to your immediate concern. Then begin reading your way to better management of your allergies and asthma.

Part I
Allergy and Asthma Basics

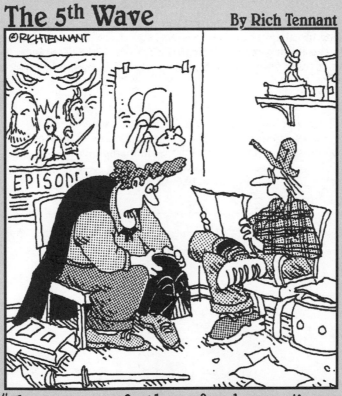

The 5th Wave   By Rich Tennant

"For years my family confused my asthma for a bad cold, bronchitis, or an obsessive need to do Darth Vader impersonations."

In this part . . .

You're experiencing symptoms that indicate you may have allergies or asthma, but you're not sure what your problem is. How do you figure out what's ailing you?

This part helps you determine what may be affecting you by explaining the signs and symptoms of allergies and asthma, the underlying mechanisms involved in allergic ailments, and how you can — as well as why you should — get a proper diagnosis of your condition.

Chapter 1

Knowing What's Ailing You

*I*f you wonder why this book covers both allergies and asthma, let me assure you that I don't cover both of these topics just because they begin with the same letter of the alphabet. In fact, allergies and asthma are like apples and oranges. Yes, you read that right: Apples and oranges are distinct, separate entities, but both are fruits, both grow on trees, and both share many other attributes as well. A similar relationship exists between allergies and asthma. In this chapter, I explain that relationship and also provide an overview of allergy and asthma conditions that I cover throughout this book.

Understanding How Allergies and Asthma Relate to Each Other

Allergy is a descriptive term for a wide variety of hypersensitivity disorders (meaning that you are excessively sensitive to one or more substances to which most people do not normally react), while *asthma* denotes a specific disease process of the lungs. Although they're two distinct topics with different definitions, allergy and asthma share a strong bond, often coexisting as partners in disease. Fully understanding either topic requires understanding them both.

Think of allergy and asthma as two distinct avenues with major intersections, like Broadway and 42nd Street or Hollywood and Vine. In order to be an aware and involved patient, you often have to travel down both pathways.

Living a healthy, fulfilling life with allergies and/or asthma involves many of the same general diagnostic, treatment, and preventive measures that I explain throughout this book. In fact, the symptoms of seemingly disparate ailments such as allergic rhinitis (hay fever), most cases of asthma, atopic dermatitis (allergic eczema), and other allergic conditions basically result from your immune system's similar, hyperreactive response to otherwise harmless substances that doctors refer to as *allergens*.

The word *allergy* is the ancient Greek term for an abnormal response or over-reaction. Contrary to popular belief, weak or deficient immune systems don't cause asthma or allergy ailments. Rather, your body's defenses work over-time, making your immune system too sensitive to substances that pose no real threat to your well-being. That's why physicians often use the term *hyper-sensitivity* to refer to an allergy.

These are the main points to keep in mind when dealing with asthma and allergies:

- ✔ Allergies aren't just hay fever. In addition to affecting your nose, sinuses, eyes, and throat (as in typical cases of allergic rhinitis), exposure to allergy triggers can also cause symptoms that involve other organs of your body, including your lungs, skin, and digestive tract. Figure 1-1 shows all the organs in your body that allergies and asthma can affect.

- ✔ These ailments are not infectious or contagious. You don't catch an allergy or asthma. However, as I explain in "Sensitizing your immune system," later in this chapter, you may inherit a genetic predisposition to develop hypersensitivities that can eventually appear as allergies and/or asthma.

- ✔ Allergies and asthma aren't like trends or shoe sizes. You don't really outgrow them. Extensive studies over the past 15 years show that although your ailment can certainly vary in character and severity over your lifetime, it's an ongoing physical condition that is most likely always present in some form.

- ✔ Allergy and asthma triggers include allergens such as pollens, animal dander, dust mites, mold spores, various contact allergens, and certain foods, drugs, and venom from stinging insects. (See "Sensitizing your immune system," later in this chapter, for more detailed classifications of these items.)

- ✔ Asthmatic reactions can also result from nonallergic triggers that act as irritants, including tobacco smoke, household cleaners, aerosol products, solvents, chemicals, fumes, gases, paints, smoke, and indoor and outdoor air pollution.

✔ Other forms of nonallergic triggers that primarily affect people with asthma are known as *precipitating factors* and include other medical conditions such as rhinitis, sinusitis, gastroesophageal reflux (GER), and viral infections (colds, flu); physical stimuli such as exercise or variations in both air temperature and humidity levels; and sensitivities to food additives such as sulfites, drugs such as beta-blockers (Inderal, Lopressor, Corgard, Timoptic), and aspirin and related over-the-counter nonsteroidal anti-inflammatory drugs (NSAIDs) such as ibuprofen (Advil, Motrin), ketoprofen (Actron, Orudis), naproxen (Aleve), and newer prescription NSAIDs known as COX-2 inhibitors, including celecoxib (Celebrex) and rofecoxib (Vioxx).

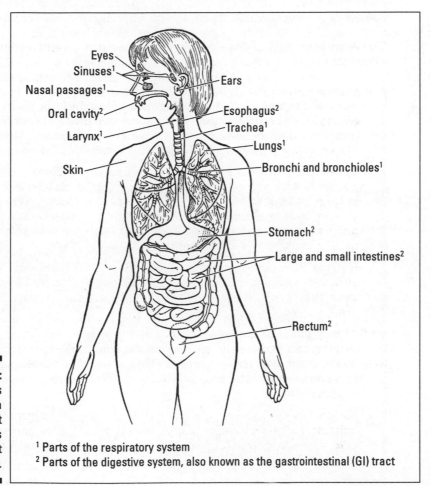

Figure 1-1: Allergies and asthma can affect organs throughout your body.

Eyes
Sinuses[1]
Nasal passages[1]
Oral cavity[2]
Larynx[1]
Skin
Ears
Esophagus[2]
Trachea[1]
Lungs[1]
Bronchi and bronchioles[1]
Stomach[2]
Large and small intestines[2]
Rectum[2]

[1] Parts of the respiratory system
[2] Parts of the digestive system, also known as the gastrointestinal (GI) tract

✔ Allergies and asthma aren't mutually exclusive conditions. Having one type of hypersensitivity doesn't prevent you from developing others. You can have multiple sensitivities to different types of allergens, irritants, and precipitating factors. Many researchers (including myself) consider allergic disorders a continuum of disease that can appear in many ways, depending on the nature and degree of your sensitivities, as well as your levels of exposure to triggers.

✔ All that sneezes, drips, runs, congests, wheezes, waters, coughs, itches, erupts, or swells is not always due to an allergic reaction. That's why, as I explain in "Diagnosing and Treating Your Allergies and Asthma: The Basics" (later in this chapter), the first step to effectively treating the underlying cause of your symptoms is properly diagnosing your ailment.

✔ Although the majority of people with asthma also have allergies (and allergic rhinitis in most cases), some manifestations of asthma seem to develop without an allergic component. In cases of adult-onset asthma, which often develops in people over 40 and is less common than child-onset asthma, *atopy* (a genetic tendency toward developing allergic hypersensitivity; see the next section) doesn't appear to play an important role. Instead, precipitating factors such as sinusitis, gastroesophageal reflux (GER), nasal polyps, and sensitivities to aspirin and related NSAIDs are more likely to trigger this condition.

Triggering Allergic Reactions

Your immune system acts as your second line of defense against foreign substances. The main barrier against foreign substances is your largest organ — your skin. (Remember that for your next appearance on *Who Wants to Be a Millionaire?*)

Usually your immune system protects you against infectious bacteria, viruses, parasites, and other harmful agents by producing antibodies that learn to recognize the invaders and subsequently fend them off without too much fuss. In fact, most of the time, as long as your immune system works well, you may not even know that this constant, ongoing process takes place to ensure your survival and good health.

However, with an allergic condition, your immune system overproduces antibodies against typically harmless or inoffensive substances such as pollens. *Atopy* (the genetic susceptibility that can predispose your immune system to develop hypersensitivities) is the inherited characteristic that usually determines why some people's immune systems overreact and mount full-scale assaults when exposed to allergens, while others can ignore or innocuously eliminate these substances.

All in the atopic family

Your genetically-determined allergic predisposition (atopy) may present itself through different allergic conditions and target organs. This predisposition and a family history of allergies are the strongest predictors that you may develop asthma and/or other allergic conditions such as allergic rhinitis (hay fever), atopic dermatitis (allergic eczema), and food or drug hypersensitivities.

For example, your Uncle Ed may have allergic rhinitis, your sister may suffer from recurrent sinus and ear infections, and cousin Al may have a childhood history of atopic dermatitis. Some of your especially unlucky relatives may even be "blessed" with a combination of all these allergic conditions, plus asthma, over the course of their lifetime. (If you want to be the most popular member of your family, buy them a copy of this book.)

A typical atopic family history could consist of a person having atopic dermatitis as an infant, developing common atopic complications such as otitis (ear infections — see Chapter 9) as a toddler, experiencing noticeable symptoms of allergic rhinitis in later childhood, and then developing asthma as a teenager.

However, an atopic history doesn't appear to put you at greater risk than the general population for developing allergic contact dermatitis (see Chapter 17) or allergic reactions to insect stings (see Chapter 21). These conditions seem to affect nonallergic and allergic people alike, for reasons that I explain in Chapter 2.

Sensitizing your immune system

A complex sensitization process, in which your immune system responds to allergens, causes allergic reactions. Allergens that your immune system may respond to include the following:

- ✔ Dust mites (see Chapter 5).

- ✔ Pollens from certain grasses, weeds, and trees (see Chapter 5).

- ✔ Mold spores (see Chapter 5).

- ✔ Dander from many animals, including cats, dogs, rabbits, birds, and horses, as well as gerbils and other pet rodents (see Chapters 6 and 11).

- ✔ Foods, including peanuts, fish, shellfish, and tree nuts (in adults) and milk, eggs, soy, and wheat (primarily in children). See Chapter 19 for more details.

- ✔ The venom of stinging insects, including honeybees, wasps, yellow jackets, hornets, and fire ants, all of which belong to the *Hymenoptera* order of insects (see Chapter 21).

✔ Drugs, including penicillin and cephalosporins (see Chapter 20).

✔ Contact allergens (see Chapter 17) such as poison ivy, oak, and sumac, as well as allergenic substances such as latex, nickel, and formaldehyde, which you can find in many everyday items. (See "Allergic contact dermatitis: Touching experiences," later in this chapter.)

Developing an allergic reaction

If you're predisposed to developing allergies, here's how a typical sensitization process and allergic reaction can develop, using ragweed pollen, one of the most common triggers of allergic rhinitis, as an example (you can find more details about this process in Chapter 2):

1. Ragweed pollen enters your body, usually as a result of inhaling it through your nose.

2. Your immune system detects the presence of these foreign substances in your body and stimulates the production of *IgE antibodies,* a special class of antibodies.

3. IgE antibodies attach themselves to the surfaces of mast cells that line tissues throughout your body, especially in your nose, eyes, lungs, and skin.

4. Your body designs IgE antibodies to counter specific substances.

   Your immune system is a magnificent memory machine: Unlike you or me, it hardly ever forgets a face. After sensitization occurs, you'll likely experience allergies to that substance for most of your life. With ragweed, for example, your immune system produces specific IgE antibodies with receptor sites that allow ragweed allergens to cross-link two of the IgE ragweed-specific antibodies. The IgE antibodies work like a lock on the mast cell surface, and the allergen is the key. When the ragweed allergen connects with two IgE antibodies on the mast cell surface, the bridging or docking mechanism unlocks the mast cell.

5. Unlocking the mast cell initiates the secretion of histamine, leukotrienes, and other potent chemical mediators of inflammation as a defensive response to the allergen. In turn, the actions of these chemicals trigger the swelling and inflammation that result in familiar allergy symptoms.

Doctors frequently use antihistamines to relieve allergy symptoms because histamine plays such an important role in the inflammatory process. In addition, as I explain in Chapters 7 and 12, in the last two decades, government-funded and pharmaceutical researchers have developed more specialized drugs to counter and/or inhibit some of the more fundamental allergic processes. In particular, inhaled topical corticosteroids, mast cell stabilizers, and leukotriene modifiers provide new therapeutic approaches to preventing and controlling symptoms of allergic and asthmatic reactions.

Managing Allergic Disease Effectively

In most parts of the world, allergies and asthma cause a wide range of problems for millions of people. Allergy and asthma problems can involve occasional minor symptoms, serious episodes and attacks, and even potentially life-threatening reactions (in the most severe and rare cases).

However, thanks to recent medical breakthroughs in our understanding of the underlying allergic and immunological factors involved in allergic reactions, it's now possible in most cases to properly diagnose what's ailing you and to develop an appropriate and effective treatment plan for controlling your symptoms and managing your condition.

Effectively managing allergic conditions — particularly asthma and allergic rhinitis — frequently requires dealing with an assortment of symptoms, treatments, and preventive measures, because allergies and asthma tend to be ailments with many faces. Think of a typical Chinese restaurant menu: You may need to order dishes from different columns in order to have a complete meal.

Previewing Allergic Conditions

Consider this part of the chapter a preview of coming reactions. In the following sections, I summarize the significant features of the most common allergic diseases and provide important details about distinguishing them from nonallergic conditions that are similar. I also include references to the chapters where I discuss these ailments in more extensive detail.

Allergic rhinitis: Running away with your nose

Frequently referred to as *hay fever,* allergic rhinitis is the most common allergic disease in the U.S. As many as 45 million Americans or more suffer from some form of this allergy. Trademark symptoms of allergic rhinitis include runny nose with clear, watery discharge; stuffy nose; sneezing; postnasal drip; and scratchy nose, ears, palate, and throat. In addition, itchy and watery eyes, symptoms of *allergic conjunctivitis,* are often associated with allergic rhinitis. Infections of the middle ear (otitis media) and of the sinuses (sinusitis) are frequent complications of allergic rhinitis.

Part II includes several chapters on the many forms of allergic and nonallergic rhinitis, as well as the ways doctors diagnose and treat these ailments (including allergic conjunctivitis), important tips on avoiding triggers of various types of rhinitis, details on medications, and information on the complications of allergic rhinitis symptoms.

Asthma: Breathing and wheezing

The most fundamental definition of *asthma* is: a chronic, inflammatory airway disease of the lungs that causes breathing problems. However, in practice, asthma has many faces and is often difficult to recognize and properly diagnose. As a result, even though currently available prescription medications offer effective ways of relieving, preventing, and controlling the symptoms and underlying *inflammation* (redness, swelling, congestion, and disruption of normal processes of the airways of your lungs) that characterize asthma, the disease continues to cause serious problems for many people worldwide.

Inflammation of the airways (bronchial tubes) is the most important underlying factor in asthma. In the vast majority of cases, if you have asthma, your symptoms may come and go, but the underlying inflammation usually persists.

Asthma's characteristic symptoms are coughing, wheezing, shortness of breath, chest tightness, and productive coughs (coughs that produce mucus). Important symptoms of asthma in infancy and early childhood include wheezing, persistent coughing, and recurring or lingering chest colds. (Because of its symptoms, asthma in children is often misdiagnosed as recurring bronchitis, recurring chest colds, or lingering coughs.)

As I mention in the first part of this chapter, asthma and allergies resemble avenues and streets that frequently intersect. In an overwhelming number of cases, asthma — like most allergies — is a manifestation of *atopy* (the genetic tendency toward developing hypersensitivity to allergens). In fact, many people with asthma also have allergic rhinitis.

The hyperreactive response of the sensitized immune system to asthmatic triggers (typically inhalant allergens, such as dander and dust mites, as well as other substances, including irritants, that also trigger allergic rhinitis symptoms) is usually the main factor in aggravating the underlying airway inflammation (see Chapter 10 for a detailed explanation of this process).

I devote Part III of this book to extensive discussions of asthma, including diagnosis, treatment, avoiding asthma triggers, asthma medications, long-term asthma management, and special considerations involving asthma during pregnancy and childhood.

Atopic dermatitis: Scratching your itch

Also described as *atopic eczema* or *allergic eczema,* atopic dermatitis is an allergic condition that targets your body's largest organ — your skin. The simplest way to define this non-contagious skin condition is the itch that scratches (or the "itch that rashes").

It's in your airways, not in your head

For centuries, many people believed that psychological factors such as anxiety, emotional disorders, or stress caused asthma. However, although these problems can *aggravate* asthma or allergies, they do not *cause* asthma or allergies.

Unfortunately, I still hear about the friends and family of asthmatics who claim that asthma is all in the patient's head. Some of these people insist that if the person would just calm down, his or her condition would go away. Actually, instead of stress causing asthma, it can be the other way around: Breathing problems can cause stress. Stressing out because you can't breathe is a perfectly normal and understandable response.

Therefore, a proper diagnosis of asthma and/or allergies and early, aggressive treatment for these conditions are crucial. In most cases, you should be able to control your asthma and allergy condition so that it doesn't control you, thus enabling you to lead a full and active life. Forget the negative stereotypes of asthmatics and people with allergies as nerdy, weak, anxious types, forever coughing and blowing their noses. Asthma and allergies can affect anyone: from the captain of the school chess team to the captain of the football team, as well as everybody in between.

"The itch that scratches" refers to the itch-scratch cycle, the hallmark of atopic dermatitis. Scratching your dry skin causes more irritation and inflammation, further damaging your skin and making it even itchier — resulting in more scratching and increasingly irritated skin. Eventually, fissures and cracks can develop on your skin, allowing irritants, bacteria, and viruses to enter, often leading to complicating infections.

Atopic dermatitis frequently occurs with allergic rhinitis and can also precede other allergic symptoms. As such, atopic dermatitis can provide an early clue that you're at risk of developing other allergies and asthma.

This section just scratches the surface of information on atopic dermatitis. If you're itching for more, see Chapter 16.

Allergic contact dermatitis: Touching experiences

Although you may not know it, you're probably already familiar with allergic contact dermatitis, because one of the most common triggers of this condition is poison ivy and other related plants of the *Toxicodendron* family. Other important triggers include latex, nickel, and formaldehyde.

The characteristic signs of allergic contact dermatitis include a red rash, swollen pimples, blisters, and itchy skin. These symptoms may appear hours to days after your skin contacts an allergen, and they usually develop where the allergen touches the skin. As you may expect, the point of allergen entry is where the skin usually shows the most severe inflammation. Chapter 17 provides more detailed information on diagnosing and treating allergic contact dermatitis, avoiding triggers of this allergy, and preventing poison ivy from ruining your picnic or camping trip.

Urticaria and angioedema: Breaking out and swelling up

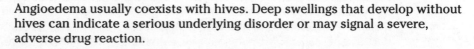

Urticaria and *angioedema,* better known as hives and deep swellings, can present perplexing problems. Figuring out why hives happen could give you hives — if that weren't one of the most common misconceptions about these skin eruptions. In fact, contrary to popular belief, stress and other psychological factors are not the primary causes of hives but may possibly aggravate a pre-existing condition.

Another common myth is that hives and angioedema (deep swellings) always result from allergic reactions. In fact, although allergies can cause some cases of *acute* (rapid onset) hives and angioedema, more often these eruptions occur as a result of nonallergic mechanisms, especially in cases of chronic hives.

Angioedema usually coexists with hives. Deep swellings that develop without hives can indicate a serious underlying disorder or may signal a severe, adverse drug reaction.

The most common allergic triggers of hives and angioedema are

- Food hypersensitivities, especially to peanuts, tree nuts, milk, eggs, fish, shellfish, soybean, and fruits such as melons and berries. (See Chapter 19 for more information on food allergies.)

- Insect stings from insects of the *Hymenoptera* order (honeybees, yellow jackets, wasps, hornets, and fire ants) can often cause small, localized hives that develop into blisters if you're sensitized to the venom of these insects. In rare cases, *anaphylaxis,* a life-threatening reaction that affects many organs simultaneously (see "Anaphylaxis: Severe systemic symptoms," later in this chapter), can follow an insect sting. See Chapter 21 for more information on insect stings.

- Medications, including penicillin, sulfa drugs, and other antibiotics; aspirin and nonsteroidal anti-inflammatory drugs (NSAIDs); insulin; narcotic pain relievers; muscle relaxants; and tranquilizers can trigger systemic hives and angioedema if you have sensitivities to allergens in these products. (See Chapter 20 for more information on drug reactions.)

Chapter 18 goes into much deeper detail about hives and angioedema.

Food hypersensitivities: Serving up allergens

Most adverse food reactions aren't the result of true *food hypersensitivities* (the more precise term for food allergies). In fact, various forms of food intolerance, food poisoning, and other nonallergic mechanisms cause the majority of reactions that most people blame on food allergies.

The most frequent triggers of actual food hypersensitivities are proteins in the following foods:

✔ Peanuts and other legumes, including soybeans, peas, lentils, beans, and foods containing these ingredients

✔ Shellfish, including shrimp, lobster, crab, clams, and oysters

✔ Fish, both freshwater and saltwater

✔ Tree nuts, including almonds, Brazil nuts, cashews, hazelnuts, and walnuts

✔ Eggs, especially egg whites

✔ Cow's milk, including products that contain casein and whey

✔ Wheat and other grains and cereals, such as corn, rice, barley, and oats

In cases in which mouth and lip swelling, wheezing, or hives occur immediately after consuming a particular food (peanuts, for example), you may easily deduce that an allergic process caused your reaction. However, in many other instances, distinguishing between food intolerance and true food hypersensitivity can require more extensive diagnostic procedures. If you're hungry for more information on adverse food reactions, see Chapter 19.

Drug hypersensitivities: Taking the wrong medicine

Certain drugs are prone to produce allergic reactions in susceptible individuals. The most frequent type of adverse allergic reactions to medications occurs with penicillin and its related compounds. Aspirin and related nonsteroidal anti-inflammatory drugs (NSAIDs) — including newer prescription NSAIDs, known as COX-2 inhibitors, such as celecoxib (Celebrex) and rofecoxib (Vioxx) — and other drugs can also trigger adverse reactions. As with adverse food reactions, most adverse drug reactions result from nonallergic mechanisms, as I discuss in Chapter 20.

Although drug hypersensitivity reactions most frequently target the skin, adverse allergic reactions to drugs can affect any organ system in your body, including mucous membranes, lymph nodes, kidneys, liver, lungs, and joints. These reactions can include skin rashes, hives and angioedema, respiratory symptoms such as coughing or wheezing, fever (sometimes resulting in drug fever, occasionally with shaking chills and a skin rash), and low blood pressure and/or anemia, resulting from an adverse reaction that destroys your red blood cells.

In less frequent but more serious cases, an adverse drug reaction can result in *anaphylaxis,* a severe, potentially life-threatening response that affects many organs simultaneously (see "Anaphylaxis: Severe systemic symptoms," later in this chapter). In fact, penicillin injections cause most drug-related anaphylactic deaths in the U.S. (Fortunately, the use of penicillin shots has significantly decreased in recent years.) For more information on drug hypersensitivities, see Chapter 20.

Stinging insects: The wrong kind of buzz

The venom of stinging insects from the *Hymenoptera* order (honeybees, yellow jackets, wasps, hornets, and fire ants) can trigger allergic reactions in people who are sensitized to those allergens. Reactions range from discomfort, swelling, itching, and hives to, in rare cases, potentially life-threatening anaphylaxis.

Like allergic contact dermatitis, insect-sting hypersensitivities are equal-opportunity allergies. Having other allergic conditions, such as allergic rhinitis, asthma, atopic dermatitis, or food allergies, or a family history of atopy puts you at no greater risk than anyone else for experiencing an allergic reaction to stings from these insects.

In Chapter 21, I provide extensive details on these insects and how you can avoid venomous encounters with them.

Anaphylaxis: Severe systemic symptoms

Anaphylaxis, an ultimate but thankfully rare form of allergic reaction, involves a severe, potentially life-threatening response that affects many organs simultaneously. The characteristic signs of anaphylaxis include

- ✔ Flushing (sudden reddening of skin)
- ✔ Dramatic itching over the entire body
- ✔ Itchy rash or hives
- ✔ Nausea, vomiting, abdominal pain, and/or diarrhea

> ✔ Swelling of the throat and/or tongue (limbs may also swell)
>
> ✔ Difficulty breathing
>
> ✔ Dizziness or fainting
>
> ✔ Severe drop in blood pressure

The most frequent causes of anaphylaxis in the U.S. are extreme allergic reactions to the following allergens:

> ✔ Venom from stinging insects of the *Hymenoptera* order
>
> ✔ Drugs such as penicillin and related compounds
>
> ✔ Foods — particularly peanuts and shellfish

In addition, *pseudoallergic reactions* (see Chapter 20) caused by drugs such as aspirin or related over-the-counter nonsteroidal anti-inflammatory drugs (NSAIDs) like ibuprofen (Advil, Motrin), ketoprofen (Actron, Orudis), naproxen (Aleve), and newer prescription NSAIDs, known as COX-2 inhibitors, including celecoxib (Celebrex) and rofecoxib (Vioxx), can (in some cases) lead to severe, potentially life-threatening reactions referred to as *anaphylactoid reactions.* These reactions are immediate, systemic reactions that closely resemble anaphylaxis but are not caused by IgE-mediated allergic responses.

If you are at risk for anaphylaxis, you should be prepared to take emergency measures to prevent this type of extremely serious reaction. Consult with your doctor about prescribing an emergency kit (such as EpiPen or AnaKit) that contains an injectable dose of epinephrine.

Dyeing your allergies

Inhaled topical corticosteroids, which are often used as asthma and allergy treatments — including beclomethasone (Vanceril, Vancenase), fluticasone (Flovent, Flonase), and other inhaled topical corticosteroid products that I list in Chapter 12 — are extremely effective in suppressing the inflammatory process. Keep in mind, however, that most asthma and allergy drugs treat the end result of a long, complex chain of immune system reactions but don't fundamentally prevent the underlying process causing your ailment. Therefore, if you stop taking your prescribed medications, the underlying disease process most likely restarts and your clinical symptoms reappear.

I compare this process to dyeing your hair. You can change your hair color, but if you don't continue coloring it (like treating your asthma and allergies with your prescribed medicine), your new hair growth comes in with its original color, because you haven't really altered its underlying, genetically determined characteristics.

Make sure that your doctor shows you how to use the kit. Learning the proper technique for administering epinephrine in your physician's office is much more effective than trying it out for the first time while you're having a reaction.

Because anaphylaxis is such a serious issue and can result from various types of exposures, I address it throughout the book, wherever applicable.

Diagnosing and Treating Your Allergies and Asthma: The Basics

The basic components of effectively managing asthma and allergies include the following steps:

- **Getting a proper diagnosis of your condition.** Identifying the specific allergens, irritants, and/or precipitating factors that may trigger your ailment is a critical component of your diagnosis. Cough medicine is not the treatment for your cough if you have asthma. First finding out *why* you're coughing (cough may be the only obvious symptom of underlying asthma in certain patients) is vital so you can then take appropriate steps to effectively control and manage your condition.

- **Avoiding or reducing exposures to allergens, irritants, and precipitating factors that may trigger your asthma and/or allergies.** Effective avoidance and allergy-proofing measures (see Chapters 6 and 11) can significantly improve your quality of life and often reduce, or in certain cases eliminate, your need for medication.

- **Taking long-term preventive medications to control your underlying condition while appropriately using short-term medications when you experience flare-ups, episodes, or attacks.** (I provide extensive information on prescription and over-the-counter allergy and asthma products in Chapters 7 and 12.)

- **Evaluating and monitoring your condition.**

- **Adhering to your treatment plan and keeping yourself informed about all aspects of your condition.**

- **Keeping yourself in good general health to avoid developing more severe symptoms or potential complications of your ailment and to help you enjoy the highest quality of life possible.**

Chapter 2

Understanding Allergy and Asthma

* *

In This Chapter

▶ Understanding the immunologic basis of your allergic condition

▶ Sensitizing your immune system

▶ Classifying your immune system's allergic responses

▶ Testing for potential immunodeficiencies

▶ Improving your quality of life with immunotherapy

* *

*I*n terms of germs, the world can still be a rough place. Despite major advances during the last 100 years in fighting infectious diseases and providing effective medical care for increasing numbers of people, viruses, bacteria, fungi, and other potentially harmful agents remain constant threats to your health. That's why your body's defense network is so important to your well-being.

As I mention in Chapter 1, your front-line defense against potentially infectious intruders is the physical barrier formed by your body's largest organ — your skin. (Your mucus membranes, as well as the highly acidic digestive juices of your stomach, the beneficial bacteria in your gut, and certain nonspecific cells, also act as immediate defenders against uninvited guests.) The second, far more complex and fundamental defense apparatus in your body — and one of the most important keys to the survival of the human species — is your immune system.

Because numerous immune system processes can play important roles as underlying factors in allergy and asthma (as well as in many other diseases), doctors frequently need to apply their understanding of *immunology* (the science of immunity) when evaluating and treating allergic conditions.

I devote this chapter to explaining the immunologic basis of allergic reactions so that you can have a better understanding of what may be at the root of your ailment and to review with you what your physician considers when diagnosing and treating your condition.

Protecting Your Health: How Your Immune System Works

The most basic function of your immune system is to distinguish between your body (self) and potentially harmful (non-self) agents. Your immune system performs the following functions to protect you:

- ✔ Recognizes foreign (therefore, potentially harmful) microorganisms, their products, and toxins, all known generally as *antigens*. These substances can stimulate a response from your immune system and react with an antibody or a sensitized *T-cell* (a specialized immune system cell involved in cell-mediated immunity, as I explain in "Reacting to allergen exposures," later in this chapter). Allergens, which usually consist of proteins, are particular types of antigens, which initiate an allergic response.

- ✔ Identifies self antigens. These antigens are usually damaged and improperly functioning cells in your body. Malignant cells that can develop into tumor-causing cancerous cells are an example of self-antigens.

- ✔ Assists in removing antigens from your body.

The immune system defense is vital to the survival of all animals. If your immune system functions properly, its protective function is an underlying, ongoing, and generally imperceptible aspect of your everyday existence.

Your immune system can work as a double-edged sword, however. In some cases, it deploys its defensive functions too zealously while trying to protect your body against any type of perceived threat. In such cases, rather than preventing infections, your immune system can actually instigate certain types of health problems, including

- ✔ **Autoimmune disorders:** These disorders include serious diseases such as rheumatic fever, a rare complication of an inadequately treated strep infection of the upper respiratory tract (strep throat), in which the immune system can attack heart tissue cells that cross-react with *Streptococcus* bacterial antigens. This kind of complication is why it's so important that you take the full course of antibiotic therapy your doctor prescribes for strep throat and that you return to your doctor's office for a repeat throat culture to make sure that your infection has completely resolved. (For more information on cross-reactivity, see Chapter 6.)

In other cases, the immune system (for reasons we're still working to discover) loses its ability to distinguish between certain self and non-self substances. This inability to make that distinction can cause diseases such as systemic lupus erythematous, psoriasis, rheumatoid arthritis, and some forms of diabetes, when your immune system perceives otherwise functional and vital cells in your body as antigens and turns its firepower on them.

✔ **Rejection of organ transplants:** Doctors usually try to find a close genetic match between patient and organ donors to reduce the risk of the patient's immune system rejecting the donated organ. In many cases, however, physicians still need to administer drugs to suppress the patient's immune system and prevent organ rejection. This suppression of the immune system can then increase the risk of opportunistic infections, potentially harming the patient.

✔ **Allergic conditions:** If you have allergies or asthma, you almost certainly have an immune system that works too well or overreacts. As I explain in Chapter 1, doctors use the term *hypersensitivity* to refer to allergies because your immune system is overly sensitive to substances such as pollens, animal dander, and other types of allergens that offer no real threat to your health. With hypersensitivity, your immune system acts sort of like an alarm system that summons a SWAT team regardless of whether a cat burglar or just a cat is intruding on your property.

Classifying Immune System Components and Disorders

Your immune system consists of several related processes. Think of these processes as a civil defense network of arsenals, supply lines, logistical support, and command and control centers for the cells that actually defend your body. The most important organ and tissue components of your immune system include the following:

✔ **Bone marrow:** This is where stem cells (early, non-specific types of cells) originate, developing into *B-cells* (specialized types of plasma cells) that subsequently secrete distinct forms of plasma proteins, known as *antibodies*. These antibodies are divided into the following five classes of *immunoglobulins* (identified by the prefix Ig):

- **IgG:** The major component of gammaglobulin used for treating certain types of immune deficiencies, IgG antibodies account for at least three-quarters of the antibodies in your body. This class of antibodies, together with IgM antibodies, in cooperation with your white blood cells, are vital in defending you against bacterial infections. IgG antibodies also play an important role in preventing allergens from initiating an allergic reaction. As a response to *immunotherapy* (allergy shots), the production of IgG antibodies is believed to work by blocking IgE antibodies from binding to mast cells, thus preventing the subsequent release of chemical mediators of inflammation that produce allergy and asthma symptoms. (See "Reacting to allergen exposures," later in this chapter, for more information.)

- **IgM:** About 5 percent of your antibodies belong to this class, which plays a role in the primary immune response and also enhances the role of IgG antibodies.

- **IgA:** The primary antibody in your mucus membrane surfaces, IgA antibodies reside in your saliva, tears, and in the secretions of the mucosal surfaces of your respiratory bronchi, gastrointestinal, and genital tracts, where these antibodies protect against infection. They're also present in mother's milk for the first few days after giving birth, thus providing antibody protection for breast-fed newborns.

- **IgD:** This antibody class, which works with the antigen at cell surface contact, seems to exist in very small quantities and plays a non-specific role in the immune process.

- **IgE:** Although present in only minute quantities in your body, IgE antibodies (also known as *reaginic antibodies*) are key players in allergic reactions (hence the longer paragraph; these antibodies are probably the reason you're reading this book). Although everyone produces IgE antibodies, allergy sufferers have an inherited tendency to overproduce these agents. IgE antibodies can induce other cells, particularly mast cells and basophils (special sentinel cells, as I explain in "Reacting to allergen exposures," later in this chapter), to set in motion a complex chain reaction that culminates in your allergy and asthma symptoms.

  Mast cell surfaces have special IgE receptor sites. Two allergen-specific IgE antibodies linking to an allergen (such as pollen, animal dander, molds, dust mite allergens, insect sting venom, and certain foods and drugs) on the surface of the mast cell can trigger a Type I allergic reaction (see "Classifying Abnormal Immune Responses," later in this chapter).

✔ **Thymus:** Secretions of special hormones (such as thymosin) from this gland are vital for regulating your immune system's functions. The thymus also helps "educate" (encode) certain T-cells, which then play a key role in developing antibodies against antigens.

✔ **Lymph nodes:** The lymphatic system provides drainage for your immune system. Your lymph nodes filter out material that is the result of a local inflammatory reaction. If you seem to have, for example, strep throat, your doctor checks for swollen lymph nodes downstream from the infected area (under your throat) as an indication of infection.

✔ **Spleen:** This organ filters and processes antigens in your blood.

✔ **Lymphoid tissues:** These important immune system participants, which include your tonsils, adenoids, appendix, and parts of your intestines, help process antigens.

Inflaming you for a good reason

You may wonder why you're equipped with IgE antibodies if they're so problematic. This seemingly bothersome immunoglobulin is actually a significant part of the reason the human species made it to another millennium. During prehistoric days, in addition to the challenges of hunting and gathering our daily meal (and trying not to become another animal's chow in the process), we also had to contend with all sorts of infectious agents, especially parasites.

The potent inflammatory action triggered when a parasite-specific antigen would bind with cell-bound IgE antibodies probably insured that parasitic infections couldn't affect enough humans to endanger our species. In fact, IgE antibodies remain important players in the immune responses of some people in less-developed regions of the world, where parasites continue to pose threats to human health.

Occasionally, I see patients who have recently arrived from less-developed countries and who have highly elevated IgE and eosinophil levels in their blood tests. In those cases, I rule out parasitic infections before moving on to a more likely diagnosis of an allergic condition. However, because parasites are such an extremely rare problem in the U.S. population, elevated IgE and eosinophil levels are almost always a sign that I'm dealing with an allergic patient in my practice.

In most modern-day humans, IgE antibodies play a role similar to that of fat cells. In prehistoric days, humans needed fat cells to store food and stave off hunger when their hunting and gathering was less than productive. Now human fat cells turn into love handles, and IgE antibodies trigger allergies.

Protecting and serving in many ways

The protective mechanisms of your immune system consist of four basic components. Think of these components as separate armed forces branches that use different but related means to accomplish the immune system's overall defense mission. The four basic components are

- **Humoral immunity:** This component (which is not a vaccine against stand-up comedians) acts similarly to an internal air force, using *B cells* (see "Classifying Immune System Components and Disorders") to produce and deploy antibodies (the immune system's equivalent of high-tech weaponry). This component provides your body with its primary defense mechanism against bacterial infection and also plays a major role in developing allergies in people with a family history of *atopy* (the genetic susceptibility that can predispose the immune system to develop hypersensitivities and produce antibodies to otherwise harmless allergens).

- **Cell-mediated immunity:** This component uses *T cells* (see "Protecting Your Health: How Your Immune System Works") and related cell products (sort of like the army, battling in the trenches), rather than antibodies, to directly protect you against viruses, fungi, intracellular organisms, and tumor antigens.

- **Phagocytic immunity:** The function of this component is similar to a mop-up squad (or vultures and other scavengers), because it uses so-called *scavenger cells* (macrophages) that circulate throughout your body, looking for debris to clean up. This form of immunity doesn't play a significant role in the allergic process.

- **Complement:** This term describes a composite system of plasma and cell membrane proteins that interact with one another, as well as with antibodies, and serve as important mediators in your civil defense system, protecting the home front like the Coast Guard. Diseases associated with complement deficiency vary depending on which component of the complement system is lacking. Some people may have an increased susceptibility to infection, some may experience a rheumatic disorder (such as lupus erythematous or rheumatoid arthritis), and some may have hereditary angioedema (deep swellings) that occur without hives and can potentially cause life-threatening symptoms (Chapter 18).

Distinguishing between immune deficiencies and allergic conditions

Years ago, when I mentioned *immune deficiency,* people needed an extensive explanation of the subject. Now I spend most of my time clarifying that immunodeficiency isn't synonymous with AIDS (Acquired Immunodeficiency Syndrome), but rather that AIDS represents just one out of a whole multitude of immune deficiency diseases.

If your doctor advises testing for immune deficiency, he or she isn't necessarily ordering an AIDS test. Instead, your physician is most likely ordering immune deficiency tests to rule out other types of diseases.

Although allergy and asthma conditions are almost always synonymous with a hyperreactive immune system, rare cases exist in which people with IgA deficiencies, who have recurring infections, may also have allergic conditions. However, immune deficiencies of any type are very rare when compared to the overall incidence of allergies and asthma.

Keep the following important points about immunodeficiencies and allergy and asthma in mind:

- ✔ In most cases, if you have allergies and asthma and a medical history of recurring infections, your over-responsive immune system is actually swamping your system with excess mucus that gets infected and indirectly causing your infections such as sinusitis (Chapter 9) or bronchitis (Chapter 10).

- ✔ In over 20 years of treating thousands of patients referred to me for recurring infections, I've seen only a handful of patients with immune deficiencies. In the vast majority of cases, I found that these patients actually had allergies and/or asthma.

- ✔ If you have a bacterial infection such as sinusitis or bronchitis, your physician should evaluate whether your infection is a complication of allergic rhinitis and/or asthma before checking for much less common immune deficiencies.

- ✔ Doctors can rule out the vast majority of immune deficiency syndromes by using simple blood tests that measure your blood count and antibody levels. For this reason, I strongly advise against indiscriminately receiving gammaglobulin therapy unless you first have an immune work-up that reveals a significant deficiency requiring this kind of treatment.

Immunizing and immunology

You often hear that life is a constant learning process. This statement is especially true for your immune system. In fact, your immune system is a seemingly limitless learning machine that constantly memorizes the characteristics of countless antigens in order to create memories of these encounters that allow your defenses to react to exposures in the future.

The memory chips of any computer that you or I are liable to use in our lifetimes pale in comparison to the virtual total recall of the immune system. Through the humoral component (see "Protecting and serving in many ways," earlier in this chapter), your immune system can recognize hundreds of trillions of antigens and produce specific antibodies against each and every one of these substances. Compare this feat to remembering the name, looks, and characteristics of every single person, animal, and plant that you encounter throughout your lifetime (which could come in handy at your high school reunion).

Memorizing menaces to your health

Your immune system's phenomenal capacity to memorize explains how having a particular viral infection usually enables you to acquire an immunity to that specific virus for the future. Your immune system usually recognizes the antigen on subsequent exposure, thus triggering a rapid response from its specialized mechanisms and cells, which neutralize and dispose of the offending virus before it can adversely affect you.

Many ancient cultures recognized that people who survived infectious diseases were usually immunized against catching the same ailment again. In fact, ancient Chinese and Egyptian doctors practiced limited forms of immunization.

Fooling your immune system for your own good

Immunization tricks your immune system into thinking that you've actually had a full-blown infection, without risking the potentially life-threatening consequences that a disease such as polio can cause. Your immune system's reaction to the perceived infection insures that if you ever receive exposure to that same virus, your defensive mechanisms will respond rapidly and effectively, thus protecting your health.

Vaccines developed thanks to advances in immunology are the main reason that parents in the United States and many other parts of the world no longer need to worry about their children succumbing to a summer epidemic of polio. Other diseases that medical science has successfully brought under control as a result of immunizations include smallpox, diphtheria, pertussis (whooping cough), tetanus, chicken pox, measles, German measles (rubella), and mumps, as well as forms of hepatitis and meningitis.

In fact, stimulating your immune system into producing a protective immune response against allergens is the underlying basis of immunotherapy (allergy shots), as I explain later in this chapter.

Classifying Abnormal Immune Responses

As I mention earlier in this chapter, your immune system can cause you trouble when it malfunctions, either because of a deficiency or by doing its job too well. Scientists refer to these abnormal responses according to four distinct classifications of reactions.

Although allergic responses can involve aspects of all four types of these mechanisms, Types I and IV, which process and memorize previous antigen encounters, are most important in the vast majority of allergic conditions.

IgE-mediated reactions (Type I)

IgE-mediated reactions (Type I) result in immediate allergic reactions. Also known as *immediate hypersensitivity,* they often result from an insect sting or the injection of a drug such as penicillin in people who have extreme sensitivities to these triggers. The most dramatic and dangerous Type I reaction is anaphylaxis (see Chapter 1).

Allergic rhinitis (hay fever), allergic asthma, and certain types of drug allergies are other examples of this type of immune mechanism. Because of the sudden onset of the allergic reaction in cases of immediate hypersensitivity, allergy skin testing (see Chapter 8) can provide quick results in identifying the triggers of those conditions in many cases. For a more in-depth explanation of Type I reactions, see "Developing an Immediate Hypersensitivity," later in this chapter.

Cytotoxic reactions (Type II)

Cytotoxic reactions (Type II) involve destruction of cells, such as the reactions that result in the breakdown of red blood cells. This mechanism can potentially lead to anemia and fewer platelets in the blood, a situation that decreases your blood's ability to clot.

Certain drugs such as penicillin, sulfonamides, and quinidine can trigger cytotoxic reactions. Type II reactions play a role in Rh-factor anemia and jaundice in newborns and are also the way a patient's body may reject an organ transplant.

Immune complex reactions (Type III)

Manifestations of *immune complex reactions (Type III)* include fever, skin rash, hives, swollen, tender lymph nodes, and aching or painful joints. These types of reactions are among the ones that physicians usually refer to as *serum sickness.* Typically, these symptoms appear one to three weeks after taking final doses of drugs such as penicillin, sulfonamides, thiouracil, and phenytoin.

Type III reactions also play a role in the development of autoimmune disorders, such as systemic lupus erythematous, psoriasis, rheumatoid arthritis, some forms of diabetes, and certain types of kidney disease.

Cell-mediated reactions (Type IV)

Allergic contact dermatitis is one of the primary examples of *cell-mediated reactions (Type IV),* a localized, non-systemic reaction (Chapter 17). Doctors also use the term *delayed hypersensitivity* to describe this process, in which contact with an allergen results in an allergic reaction hours or even days later. (For example, if you have allergic contact dermatitis, you may not realize that you've contacted poison ivy until you're driving home from your weekend camping trip.)

Although the delayed reaction is rarely life-threatening, in some cases it may take longer to subside or disappear than reactions involving atopic conditions, such as immediate hypersensitivity (see "IgE-mediated reactions (Type I)" at the beginning of this section).

Developing an Immediate Hypersensitivity

Type I allergic reactions involve numerous complex processes, with many players taking part in various ways. This section explains the roles that the most important cells and chemicals play in developing your sensitivities and triggering your reactions. Likewise, this chapter summarizes the sequence of events involved in sensitizing your immune system and triggering subsequent allergic reactions.

Setting the stage for allergic reactions

Significant cell participants in Type I reactions include the following:

- **Mast cells:** These connective-tissue cells play a pivotal role in allergic disease processes. Mast cells are primarily located near blood vessels and mucus-producing cells in the tissues that line various parts of your body. With allergies and asthma, doctors concern themselves with your mast cells' actions in the lining of your eyes, ears, nose, sinuses, throat, the airways of your lungs, your skin, and your gastrointestinal (GI) tract.

- **Basophils:** These cells live in your bloodstream near the surfaces of tissues and are important players in late-phase reactions. (See "Reacting to allergen exposures," later in this chapter, for more information.)

Mast cells and basophils are among the first cells that antigens encounter when entering your body. These sentinel cells are coated with numerous IgE receptor sites that can accommodate IgE antibodies that are specific to various allergens (corresponding, for example, to different pollens and animal dander).

These cells also contain potent chemical mediators of inflammation that are released when IgE and a specific allergen cross-link and activate them, resulting in the inflammation that leads to allergy and asthma symptoms.

✔ **Eosinophils.** Other mediators attract these white blood cells to the site of an allergic reaction and generate an array of other inflammatory mediators, including enzymes that can cause tissue damage. Eosinophils also play prominent roles in late-phase reactions that affect some people with allergies and asthma, particularly with symptoms of nasal congestion that can occur hours after an initial episode of allergic rhinitis. (See "Reacting to allergen exposures," later in this chapter.) If you have uncontrolled asthma, constant eosinophil activity may lead to *airway remodeling* — the replacement of healthy tissue with scar tissue — and can potentially cause irreversible loss of lung function.

Preventing this type of serious lung damage is one of the main goals of treating asthma early and aggressively, particularly with inhaled topical corticosteroids. (See Chapter 12 for an extensive survey of asthma medications.) Because eosinophils tend to accumulate in your nasal passages if you have allergic rhinitis, your doctor may use a nasal smear (Chapter 3) to check for the presence of eosinophils when diagnosing your condition.

Histamine and leukotrienes (which I refer to in many other parts of this book) are just two of the vast array of potent chemical mediators of inflammation released from mast cells and basophils during allergic reactions. This multitude of mediators can induce the following actions in your body:

✔ Dilate your blood vessels, leading to increased fluid leakage, which increases inflammatory action.

✔ Increase mucus secretions, resulting in a runny nose, watery eyes, and airway congestion, depending on where the trigger causes the allergic reaction.

✔ Activate your sensory nerves, causing increased itching. (If you have allergic rhinitis, your nose may feel itchy when you experience other allergy symptoms because these mediators activate your sensory nerves.)

✔ Cause tissue damage, often with accompanying pain and discomfort.

✔ Promote the production of IgE and activation of eosinophils, thus supporting allergic inflammation.

✔ Attract other inflammatory cells to the area to amplify the inflammatory reaction.

✔ Cause constriction of the smooth muscles of your respiratory airways.

Reacting to allergen exposures

This section shows you how the players I describe in the preceding section interact. A typical sequence of reactions in an IgE response (immediate hypersensitivity) consists of the following steps:

1. **Your immune system receives exposure to an allergen.**

   Allergen exposures can result from the following occurrences:

   - **Inhaling:** Inhalant allergens (or *aeroallergens*) such as pollens, molds, dust mite allergens, and animal dander often pass through your nose and/or your mouth, putting the allergens in contact with immune cells lining your nose, mouth, throat, and airways of the lungs. Common symptoms of these exposures include runny nose, sneezing, watery eyes, stuffy nose, postnasal drip, coughing, chest tightness, wheezing, and shortness of breath.

   - **Ingesting:** You may swallow allergens, such as those contained in peanuts, shellfish, eggs, milk, or in drugs such as penicillin. These exposures can trigger oral symptoms such as itching and swelling of the tongue, lips, and throat; GI tract symptoms such as nausea, stomach cramps, vomiting, and diarrhea; skin reactions such as hives and angioedema (deep swellings); and respiratory symptoms such as coughing, wheezing, and shortness of breath.

   - **Touching (direct contact):** Direct contact exposures typically involve Type IV delayed hypersensitivity responses, including reactions to poison ivy, nickel, and latex, among numerous others (Chapter 17). Symptoms from direct contact usually result in localized, topical reactions such as skin rashes.

   - **Injecting:** Medical syringes and insect stingers are vehicles for injecting allergens. Injections can cause particularly severe reactions because allergens go directly into your bloodstream, which can spread the allergens rapidly to organs throughout your body. Penicillin shots are the most dramatic (and often severe) examples of drug-related anaphylaxis in people with penicillin hypersensitivities. The venom from stinging insects can also cause potentially life-threatening reactions.

2. **Your body develops an IgE antibody response to the allergen.**

   If you have an atopic predisposition for developing allergies, scavenger cells (macrophages) that usually rid your body of foreign proteins (such as allergens) act as antigen- (allergen-) presenting cells. This setup triggers T cells (other specialized immune system cells) to recruit B cells that develop into plasma cells. This process culminates in the production of specific IgE antibodies designed against the allergen (see Figure 2-1).

3. **Allergens bind to specific IgE antibodies attached to the surface of mast cells or basophils.**

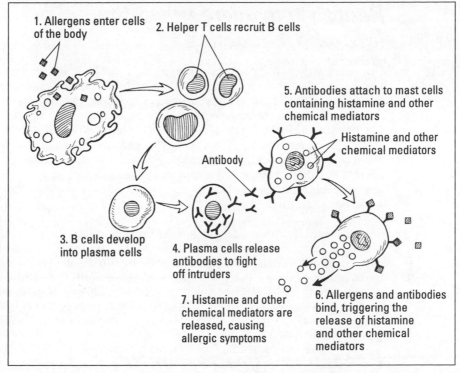

1. Allergens enter cells of the body

2. Helper T cells recruit B cells

5. Antibodies attach to mast cells containing histamine and other chemical mediators

Histamine and other chemical mediators

Antibody

3. B cells develop into plasma cells

4. Plasma cells release antibodies to fight off intruders

7. Histamine and other chemical mediators are released, causing allergic symptoms

6. Allergens and antibodies bind, triggering the release of histamine and other chemical mediators

Figure 2-1:
The allergic inflammatory response is a complex process involving many types of cells.

The first time you're exposed to the allergen, you don't typically experience a reaction. However, you produce specific IgE antibodies that bind to receptor sites on mast cells. Thus your immune system is *sensitized,* and further exposure to that allergen initiates an allergic response.

4. You're re-exposed to the allergen. The allergen attaches to two specific IgE antibodies on the surface of the mast cell in a lock-and-key arrangement.

5. This cross-linking of the allergen to two specific IgE antibodies on the surface of the mast cell activates the mast cell to release its potent chemical mediators of inflammation, which affect various organs and trigger your allergic symptoms.

In some cases, particularly with reactions to insect stings and penicillin, you may think that your allergic reaction was the result of just a single exposure. In most instances, however, you received a prior, sensitizing exposure, perhaps in one of the following ways:

- With regard to insect stings, you may have been stung as a child. If that experience wasn't traumatic and resulted only in a minor, localized reaction, you may have forgotten about it.

- Your first exposure to penicillin allergens may be even less memorable: The cow's milk or beef that you eat can include this antibiotic from the animal's feed.

Doing it one more time: The late-phase reaction

The allergic response consists of two phases involving inflammatory cells and potent chemical mediators of inflammation. The immediate, early phase occurs within one hour of initial allergen exposure. An additional, late-phase reaction can occur in some people anywhere from three to ten hours after the initial allergic response. Basophils influence eosinophils (see "Setting the stage for allergic reactions," earlier in this chapter) to stage a second, rallying effort against the allergen, hours after you think you're recovered from an allergic episode. In some cases, this late-phase reaction can actually be more severe than the initial reaction. Congestion is often a prominent symptom of a late-phase response.

Because antihistamines and quick-relief bronchodilators are only effective for dealing with early-phase reactions, your doctor may need to prescribe oral corticosteroids (such as Prednisone or Medrol) to control late-phase symptoms. Immunotherapy (allergy shots) is a unique form of treatment that helps decrease both early- and late-phase reactions to allergen exposures, as I explain in "Reaping the Benefits of Immunology," later in this chapter.

Becoming hyperresponsive

Typically, if you're consistently exposed to an indoor allergen — for instance, animal dander — you may find that during ragweed season, your symptoms appear to become more bothersome even at lower levels of exposure than you have experienced previously. By increasing your *allergen load* (your total level of exposure, at any one time, to any combination of allergens that trigger your allergies — see Chapter 6), other allergens and irritants may be more likely to also cause problems for you. In this case, eliminating animal dander from your home could result in fewer allergy symptoms during ragweed season.

Conversely, although your friend's cat might not be an issue for you most of the year, Fluffy's dander may trigger your allergic rhinitis and/or asthma symptoms during ragweed season. That's because exposure to the pollen causes you to develop a lower threshold for allergy symptoms (making you *hyperresponsive*) when exposed to this friendly feline.

Reacting non-specifically

Another reaction complication that occurs is non-specific reactivity. *Non-specific reactivity* develops when your nasal passages and breathing airways become so inflamed and sensitized by repeated, constant exposure to triggering allergens that nonallergic irritants also cause reactions. Non-specific irritants often include:

- Tobacco smoke (from cigarettes, cigars, pipes)
- Fumes and scents from household cleaners, strongly scented soaps, and perfumes and colognes; from glues, solvents, and aerosols; and from unvented gas, oil, or kerosene stoves
- Smoke from wood-burning appliances or fireplaces
- Air pollution
- Gases, from chemicals found primarily in the workplace

Although the reactions triggered by irritants are not IgE-mediated, they still increase injury to already sensitive areas. If you're continuously exposed to allergens and irritants, a vicious cycle can develop, and the damage that allergic reactions cause is compounded by irritants, thus aggravating your affected areas further and increasing their sensitivities, resulting in more symptoms and further injury to your airways.

Reaping the Benefits of Immunology

Immunology provides great benefits for treating allergy and asthma conditions, enabling doctors to modify your immune system's reactions to allergy and asthma triggers with immunotherapy (allergy shots). The immunologic response that results from immunotherapy triggers promotes immune system actions that protect rather than damage your body, as I explain in Chapter 8.

Immunotherapy is the most effective way, in most cases, to treat the underlying causes of allergic ailments such as allergic rhinitis (and allergic conjunctivitis), allergic asthma, and allergies to insect stings (with venom immunotherapy, or VIT, as I explain in Chapter 21).

BERGER BIT

Enhancing your future with immunology

The advances that medical science has made with immunology during the last century are among the greatest human achievements in the history of mankind, producing medical miracles for the entire world that would have seemed like sheer fantasy 100 years ago. I believe that the continued progress in our understanding of immunology will enable medical researchers to find far more effective ways of preventing infectious diseases that continue to cause serious problems for many people around the world. Immunologic research has already helped control some forms of cancer with the use of interferons, anti-tumor antibody therapy, and other immunologic interventions.

In the quest for more effective medications to control allergy and asthma symptoms, immunology has been the key to developing a new and innovative medication, based on using a high-tech antibody known as *recombinant human monoclonal antibody* (rhuMab), which is an anti-IgE antibody. This new drug is designed to immunologically bind with circulating IgE. This binding prevents the binding of IgE to mast cells, thus blocking the initiation of the allergic reaction.

The study of immunology matters a great deal to the whole human race. As physicians and scientists, we must continue to advance our knowledge about our immune system and unlock the secrets it holds for a healthier future. I feel confident that the 21st century will see the development of vaccines for many serious diseases such as herpes; respiratory syncytial virus (RSV) infections, which cause bronchiolitis in infants (see Chapter 14); and the worldwide scourge of AIDS. Likewise, I think that the 21st century will also result in the development of more effective forms of immunotherapy for allergies. Immunologic research may one day even produce a vaccine against allergy and asthma. (If that happens, and my patients no longer need my care, maybe I could fulfill my fantasy of trying out for a spot on the Senior Golf Tour.)

Chapter 3

Dealing with Doctor Visits

· ·

In This Chapter

▶ Preparing for your first allergy or asthma appointment

▶ Filling out forms

▶ Getting the most out of your doctor visits

▶ Understanding insurance issues and paying for treatment

▶ Knowing what to expect from your physician

· ·

*S*eeing a doctor, whether an asthma or allergy specialist or your own family practitioner, is something you should take seriously. You and your physician are partners in treating your medical condition. Developing and maintaining that partnership is one of the most important aspects of effectively managing and treating your allergies, asthma, or any other serious ailment.

The effectiveness of your treatment depends not so much on the *length* of time you spend in your doctor's office, but rather on the *quality* of that time. As much as I enjoy seeing my patients and as much as they may delight in my winning personality, the real reason they're in my office is to get better. In my experience, patients who derive the greatest benefit from treatment are those who understand how to get the most out of their doctor visits. Some tips for getting the most out of your doctor visits include:

✔ Preparing ahead of time for your doctor visits (as I explain in the next section of this chapter).

✔ Communicating well with your doctor about your condition and the effects of your treatment.

✔ Understanding all aspects of your treatment plan, including the medications your doctor prescribes, and learning the most effective ways of avoiding allergy and asthma triggers. (Chapters 6 and 11 offer more information on avoiding allergy and asthma triggers.)

✔ Participating in developing treatment goals with your doctor and making sure that you can openly communicate with him or her about the effects and results of your treatment.

✔ Adhering to your treatment plan. You are the most important factor in your own treatment process. Your good health and your quality of life clearly depend on your full and active participation in the treatment process.

Preparing for Your First Visit

When it comes to making a proper diagnosis of allergies and asthma, your primary care physician may refer you to a specialist, such as an allergist (see the sidebar "Seeing a specialist") and/or a pulmonologist (lung doctor). Your first visit will likely cover the following items:

✔ Taking a thorough medical history (see the next sections), covering any and all ailments in your life, not just those that you think involve allergies or asthma.

✔ Performing a physical examination. Depending on your condition, your past medical history, and especially on why your primary care physician referred you, your physical exam may focus only on the areas that your allergy or asthma symptoms affect, or your exam may also include a more comprehensive evaluation. (See "Getting physical," later in this chapter, for more information on the signs and symptoms your doctor may be looking for, depending on your medical history.)

✔ Allergy skin testing (depending on your medical history and medical exam) for specific allergic sensitivities and/or other appropriate tests and lab procedures (such as pulmonary function tests for asthma, as I explain in "Assessing Asthma with Spirometry" later in this chapter).

✔ Prescribing and teaching you how to use appropriate medications and/or instructing you about effective environmental control steps that you can take to avoid or reduce exposure to your allergy or asthma triggers, thus reducing your symptoms.

Doing your homework

Identifying the underlying cause of your allergy or asthma provides the best approach to effectively treating your ailment. However, as I explain in Chapter 2, because of the complexity of allergic diseases, getting to the root of what's ailing you is usually more than a matter of just performing medical tests (such as blood tests or X-rays) and interpreting the results.

Although we've seen impressive breakthroughs recently in diagnosing and treating various diseases (especially with ongoing research in developing new medications), the first step an allergy or asthma specialist still takes to treat your condition is obtaining your complete medical history. The specialist uses your medical history as the foundation of your medical evaluation.

BERGER BIT

Seeing a specialist

I recommend that you or your physician consider consulting an asthma and allergy specialist, such as an allergist or pulmonologist (lung doctor), when:

✔ **Your diagnosis is difficult to establish.** Chronic coughing and/or a runny nose that don't respond to initial treatment, such as cough or cold medications, are two of the most frequent reasons why your primary care physician may refer you to an asthma and allergy specialist.

✔ **Your diagnosis requires specialized testing.** In some cases, your primary care physician may refer you to a specialist for allergy skin testing to confirm his or her suspicion of an underlying allergy, such as allergic rhinitis (hay fever), asthma, atopic dermatitis (eczema), hypersensitivities to certain foods, or allergic insect sting reactions. Other types of specialized tests that involve referring you to a specialist can include

diagnostic procedures for asthma, such as spirometry or complete pulmonary function studies, bronchoprovocation or bronchoscopy (see Chapter 10), and/or further evaluation of your rhinitis with rhinoscopy.

✔ **Your doctor advises you to consider immunotherapy (allergy shots).** See Chapter 8 for more information on immunotherapy.

✔ **Other conditions complicate your condition or its diagnosis.** Those conditions may include sinusitis, nasal polyps, severe rhinitis, gastroesophageal reflux (GER), chronic obstructive pulmonary disease (COPD), vocal cord problems, or aspergillosis (a fungal infection that can affect your lungs).

✔ **You've experienced a previous emergency room visit or hospitalization for asthma (see Chapter 10) or anaphylaxis (see Chapter 1).**

The doctor you're consulting for your allergy and/or asthma condition usually requests that you provide very specific medical information at your first visit. After taking your medical history, your specialist may also perform an appropriate medical exam. Subsequently, he or she may also order tests and procedures to confirm your diagnosis and to more precisely identify the specific triggers of your allergy symptoms, as well as to determine your sensitivity levels to those triggers.

TIP

Preparing for an initial consultation with a specialist shouldn't stress you out the way school exams or job interviews may sometimes affect you. However, you need to spend some time before your appointment gathering and reviewing information that your specialist needs in order to make a specific diagnosis of your condition. Prepare to provide your doctor with and to discuss in detail during your consultation the following key information:

✔ Your symptoms, both those that seem to be caused by an allergic condition and any others, even if they seem unrelated.

- Any other medical conditions for which you've been treated or are presently being treated.
- Any medications you're taking, whether prescription or over-the-counter.
- Your medical history, as well as that of your family.
- Details about other factors, such as your home, work, or school environment, that may contribute to your medical condition.

I provide detailed examples of the information your doctor will request, based on these general categories, in the next section of this chapter.

You may also have questions about your medical condition. Asking your physician about your concerns during your initial consultation is certainly appropriate. Remember, there's no such thing as a stupid question when you are asking about your medical history, diagnosis, or treatment.

You may think that an issue you raise is obvious, insignificant, or irrelevant, but bringing it up may further clarify the nature of your ailment for your doctor. The best way to find out is to go ahead and ask him or her. A good physician appreciates the fact that you've taken the time to formulate your own questions. I advise writing down your inquiries ahead of time and giving them to your doctor at the beginning of your appointment, so that he or she can focus on the most important issues affecting your health during your office visit.

Filling out forms ahead of time

Many doctors (including myself) send patients a questionnaire to fill out prior to their initial consultation. The level of detail that these questionnaires require varies, depending on the symptoms you experience and the type of consultation you seek. Doctors don't send out these forms because they love paperwork, but rather because they want to insure that your first appointment is most productive.

In most cases, you can expect to spend between one and two hours at your first appointment. You may have a hectic life, but it's important to plan your schedule so that you can arrive at your physician's office on time. Remember to bring all requested forms, documents, and other materials, including your insurance and/or other payment information. (See "Paying for Your Care," later in this chapter.)

Telling your story

Whatever way it's gathered, you probably need to provide the following information at your first appointment with your asthma and allergy specialist:

Patient, know thyself

Providing your doctor with the information that he or she requests about your medical history enables you to take part in the process of diagnosing and treating your medical problems. While assembling their medical histories and related details, many of my patients have discovered patterns and connections between symptoms, triggers, and precipitating factors that they hadn't realized before.

Gaining this type of self-knowledge not only helps your physician make a diagnosis, but it can also help you make more informed choices about your treatment options, as well as assist you in avoiding the triggers and precipitating factors of your allergies or asthma.

- ✔ Your name, address, telephone number, and other contact information.

- ✔ Your age, gender, and occupation. (If you're making an appointment for your child, list your own and your spouse's age and occupation.)

- ✔ The name of your referring physician (or other person who referred you).

- ✔ The major medical problems that affect you and their duration.

- ✔ The symptoms you're experiencing and the specific areas or organs of your body that are affected. Providing details of when and in what circumstances these symptoms occur is often vital to establishing an accurate diagnosis.

- ✔ For women, let your physician know if you think or know you are pregnant or if you are planning to become pregnant.

- ✔ Aggravating factors that seem to make your condition worse. For example, if you notice that your respiratory symptoms — such as coughing, wheezing, or shortness of breath — are more severe when you visit people who have pets or when you're around smokers, make sure you tell your physician.

- ✔ The names of all the medications you're currently taking, including products that you use specifically for your condition, as well as other drugs, such as over-the-counter (OTC) preparations or herbal remedies, that you take to relieve minor aches and pains. (I advise bringing a list of medications you're currently taking.) If you're unsure of the actual drugs that you use (perhaps the label is difficult to decipher), bring the medication with you in its original container. Also, ask your pharmacist, primary care physician, or other doctors for a list of medications they've prescribed for any of your medical conditions. Because gathering this information all at once can be a challenge, I advise keeping a drug record that you can refer to when consulting with a new doctor, as I explain in "Recording your symptoms and medications," later in this chapter.

✔ If you've been treated or evaluated previously for the same condition, provide your new doctor with information on the results of these consultations and treatments. (Bringing the results from any tests you've had in the past may also save you the trouble — and cost — of repeating those procedures.)

✔ Providing accurate information on any other illnesses and related treatments you've had is also vital to evaluating your current condition.

✔ Your family history is very important in determining your diagnosis, so take time to list this information to the best of your ability (see "Taking your family history," later in this chapter). Likewise, if you fill out this form for a child, provide information on specific childhood factors, such as birth history, immunizations, and childhood illnesses (for example, bronchiolitis and/or croup).

✔ Your career, occupation, the school (or day care for children) you attend, and your hobbies or recreational activities are also important factors in figuring out what's ailing you.

✔ Your dietary history, including any special diets you follow, major food groups you avoid, and whether you've been diagnosed with any food allergies.

✔ Doctors aren't census-takers (or private detectives, for that matter), but your specialist needs to know about your home because many things in your domestic environment can trigger or aggravate allergy and/or asthma symptoms, particularly dust, animal dander, molds, and tobacco smoke. Therefore, you should provide your doctor with information on the following items:

- A list of the people living with you and any habits they may have, such as smoking or keeping pets, that can affect your condition.

- If you have plants in your home, make sure you can identify them for your doctor.

- In addition, although specialists are also not contractors, realtors, architects, or interior decorators, they generally try to assess the condition of your home including its location, age, the principal construction materials, the building's air circulation system, the condition of the basement and the type of carpets and furnishings you have. Your doctor may also ask about your yard, garden, and surrounding vegetation.

- Your doctor usually asks about your bedroom also. Don't worry; he or she isn't getting personal. However, because the bedroom is where you most likely spend the majority of your life (even more time than on the golf course, in my case), exposure to allergens in your bedroom can often play a significant role in the severity of your allergy or asthma symptoms.

Recording your symptoms and medications

Keeping a daily symptom diary can provide valuable information that your physician can use when assessing your condition. A typical daily symptom diary is usually a table with columns and rows where you can record items, such as your daily symptoms, medications you take, your peak expiratory flow rate (PEFR, to monitor asthma; see Chapter 13), and your observations about possible triggers or suspected exposures.

In addition to keeping a symptom diary, I also recommend establishing a medication record that lists all the drugs — prescription, over-the-counter, and herbal remedies— that you take over your lifetime. Recording your medications is similar to recording checks in your check register.

If you think that you may suffer from drug hypersensitivity (see Chapter 20), this medication record can also greatly help your doctor diagnose the problem. Your medication record should include the brand and generic names of *all* drugs you've used and currently take, including OTC vitamins and supplements — some of which are as potent as conventional medical products that the Food and Drug Administration (FDA) regulates and which are available only by prescription. In addition, you should also note the conditions you treat or have treated with particular drugs and the effectiveness and/or results of taking those products.

Focusing on foods

In addition to causing digestive problems such as nausea, vomiting, or diarrhea, *hypersensitivities* (allergies) to certain foods can trigger symptoms throughout your body. Food hypersensitivity symptoms can include stuffy nose, skin rashes and hives, headaches, respiratory problems (such as coughing, wheezing, and shortness of breath), and general fatigue.

If your doctor suspects that food hypersensitivity causes your symptoms, he or she may advise you to keep a detailed food diary to bring to your initial specialist consultation. Your food diary can help your specialist determine whether your problem is a food allergy or the result of another type of adverse food reaction, such as a food intolerance (see Chapter 19 for information on keeping a food diary).

Taking your family history

Because heredity often plays an important role in determining your likelihood of developing allergies, your physician usually asks about your family medical history. You don't need to become the next Alex Haley to research this information, but you should make sure that you know which relative (mother, brother, uncle, and so on) had a particular disease or condition. Letting your doctor know whether your parents, siblings or close relatives have had allergic conditions such as asthma, allergic rhinitis (hay fever), atopic dermatitis (eczema), and food or drug allergies is especially important.

In addition, because other medical conditions that run in families can influence your treatment, your physician also needs to know whether any of your family members suffer from (or had) illnesses such as diabetes, high blood pressure, heart disease, cystic fibrosis, and cancer.

Looking for signs of asthma and allergies

After discussing your medical history, your physician will also probably examine you for physical signs of your allergies or asthma. The areas that your doctor usually checks vary based on your medical history, as well as the type of symptoms you have. Areas that your doctor may investigate include the following:

- ✔ Eyes, ears, nose, throat, and sinuses. Physicians often check for redness and watering of eyes; appearance of your eardrums; swelling of your nasal lining; amount and character of nasal discharge; presence of nasal polyps; size and color of tonsils; tender or swollen lymph nodes in your neck area; and possible tenderness over your sinus areas.

- ✔ Your chest and torso, to look for expanded or over-inflated lungs and hunched shoulders, which can signal breathing difficulties.

- ✔ Your lungs (with a stethoscope), to check for wheezing, other abnormal breath sounds, and the character of your airflow.

- ✔ Your skin, to check for dry, red, itchy, and damaged skin (such as seen in atopic dermatitis — eczema), which can often indicate your predisposition to allergies.

- ✔ If your doctor suspects allergic rhinitis (hay fever) as part of your problem, he or she may also look for distinctive combinations of gestures and facial features, particularly in children and adolescents, as I detail in Chapter 4.

Allergy testing and other diagnostic studies

In order to confirm or more precisely identify the underlying cause of your symptoms, your doctor may advise certain tests and procedures. The types of diagnostic studies that your specialist performs depend on your medical history and the results of your physical examination. In the following sections, I provide an overview of the most frequently used tests and procedures.

Allergy skin testing

Allergists consider skin testing the gold standard for identifying sensitivities to certain types of allergens. In some cases, allergy skin testing can also indicate your level of sensitivity to the particular allergen. Allergy skin tests are usually most useful for identifying sensitivities to pollen, dust mites, molds, animal dander, insect stings, food hypersensitivities, and, if necessary, for penicillin hypersensitivities

Skin testing for allergies in the doctor's office generally involves placing a drop of a suspected allergen on your skin and then pricking, puncturing, or scratching your skin with a device to see whether the allergen produces a reaction. If you're allergic to the administered allergen, your skin usually reacts in a way that resembles a mosquito bite or small hive.

A positive reaction can help identify the cause of your allergic reactions and may also indicate your sensitivity level to that allergic trigger. (See Chapter 8 to find out more about allergy skin testing.)

Using RAST for allergy testing

Your allergist may recommend using *radioallergensorbent testing* (RAST) for diagnosing your allergic sensitivities. Although RAST is not as precise, practical, comprehensive, or cost-effective as allergy skin testing, your doctor may advise using this procedure under specific circumstances. See Chapter 8 for more information on RAST.

Assessing asthma with spirometry

If your symptoms include coughing, wheezing, and shortness of breath, your doctor should assess your lung functions with spirometry to evaluate whether asthma is the underlying cause of your condition.

A *spirometer* is a sophisticated machine that measures airflow from your large and small airways before and after you inhale a short-acting bronchodilator. For adults and children over age 4 or 5, this procedure provides the most accurate way of determining whether airway obstruction exists and whether your condition is reversible (meaning that it improves after taking appropriate medication). Your doctor may also advise other lung function tests if he or she suspects that other coexisting respiratory conditions may cause or affect your symptoms (see Chapter 10).

Other procedures for diagnosing allergies and asthma

Confirming an allergy or asthma diagnosis may also involve additional studies and tests, such as:

- **Rhinoscopy:** This technique is useful for investigating causes of nasal obstruction or blockage, postnasal drainage, and the condition of the sinuses.

✔ **Nasal smear:** Although not considered a definitive diagnostic test, a nasal smear can help your doctor determine whether you suffer from allergic rhinitis. This procedure generally involves taking secretions from your nose, usually with a flexible, plastic device, which your doctor then examines under a microscope for levels of *eosinophils* (a type of white blood cell — see Chapter 2). Elevated counts of eosinophils can indicate an allergic condition.

✔ **A chest and/or sinus X-ray or a CAT scan of the sinuses (see Chapter 9):** Your doctor may also order these types of imaging tests to determine whether other disorders, such as chronic bronchitis and emphysema — collectively referred to as *chronic obstructive pulmonary disease (COPD)*, pneumonia, or sinusitis (sinus infection) may be part of your medical condition.

✔ **Bronchoprovocation:** In some cases, spirometry may indicate normal or near-normal lung functions, although asthma nonetheless seems the most likely cause of your symptoms. Therefore, your doctor may advise bronchoprovocation to more precisely diagnose your condition. These types of tests usually involve exercising for several minutes (on a stationary bicycle or treadmill in your doctor's office) or inhaling a small dose of methacholine or histamine (see Chapter 10), in order to determine whether mild asthma symptoms occur as a result of bronchial constriction. This test allows doctors to diagnose individuals whose asthma is otherwise not apparent, but whose symptoms appear as a response to these challenges due to the hyperreactivity of their airways (see Chapter 10).

✔ **Tympanometry:** Doctors often use this procedure, which measures your ear drum response to various pressure levels, to determine whether you have *otitis media* (inflammation of the middle ear, often associated with ear infections) — a frequent complication of both sinusitis and allergic rhinitis.

✔ **Thyroid function test:** Because *hypothyroidism* (an underactive thyroid) can cause chronic nasal congestion similar to a severe case of allergic rhinitis, your doctor may order this test to rule out an alternate diagnosis.

✔ **Elimination diet:** If skin testing for food allergies isn't conclusive, your doctor may advise an elimination diet (which you should only undertake under your physician's supervision) to confirm what's triggering your adverse food reactions. (For more food for thought on food allergies, turn to Chapter 19.)

✔ **Oral food challenges:** These tests involve ingesting — under medical supervision — very small quantities of foods that contain suspected allergens. They should be performed only if your previous adverse food reactions haven't been life-threatening (see Chapter 19).

Following Up: Second and Subsequent Visits

Your second visit with an allergy or asthma specialist usually takes place one to two weeks after your initial consultation. This return visit is every bit as important as your first appointment, so make sure that you take with you any information, records, or documents your physician may require, based on your previous appointment.

When scheduling your follow-up visit, I suggest asking your doctor's office how much time the physician expects to spend with you, so you can plan your day accordingly.

Doctor, doctor, give me the news

During your second consultation, your doctor usually goes over the results of your tests, explains your diagnosis, and reviews your treatment plan.

Always ask for a specific diagnosis when you see a specialist.

Depending on your diagnosis and medical condition, your physician may take all or some of the following steps during your second visit (or third in some cases):

- ✔ **Review the effectiveness of medications that he or she prescribed for you at your previous visit.** In some cases, your doctor may need to adjust your medications and dosages.

- ✔ **Provide you with a summary of the most important findings of your initial consultation.** You should also ask for recommendations concerning additional educational materials (such as this book!)

- ✔ **Provide you with a written treatment plan.** Make sure that you understand this plan and can adhere to it. If you have concerns or questions about your advised treatment, inform your physician.

- ✔ **Give you handouts with written instructions on avoiding the allergens, irritants, and/or precipitating factors that may trigger your asthma or allergies.**

Considering allergy shots

If your medical history and skin testing provide clear evidence that you're allergic to certain allergens, your doctor may advise you to consider immunotherapy (allergy shots). If your physician suggests immunotherapy, he or she should make sure that you understand the commitment that this treatment requires.

Immunotherapy is not a quick fix, and it requires a significant investment of time on your part. For inhalant allergens and insect stings (using venom immunotherapy, or VIT, as I explain in Chapter 21), it may take up to one year of allergy shots before you and your doctor can determine whether you are clearly benefiting from the therapy. Your adherence to the program is the key for effective immunotherapy, meaning that you need to maintain the injection schedule that your allergist prescribes as much as possible (see Chapter 8).

Paying for Your Care

Here's the fun part: dealing with your medical bills. Make sure that you read and understand your physician's financial policy before your first appointment so that you know and understand what your payment terms are.

The terms of financial policies usually depend on the level and type of health insurance you carry. If you're covered by Medicare or a contracted insurance plan, such as a health maintenance organization (HMO), you generally aren't billed, although you may need to make a small co-payment at the time of your visit (usually between $5 and $20).

However, you may need to pay out-of-pocket for your first office visit (at the time of your appointment) if any of the following applies to you:

✔ You don't carry health insurance.

✔ You have a private health insurance policy.

✔ You aren't covered by an insurance plan, such as an HMO, that contracts with your doctor's practice.

✔ You can't (or don't) provide your doctor's office with insurance information. (Make sure you have all requested health care documents and records with you when you see your physician.)

Dealing with insurance issues

With the movement toward managed care, seeing a specialist is frequently more difficult for patients. I believe that having a first-rate health insurance policy, one that provides full access to the physicians you need to see, when you need to see them, is preferable. If you have the opportunity to choose among several medical coverage plans, paying a little bit more for a policy that allows direct access to specialists when you need them is well worth the extra investment. (Just like in most other purchases, you get what you pay for!)

I strongly advise my patients not to sell themselves short by buying insurance solely on the basis of price. A low-cost plan may work just fine when you're in good health and don't really require much specialty medical care. However, if you develop a serious medical problem, you may find that many of these low-cost plans cover expert treatment only after your ailment deteriorates into a potentially irreversible or life-threatening condition.

Gatekeeping and your treatment

Good primary care practitioners on the front lines of health care are essential to the well-being of much of the world's population, especially in the United States. In the U.S., however, these doctors often work under difficult circumstances because of the limitations and deficiencies of the health insurance financing system.

In many cases, health maintenance organizations (HMOs) attempt to control their costs by providing bonuses and other incentives to primary care physicians (often known as *gatekeepers*) who limit referrals to specialists. *Capitation,* which involves giving these doctors restricted budgets for treating patients, has led to many complaints by both patients and primary care physicians alike.

According to a recent study in the *New England Journal of Medicine,* at least one-quarter of primary care physicians worry that they're treating complicated conditions that specialists could handle better. This study also found that many primary care physicians, who receive a larger proportion of their income through capitation and who serve as gatekeepers for large numbers of patients, think their practice is too broad. These doctors also report that they are often required to treat people with more complex conditions than they treated in the past.

Getting the care you need and deserve

If your primary care physician tells you that no other treatment is available for your condition, he or she may actually mean there's nothing more that can be done for you in your managed care setting. If this situation happens to you and/or you're dissatisfied with the medical care you are receiving, consider taking the following steps:

✔ **Find out whether your HMO provides bonuses or other forms of incentives for limiting referrals.** Although you may feel uncomfortable asking your primary care physician about this topic, you have a right to know about the policies that directly affect the delivery and quality of your health care.

✔ **Become your own advocate.** Read up on the current issues regarding health care and understand your rights (as well as your responsibilities) as a patient. Especially if your child has asthma, an excellent place to start is by reading *A Parent's Guide to Asthma: How You Can Help Your Child Control Asthma at Home, School, and Play,* by my friend Nancy Sander, the founder of the Allergy and Asthma Network/Mothers of Asthmatics. (I list more valuable information resources in the appendix.)

✔ **If a managed care plan that you're considering lists an impressive roster of specialists, make sure you can consult with these experts when you need them.** Some HMOs won't let you see a specialist until you're hospitalized, which is one hospitalization too many, in my opinion.

Working Well with Your Doctor

Expectations from treatment can vary from one individual to another, often depending on different people's priorities in life, so make sure you clearly communicate your own personal expectations to your doctor. Ask your doctor what you should expect to achieve from the treatment he or she prescribes for you, and participate in setting and developing your own individualized treatment goals. (If you have asthma, see the suggested goals for an effective asthma management plan, which I list in Chapter 13.)

The vast majority of people with asthma and allergies can lead normal lives. With effective, appropriate care from your doctor and your own motivated participation as a patient, your treatment plan should enable you to lead a full and active life. However, if following your plan properly doesn't allow you to participate fully in the activities and pursuits that matter to you, openly communicate your concerns to your physician and together adjust your plan to maximize the effectiveness of your treatment.

Part II
Taking Care of Your Nose

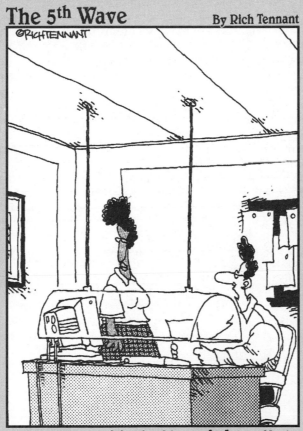

The 5th Wave   By Rich Tennant

"It's a sneeze-shield off a salad bar. My HMO won't pay for a non-sedating antihistamine."

In this part . . .

You don't need to be Cyrano de Bergerac or Jimmy Durante to know that your nose is a special organ of your body. If you have symptoms that indicate allergic rhinitis (hay fever), you need to understand that this allergy can often have more serious consequences than just annoying sneezing, a runny nose, a scratchy throat, and watery eyes.

This part discusses what may trigger your allergic rhinitis, the effects that the ailment can have on many parts of your body and how they occur, the types of complications frequently associated with the condition, and what you and your doctor can do to effectively treat your problem. Treatment measures include ways of avoiding allergens and irritants, appropriate medications you can take to control and prevent your symptoms, and using immunotherapy (allergy shots) in certain cases to manage your allergic rhinitis for the long term.

Chapter 4

Hay Fever Highlights

• •

In This Chapter

▶ Understanding hay fever

▶ Diagnosing hay fever — some telltale signs that you can use

▶ Recognizing the importance of treating hay fever

▶ Managing hay fever

▶ Considering special hay fever cases

• •

*H*ay fever is the most common allergic disease in the United States. As many as 45 million Americans may suffer from some form of this allergy, including 10 to 30 percent of all adults and up to 40 percent of all children. That's a lot of sneezing fits, runny noses, clogged sinuses, and itchy, watery eyes. Although the effects of hay fever are rarely life-threatening (even though some of us sometimes feel as if we could die when symptoms take hold), hay fever can still be a debilitating disease with serious consequences if you don't treat and manage it appropriately.

The term *hay fever* is actually a misnomer, stemming from 19th century studies of English farmers who mistakenly blamed spring hay cutting as the cause of nasal inflammatory ailments. Likewise, people in the 19th century referred to any ailment as a fever. In 1871 Charles H. Blackley identified airborne pollen from various plants — especially grasses — that depend on wind for cross-pollination as the primary causes of hay fever. The term "grass grief" didn't catch on, however, so we continue to use *hay fever* as a generic term for what doctors call *allergic rhinitis* — usually for the most common variety, *seasonal allergic rhinitis.*

Allergic rhinitis affects so many people that the estimated costs of medical treatment, absenteeism, and lost productivity from this type of allergy are perhaps as high as $11 billion annually in the United States. Studies have shown that 80 percent of people with allergic rhinitis develop the condition before their 20th birthday. U.S. schoolchildren with allergic rhinitis miss the equivalent of 1.5 million school days per year and are at an increased risk of experiencing developmental delays (such as hearing and speech difficulties); suffering from poor school performance (due to drowsiness and irritability); and developing learning disabilities (due to poor focus and concentration), as well as emotional and behavioral problems.

Rhinoids, rhinitis and rhinos: It's all Greek to your nose

Rhinitis is the medical term for inflammation of the nasal mucous membranes. The word derives from *rhin*, the ancient Greek for nose — hence the rhinoceros with horns (*keros*) on its nose — but has no relation to the Rhine, although your nose may run like a river during allergy season.

The second part of the term, *itis,* means swelling or inflammation, as in *tonsillitis* (an inflammation of the tonsils) or *appendicitis* (an inflammation of the appendix), and of course— you guessed it — *rhinitis,* an inflamed nose.

Here's some more nosy terminology that you can use to impress your friends and to better understand your doctor:

✔ **Rhinology:** The anatomy, pathology, and physiology of the nose.

✔ **Rhinoscopy:** An examination of nasal passages.

✔ **Rhinovirus:** A virus that causes respiratory disorders such as the common cold.

✔ **Rhinopharyngitis:** An inflammation that affects the mucous membranes of the nose and throat.

✔ **Rhinorrhea:** Runny nose.

Although often called "hay fever," allergic rhinitis itself doesn't cause a fever. If you do run a temperature while experiencing symptoms that resemble hay fever, you may actually be suffering from a viral or bacterial infection, such as sinusitis (see Chapter 9), influenza (flu), or pneumonia.

Catching Up with Your Runny Nose

In order to effectively and appropriately manage hay fever (allergic rhinitis), I strongly advise you to consider the following factors:

✔ **You're in it for the long-term:** This disease usually recurs persistently and indefinitely after you have become sensitized to the *allergens* (see Chapter 2) that trigger hay fever symptoms.

✔ **You need a healthy nose:** Because your nose is such a vital part of your respiratory system, your nasal health is vital to your overall wellness. Lack of treatment or ineffective or inappropriate management of allergic rhinitis can lead to complications such as nasal polyps (outgrowths of the nasal lining), sinusitis (inflammation of the sinuses; see Chapter 9), recurrent ear infections (potentially causing hearing loss; see Chapter 9), aggravation of bronchial symptoms, dental and facial abnormalities, and poor speech development in children.

Not only does your nose hold up your sunglasses, but it also provides other beneficial functions:

- Your nose helps to warm and humidify the air you breathe in.

- The interior of your nose acts to filter and cleanse the air you breathe in, through the action of the *cilia* (tiny, hair-like projectons of cetain types of cells that sweep mucus through the nose).

- Your nose is also critical for your sense of smell and the quality of your voice. For example, when your nose is stuffy or congested, your voice often sounds different (often referred to as *nasal voice*).

✔ **You need to know why you're blowing your nose:** A proper diagnosis of your allergic rhinitis condition requires a review of your medical history, a physical examination, observation, analysis, and, in some cases, skin testing to identify the allergens involved, all to help determine the most effective course of treatment.

✔ **Avoidance may be the key:** In many cases, the most effective and least expensive method of managing your allergic rhinitis is to avoid the allergens that trigger your symptoms. Although you may not be able to completely avoid all the allergens that cause your symptoms, partial avoidance may provide you with enough relief to substantially improve your quality of life (see Chapter 6 for avoidance information).

✔ **Drugs can be dangerous:** If you suffer from hay fever, you may resort to common first-generation, over-the-counter (OTC) antihistamines, decongestants, and nasal sprays to relieve your symptoms. However, many of these medications often produce significant side effects, including drowsiness (seriously limiting the safe use of these antihistamines), impaired vision, hypertension, nausea, gastric distress, constipation, insomnia, irritability — and that's the short list. Besides creating more havoc in your life than allergic rhinitis already provides, these side effects can also be potentially dangerous. Overusing OTC decongestant nasal sprays can also lead to a condition known as *nasal rebound* (see the sidebar on this topic in Chapter 7).

✔ **New and improved medication is available:** In cases where avoidance doesn't provide you with sufficient relief, newer and safer prescription drugs — including second-generation non-sedating and less-sedating antihistamines and nasal sprays — are often effective and produce fewer side effects than their OTC counterparts. However, these prescription drugs are only effective if you follow your doctor's instructions and take them properly.

Fear of flowers: Rose fever and other nose misnomers

Roses, like hay, receive a bad rap. Because these flowers tend to bloom in spring and summer when levels of wind-borne tree and grass pollens are usually at their peak, some hay fever sufferers mistakenly blame roses for causing allergy symptoms (hence the term *rose fever*). However, insects pollinate most attractive, colorful plants — including roses. In contrast to lighter tree, weed, and grass pollen and mold spores, the pollen that these plants produce is a sticky, heavier pollen that is much less likely to become wind-borne.

In fact, among the more than 700 species of North American trees, only about 10 percent release pollens that trigger symptoms of allergic rhinitis. Please note, however, that if you're a gardener and/or a florist who maintains a consistently high exposure to many types of flowers (not just roses), you can become sensitized to pollen from flowering plants, resulting in a form of occupational allergic rhinitis.

We're Not Just Making Hay

Hay fever is a common and nonspecific term for many varied types of allergic rhinitis, and it's often used in a general manner when discussing nasal inflammatory disorders — as well as for selling hay fever medications. Because the term *hay fever* describes so many different nasal inflammatory disorders, you may not be aware that allergists make distinctions between the different forms of allergic rhinitis. Allergists group these forms of hay fever according to the various types and patterns of exposure.

The three principal classifications of hay fever are

- ✔ Seasonal allergic rhinitis
- ✔ Perennial allergic rhinitis, including perennial allergic rhinitis with seasonal exacerbation (worsening — see the nearby "Chronic woes: All allergens, all the time" sidebar)
- ✔ Occupational allergic rhinitis

Seasonal allergic rhinitis

Seasonal allergic rhinitis is the most common form of allergic rhinitis, with symptoms occurring at specific times of the year when particular pollen and/or mold spore allergens are in the air. Hay fever symptoms can vary from

Allergy season

The term *allergy season* usually denotes the period from mid-spring to early summer, when a high concentration of airborne pollens and mold spores affects a significant number of sensitized people. Similarly, the period from late summer to fall, when weed pollens proliferate, is often termed *ragweed season*. However, no matter what the time of year, if enough allergenic pollen is present, it's going to be someone's allergy season. Allergists often use the term *pollination season* instead of *allergy season* to designate a period of time when significant amounts of tree, grass, or weed pollens are in the air.

year to year, however, due to climatic conditions and regional differences that affect the quality and quantity of pollen and mold spores in the environment. Hay fever symptoms can also vary because of the timing and types of exposure that you experience to these substances. The levels of wind-borne tree, grass, and weed pollens are usually at their peak in the U.S. and Canada during the following times of year:

- **Late winter (warmer climates) to late spring:** Tree pollens.

- **Late spring to early summer:** Grass pollens.

- **Mid-summer to fall:** Weed pollens, especially ragweed, which accounts for up to three-quarters of seasonal allergic rhinitis cases in the U.S. The presence of weed pollen may continue in warmer climates through December, in the absence of an early frost.

Wind-borne mold spores are present at various levels for most of the year, but they tend to cause a significant problem mostly during the late summer and fall. For more details on what's blowin' in the wind, turn to Chapter 5.

Perennial allergic rhinitis

Perennial allergic rhinitis is usually the result of your immune system becoming sensitized to a triggering agent or combination of agents that are constantly present in the environment, whether in the home, outdoors, at work or school, or other locations that you frequent. The symptoms involved in this condition can be just as severe as the symptoms of seasonal allergic rhinitis.

Chronic woes: All allergens, all the time

During allergy or ragweed season, or at other times of the year when significant quantities of allergenic material are present, if you already have perennial allergic rhinitis, you may also experience a seasonal worsening of your allergies, resulting in even more disabling symptoms. Doctors refer to this condition as *perennial allergic rhinitis with seasonal exacerbation* (worsening). In some cases, consistent and long-term exposure to multiple allergens can also lead to chronic allergic rhinitis. *Chronic allergic rhinitis* means that your allergy symptoms are severe on a constant basis.

Occupational allergic rhinitis

Occupational allergic rhinitis is more difficult to diagnose and treat because it often involves various combinations of a multitude of potential triggering agents and irritants found in many workplaces and occupations. Also, this specific type of hay fever often affects people with occupational asthma. (I provide details on occupational asthma in Chapter 11.) Your doctor should determine the following factors in the course of diagnosing occupational allergic rhinitis:

✔ Do your symptoms primarily occur at work? Or, if already present elsewhere, do your symptoms worsen while in the workplace?

✔ Do your symptoms disappear or improve after you leave work — at the end of the day; during weekends or vacations; when your work location changes; or if you take a new job?

✔ Do any of the your colleagues and coworkers experience similar allergic symptoms?

What Makes Noses Run?

In addition to wind-borne grass, weed, and tree pollens and mold spores, other allergic and nonallergic rhinitis triggers found in indoor environments include

✔ Dust mite allergens

✔ Indoor mold growths

✔ Animal dander, saliva, and urine from warm-blooded pets such as dogs and cats

✔ Waste and remains of pests, such as mice, rats, and cockroaches

- Allergens found in workplaces, schools, or other indoor or enclosed locations that you frequent

- Allergenic substances, such as fibers, latex, wood dust, various chemicals, and many other items

As I explain in Chapter 2, many substances that don't trigger an allergic response from your body's immune system can still intensify allergy or asthma conditions. Allergists refer to these substances as *irritants*. Common types of irritants include tobacco smoke, aerosols, glue, household cleaners, perfumes and scents, and strongly scented soaps.

Getting a Medical Evaluation

I strongly advise anyone who experiences significant hay fever symptoms to consult a physician to determine whether those symptoms are the result of a form of allergic rhinitis, a nonallergic type of rhinitis, a sinus infection, or a respiratory disease. A proper diagnosis is critical for the effective and appropriate management of any of these conditions.

That sneezy, itchy, runny feeling

Many allergic rhinitis sufferers mistakenly assume that they have lingering colds that afflict them every spring (or whenever the weather changes). However, even though viral infections such as the common cold and various strains of flu may follow cyclical patterns, the frequency of these illnesses is usually not as consistent or as constant as seasonal, perennial, or occupational allergic rhinitis. Symptoms associated with these forms of allergic rhinitis may often include

- Runny nose with clear, watery discharge

- Nasal congestion (stuffy nose)

- Sneezing

- Postnasal drip (nasal discharge down the back of your throat)

- Itchy, watery eyes (allergic conjunctivitis)

- Itchy nose, ears, and throat

- Persistent irritation of the mucous membranes of the eyes, middle ear, nose, and sinuses (in chronic cases)

Approximately half of all patients with allergic rhinitis experience additional clinical symptoms due to a *late-phase reaction* (see Chapter 2), occurring three to ten hours after allergen exposure, which typically leads to persistent symptoms, especially nasal congestion. The late-phase reaction is also implicated

Telltale signs: Salutes, shiners, and creases

The symptoms of allergic rhinitis that I list in this chapter often produce a distinctive combination of gestures and facial features, particularly in children and adolescents. If you or someone close to you seems to suffer from allergic rhinitis, keep these sufferer-specific characteristics in mind. These physical signs are often so unique that I can usually tell, when looking in the waiting room, who are the likely allergic rhinitis sufferers. When my children were younger, I noticed similar traits among their friends who had allergies as well. The following gestures and facial formations are characteristics that you and your doctor should look for to help diagnose your specific condition:

✔ **Allergic salute:** As tempting as it may be to consider this gesture a sign of respect for your doctor, the allergic salute actually describes the way that most people use the palm of their hand to rub and raise the tip of their nose to relieve nasal itching and congestion (and possibly to wipe away some mucus).

✔ **Allergic shiner:** Allergic rhinitis symptoms can really beat up some patients. Dark circles

under the eyes, due to the swelling and discoloration caused by congestion of small blood vessels beneath the skin in this area, can give you the appearance of having gone a few rounds with Mike Tyson.

✔ **Allergic (adenoidal) face:** Allergic rhinitis may cause swelling of the *adenoids* (lymph tissue that lines the back of the throat and extends behind the nose), resulting in a sort of tired and droopy appearance.

✔ **Nasal crease:** This line across the bridge of the nose is usually the result — particularly in children — of rubbing the nose (allergic salute) to relieve nasal congestion and itching.

✔ **Mouth breathing:** Cases of allergic rhinitis in which severe nasal congestion occurs can result in chronic mouth breathing, leading to the development of a high, arched palate, an elevated upper lip, and an overbite. (This symptom is one of the main reasons why so many teens with allergic rhinitis wind up at the orthodontist.)

in *non-specific reactivity* (increased sensitivity) of the nasal lining to nonallergic irritants (see Chapter 2).

Allergic rhinitis usually does *not* cause symptoms such as fever, achy muscles or joints, or tooth or eye pain. If you're experiencing these types of symptoms, the source of your ailment may be a type of viral or bacterial infection or the result of some physical factor, such as injury. Your doctor should evaluate your condition.

If you have a deviated (crooked) septum (the *septum* is the bony cartilage between your nostrils), it can block one or both sides of your nose, leading to a runny or congested nose. Because the resulting symptoms resemble allergic rhinitis, examination of your septum should be part of your physical examination. Surgical correction of a deviated septum may be necessary to relieve severe nasal airway obstruction.

The eyes have it: Allergic conjunctivitis

Symptoms such as redness over your eyeballs and the underside of your eyelids, as well as swollen, itchy, and tearing eyes, are characteristic of what doctors refer to as *allergic conjunctivitis*. This ailment often coexists with allergic rhinitis, and most of the same allergens as those involved with allergic rhinitis can trigger seasonal or perennial outbreaks of this conjunctivitis.

All that drips is not allergic

Many people think that runny, congested noses and sneezing are always the result of an allergic reaction. However, be aware that rhinitis also comes in nonallergic flavors, such as the following types:

- ✔ **Infectious:** Upper-respiratory viral ailments such as the common cold are often the cause of acute or chronic nasal distress.

- ✔ **Hormonal:** Women may experience severe nasal congestion while taking birth control pills, as well as during ovulation or during pregnancy — most notably from the second month to the full term. In pregnancy cases, congested nose symptoms usually disappear after delivery.

- ✔ **Emotional:** Women and men may experience runny and congested noses during sexual arousal. Other intensely emotional situations (such as laughing or crying) can also provoke your nose to run or congest.

- ✔ **Vasomotor:** The most typical examples of this form of nonallergic rhinitis are the nasal congestion, runny nose, and sneezing that can occur as a result of sudden temperature changes (for example, a blast of cold air). Exposure to bright lights or irritants, such as tobacco smoke, perfume, bleach, paint fumes, newsprint, automotive emissions, and solvents can also trigger vasomotor rhinitis.

- ✔ **Drug-induced:** Anti-hypertensives (medications for high blood pressure), as well as aspirin and NSAIDs (nonsteroidal anti-inflammatory drugs, like ibuprofen) can also induce symptoms of a runny or congested nose. Abused drugs, such as cocaine, can also produce rhinitis symptoms.

- ✔ **Gustatory:** Hot, spicy foods — especially those with serious peppers — can provoke watery eyes, runny noses, and sneezing (and temporarily clear sinuses in the process — whew!). Beer, wine, and other types of alcoholic drinks can also produce these sorts of symptoms in some people. This type of immediate, localized nonallergic reaction to certain types of cuisine and alcoholic beverages is not the same as the more complex allergic process that occurs with a food allergy, as I explain in Chapter 19.

In order to effectively diagnose your condition, a physician must review your medical history, as well as your family's history of allergies, and perform a physical examination. If your family doctor suspects a form of allergic rhinitis, he or she will probably refer you to a specialist, such as an allergist (someone like me) or an otolaryngologist (an ear, nose, and throat doctor), in the following situations:

- ✔ If clarification and identification of the triggers of your condition are needed.

- ✔ If the management of your allergic or nonallergic rhinitis isn't resulting in a substantial improvement of your condition, due to inadequate treatment and/or adverse reactions to medications.

- ✔ If you need to learn how to avoid allergens and irritants that may be triggering your symptoms (see Chapter 6).

- ✔ If your rhinitis or side effects of medications for the condition impair your abilities to perform in your career or occupation (especially in operating an airplane or motor vehicle).

- ✔ If the disease has a significant adverse effect on your quality of life by affecting your comfort and well-being.

- ✔ If rhinitis complications develop, such as sinusitis, otitis (ear inflammation), and facial signs (see the "Telltale signs: Salutes, shiners, and creases" sidebar earlier in this chapter).

- ✔ If you have coexisting conditions such as recurring or chronic sinusitis (see Chapter 9), asthma (see Chapter 10) or other respiratory condition, otitis (see Chapter 9), or nasal polyps.

- ✔ If your doctor needs to prescribe oral (systemic) corticosteroids (see Chapter 6) to control your symptoms.

- ✔ If your symptoms last more than three months.

- ✔ If your medication costs are a financial hardship.

In addition to performing a general observation to check for allergic salute, allergic shiners, allergic face, mouth breathing, and facial pallor (a pale face is often a sign of fatigue), your doctor will most likely examine the following areas:

- ✔ The front of your nose to check for an allergic crease and the condition of your septum (the "great divide" of cartilage between your nostrils).

- ✔ Your nasal passages, to check for swelling of the nasal turbinates (protruding tissues that line the interior of the nose — see Figure 4-1), nasal polyps (pale, round or pear-shaped, smooth, gelatinous outgrowths of the nasal lining), congestion, and the character, color, and amount of secretions from your nose.

✔ The inside of your mouth and the back of your throat for redness, swelling, enlarged or diseased tonsils, and to check drainage from the nasal cavity. In addition, your doctor may check for the presence of a high arched palate and/or *malocclusion* (misalignment of jaw and teeth, due to mouth breathing and tongue thrusting).

✔ Your neck and face, to check for lumps and sensitive, painful, or numb areas.

✔ Your eyes and ears, for signs of inflammation and/or infection.

✔ If indicated, further examination might include checking your vocal cords, adenoids, sinuses, and Eustachian tubes (the connection between your middle ear, nose, and throat that causes your ears to pop when descending in an airplane).

In addition to evaluating your physiological condition, your physician also attempts to determine

✔ The pattern, frequency, and seasonal variations of the allergic reactions that you experience.

✔ The types of allergens and irritants to which you may be exposed at home, work, school, friends' and relative's homes, and other locations that you frequent, such as malls, theaters, restaurants — even modes of transport, such as vehicles, trains, boats, and airplanes.

The patient's part

You can also keep track of when and where your allergic symptoms occur in order to help with the diagnostic process. For example, you may experience mild but manageable hay fever symptoms when visiting friends who have dogs and cats. However, you may find that, on occasion, your symptoms from those visits are more severe.

If you can track the times and dates of your allergic episodes, you can greatly help your doctor in determining whether the presence of seasonal allergens such as ragweed may worsen your condition by increasing your allergen load (see Chapter 6).

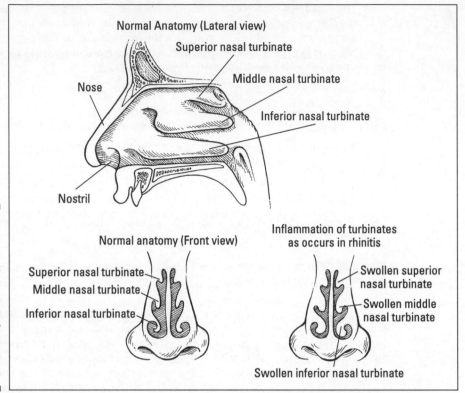

Figure 4-1:
The two cross-sections show the difference between a healthy nose and one with rhinitis.

Skin tests: The gold standard

Your doctor may also need to conduct allergy skin tests to confirm and identify the specific allergens that trigger your condition. In some cases, skin testing can also indicate your level of sensitivity to the allergens that bother you. A skin test procedure generally involves the doctor placing a drop of a suspected allergen on your skin and then using a device that pricks, punctures, or scratches the area to see whether the allergen produces a reaction. If you're allergic to that specific allergen, your skin reacts in a way that resembles a mosquito bite or hive. If you're on pins and needles to gather more information about skin tests, see Chapter 8.

Managing Rhinitis

As I note in Chapter 1, three basic approaches exist for treating and managing allergies, including forms of allergic rhinitis.

Avoidance

Benjamin Franklin once advised, "An ounce of prevention is worth a pound of cure." Eliminating (or at least lessening) your exposure to allergens and irritants can often result in less severe symptoms and less need for medication. In Chapter 6, I give you more detailed advice on what allergens and irritants to avoid and how to avoid them, especially in your home and bedroom, where most of us spend the greater parts of our lives.

Pharmacotherapy

Pharmacotherapy is the term doctors use for treating patients with medications. This form of therapy is particularly important in allergic diseases, because complete avoidance of allergens can be difficult. Therefore, your doctor may also recommend or prescribe one or more medications to help manage your condition, depending on the nature and severity of your symptoms, occupation, age, and other factors that your physician may assess. I provide an in-depth analysis of these products and their recommended uses and side effects in Chapter 7.

Immunotherapy

If your doctor concludes that avoidance and drug therapies don't provide effective results, and if the severity of your symptoms or the nature of your occupation warrants it, your doctor may advise you to consider *immunotherapy,* otherwise known as *desensitization, hyposensitization,* or just plain-old *allergy shots.* Immunotherapy treatment for allergic rhinitis generally requires at least three years of injections. (For an in-depth discussion of immunotherapy, turn to Chapter 8.)

Considering special cases

Certain groups of hay fever patients require more specialized treatment and consideration. These groups include

- **Children:** Oral antihistamines and mast cell stabilizers (nasal cromolyn, such as Nasalcrom) sprays are currently the first medication options for younger patients who experience allergic rhinitis symptoms. Your family doctor may also consider topical nasal corticosteroid sprays.

- **Elderly people:** Doctors generally advise that elderly patients use non-sedating prescription antihistamines, which produce fewer significant side effects, instead of over-the counter (OTC) antihistamine products. In addition, topical nasal corticosteroids are often recommended for elderly patients.

- **Pregnant women:** Physicians often consider mast cell stabilizer sprays (nasal cromolyn, such as Nasalcrom) as the first medication option for the relief of allergic rhinitis symptoms among pregnant women. During the first trimester of pregnancy, your doctor may advise you to avoid oral decongestants. However, after the first trimester of pregnancy, your doctor may prescribe some antihistamines such as chlorpheniramine (Chlor-Trimeton), decongestants such as pseudoephedrine (Sudafed), and topical nasal corticosteroids (Flonase).

- **Athletes:** Your doctor needs to make sure that any recommended or pre-scribed OTC or prescription product is not on any sports federation's list of banned substances. The U.S. Olympic Committee (USOC) and the International Olympic Committee ban the use of all oral and topical nasal decongestants and oral corticosteroids. In addition, some international sports federations also ban the use of oral antihistamines. Using other nasal products may require written approval by governing sports bodies. Obviously, whether the use of a product is governed or not, if you're an athlete, you need to avoid any medication that may adversely affect your performance or give you an unfair competitive advantage.

Chapter 5

Pollens, Molds, and Dust

• •

In This Chapter

▶ Understanding what you're breathing

▶ Reading pollen counts: News you can use

▶ Minding mites and other dusty denizens

• •

Something's in the air — and it may affect your allergies and asthma. Under normal circumstances, breathing is a reflex you don't even think about — as long as nothing in the air interferes with the process. However, unless you live in a bubble, every time you breathe in, you inhale more than just oxygen into your nose and lungs.

In fact, the air that most of us breathe is full of many types of airborne particles that are too small to see with the naked eye. In addition to pollutants and other airborne materials, these particles include allergenic substances, known as *aeroallergens,* that can trigger allergic reactions and significantly affect the well-being of people with asthma or allergies. The inhaled aeroallergens that trigger allergic reactions are known as *inhalant allergens.*

The following common inhalant allergens are the most frequent triggers of allergic rhinitis (also known as *hay fever;* see Chapter 4) and asthma. (See Chapter 11 for further information on what these allergens do to people with asthma.)

✔ Pollens that wind-pollinated plants produce, such as ragweed

✔ Wind-borne mold spores

✔ Household dust, which can contain various types of allergenic substances, such as dust mite allergen, dander, and other allergenic materials from household pets and pests, allergenic fibers, and indoor mold spores

At least 35 million people in the United States are allergic to wind-borne inhalant allergens. Wind-borne inhalant allergens can also enter buildings through open windows and doors, on your clothing, your pets' fur, and even on your own hair and then trigger allergic reactions indoors.

Pollens

Pollens can trigger allergic rhinitis and asthma symptoms. Plants that depend on wind rather than insects for pollination — grasses, trees, or weeds — produce pollens. These plants release their wind-borne pollens in huge quantities in order to reproduce. For example, ragweed plants may release up to one million pollen granules in a day, and the massive amounts of pollen granules that some trees release can resemble clouds.

Pollens are such universal features of life on our planet that pollen samples from excavation sites enable archaeologists and botanists to reconstruct what the natural environments of ancient times were probably like.

Pollen particulars

Seed-bearing plants reproduce by *pollination,* which involves the transfer of pollen granules — the plants' sperm cells — from male parts of a plant to receptive female reproductive sites. When pollen granules reach female sites, they produce pollen tubes that carry the sperm cells close to the female reproductive cells. (See . . . technical stuff can sometimes be exciting!)

A variety of means, including insects, animals, or the wind, can transport pollen granules. Wind-borne pollens that trigger allergic rhinitis symptoms come from three classifications of plants:

- ✔ **Grasses:** The grasses that cause most grass-induced allergic rhinitis are widespread throughout North America and were imported from Europe to feed animals and create lawns. In contrast, the many native grasses of North America produce little pollen. I provide more details on these grasses in "Allergens in the grass," later in this chapter.

- ✔ **Weeds:** The most important weeds that trigger symptoms of allergic rhinitis are those of the tribe *Ambrosieae,* known as *ragweeds.*

- ✔ **Trees:** Most trees that release symptom-causing pollens are *angiosperms* (which means "flowering seeds," although these trees don't actually flower) such as willows, poplars, beeches, or oaks, but pollen from a few *gymnosperms* (naked seeds) such as pines, spruces, firs, junipers, cypresses, hemlocks, and cedars can also trigger symptoms of allergic rhinitis.

Although these plant groups account for most cases of pollen-induced allergic rhinitis, only a small percentage of the members of each group has been shown to produce allergenic pollen.

Dead wood

Although you may experience allergy symptoms when exposed to the pollen of certain grasses, weeds, or trees, that doesn't actually mean you're allergic to the pollinating plants themselves.

If you're allergic to oak pollen, you're not allergic to the actual oak tree, you're only allergic to the pollen granules produced by the tree. Therefore, even though oak pollen may trigger your allergies, you can still use furniture made from the wood of the tree. That antique oak desk in your study won't trigger your allergies — it stopped pollinating a long time ago.

Blowin' in the wind

For certain plants, wind pollination has worked well for millions of years, enabling many plants to survive and flourish in environments that don't provide many insect or animal pollinators. Our much younger species (*homo sapiens* — you and me) has also flourished in these areas, with the result that we're often in the pollen path of wind-pollinating plants. Instead of wind-borne pollen granules reaching their intended targets, they can often end up in your eyes, nose, throat, and lungs, causing allergic reactions in susceptible individuals.

Pollens (and molds) for all seasons

Most wind-pollinating plants in the U.S. and Canada release their pollens at specific times during the year. These periods can be classified into five pollen seasons. If your allergies begin or worsen during one of these seasons, the predominance of particular pollens at that particular time of the year may cause your allergies. Here's the type of pollen (or molds) that may affect you in each of the five pollen seasons:

- If your symptoms get worse during spring, the probable cause is tree pollen.

- In late spring and early summer, grass pollen is the likely culprit.

- From late summer to autumn, weed pollen, especially from ragweed, may cause you problems.

- Especially during the summer and fall but also throughout the year except during snow cover, mold spores, particularly those of airborne molds, may trigger your allergies.

- In winter, wind-borne pollens are rarely a factor in most parts of the U.S. and Canada. However, in the warmer parts of the U.S that don't experience prolonged freezing temperatures (such as southern California), pollinating plants and molds can still release pollen and mold spores whenever there's no snow cover, thus potentially triggering allergies during the winter in southern regions.

Take my pollen, please!

The plants that are the main culprits in allergic rhinitis depend on wind pollination because they're not pretty or colorful enough to attract insects or other animals to do the pollinating. Most flowers that appeal to us — and to insects and other animals — produce heavier pollens that stick to the insects or animals that carry it to female plant reproductive sites. Therefore, you're far less likely to acquire sensitivities to pollen from roses or other attractive, colorful plants, unless you experience constant, close contact with flowers. If you do experience allergy symptoms after stopping to smell the roses, your reaction may be caused by pollens from nearby grasses, weeds, or trees.

If your allergic rhinitis symptoms follow a seasonal pattern such as those I just listed, consult your doctor to find out whether specific pollens are the problem. Also, you might ask your doctor for information on the major aeroallergens for the area 50 to 100 miles around where you live and work.

Non-natives

A list of local allergenic plants can serve as a good starting point to figuring out what plants may be affecting your allergies. However, knowing about non-native plants in your environment is also useful. Non-native plants in your environment often include trees and grasses — some of which may also produce allergenic pollen — that may have been planted around your community for decorative purposes.

Counting your pollens

Many newspapers and television and radio news programs regularly report *pollen counts*. The pollen count is the measurement of the total number of granules of a particular pollen per cubic meter per day. Pollen counters rate the resulting numbers according to five categories, ranging from absent to very high.

Bear in mind that the severity of symptoms triggered by pollens depends not only on the actual pollen count itself but also on the particular pollen being measured. In addition, the proximity of the collection station to the particular pollen being reported usually affects the actual count. Also, each region of the world has its own predominant allergy producing pollens. Table 6-1 provides the generally accepted guidelines for interpreting pollen counts for ragweed, which is the most closely followed type of pollen count in many parts of the U.S. and Canada.

Table 5-1	Ragweed Pollen Count Guidelines	
Category	*Pollen Grains Per Cubic Meter Per Day**	*Degree of Symptoms*
Absent	0	No symptoms
Low	0 – 10	Symptoms may only affect people with extreme sensitivities to these pollens.
Moderate	10 – 50	Many people who are sensitive to these pollens experience symptoms at this rating.
High	50 – 500	Most people with any sensitivity to these pollens experience symptoms.
Very High	over 500	Almost anyone with any sensitivity at all to these pollens experiences symptoms. If you're extremely sensitive to ragweed pollen, your symptoms can be severe at this level.

*These figures are averages.

Here are some other factors to keep in mind when reading a pollen count:

- ✔ Today's pollen count was collected yesterday and usually reflects what was in the air 24 hours ago.

- ✔ Rain can temporarily clear pollen out of the air. However, short thunderstorms — characteristic of late spring and summer in parts of North America — can actually spread pollen granules further.

- ✔ Hot weather increases pollination, whereas (you probably figured this one out already) cooler temperatures reduce the amount of pollen that plants produce.

Go west, young pollen!

When I was boy growing up in New York, I remember my doctor telling patients with allergies to move to Arizona because of the area's dry climate and sparse plant population. Over the years, plenty of folks have indeed moved to Arizona (and not just because of my doctor). Many of Arizona's new residents decided to plant non-native ornamental plants, such as mulberry trees, to spruce up the desert scenery. Mulberry trees thrive in the hot, dry climate and produce clouds of allergenic pollen. As a result, Phoenix and other cities in the state are now major allergy centers. In fact, some of the busiest allergists in the U.S. practice in Arizona.

✔ Pollen grains are typically at their highest concentrations from mid-morning to early afternoon.

✔ Because they're wind-borne, many pollen granules travel great distances, so the plants in your backyard or your neighbor's garden may not be what's triggering your allergies. Chopping down the olive tree in front of your house may have little, if any, effect on your allergies.

Quality, not quantity

Not all pollens are equal. Studies show that a little pollen from grasses such as Bermuda and bluegrass or trees such as oak and elm can go a long way in triggering allergies. On the other hand, your allergic rhinitis symptoms will usually only be triggered by much higher and direct exposures to pine and eucalyptus pollen (these pollens are large and heavy and don't disperse widely in the wind). Similarly, a moderate ragweed pollen count usually has far more effect than even a high English plantain count, depending especially on your sensitivity to those pollens. So knowing the types of pollens that are blowing in the wind, as well as how much of those pollens are actually in the wind, is important.

Consider the following tips to help you minimize problems during those high pollen-count days:

✔ If your community reports high counts for pollens to which you are allergic, you can take steps to avoid or reduce your exposure to those pollens. For details on how, see Chapter 6.

✔ If complete or significant avoidance isn't practical or possible, you can use pollen counts to help you determine (based on your doctor's advice) when to take medication to prevent the onset of symptoms or at least to keep those symptoms from interfering dramatically with your life. For an extensive survey of allergic rhinitis medication, see Chapter 7.

✔ The most important pollen levels for you to consider are the ones that trigger your allergies. Many of us react differently to different levels of airborne pollen, and pollens vary between regions. However, you should be concerned when pollen counts reach the moderate range, because that's generally the point at which many people with allergies start to experience symptoms.

Contact the National Allergy Bureau (NAB) of the American Academy of Allergy, Asthma, and Immunology (AAAAI) for more information on the pollens and molds in your area. Check out the NAB Web site at www.aaaai. org/nab/ or call 1-800-9-POLLEN (1-800-976-5536). In the appendix, I list additional information on organizations and health agencies that can provide you with more extensive local pollen surveys.

Allergens in the grass

Grass pollens are the most common cause of allergies in the world. Although only a small percentage of the more than 1,000 species of grasses in North America actually produce pollen that triggers allergic rhinitis and asthma, these particular species are widespread throughout the continent and release huge amounts of pollen granules into the air. Most of these allergy-triggering grasses are non-native plants that were imported to grow feed for farm animals and for planting our luscious lawns.

Wind-pollinated grasses release vast amounts of pollen granules during the late spring pollen season. The most significant allergy-symptom provoking grasses are

- Bermuda grass
- Bluegrass
- Orchard grass
- Ryegrass
- Timothy
- Fescue

Of the grasses in the previous list, Bermuda grass may be the most significant allergy trigger. Bermuda grass releases pollen almost year-round and abounds throughout the southern U.S., where the grass is cultivated for ornamental purposes and as animal feed.

Other grasses, such as rye, timothy, blue, and orchard, share allergens in common, so an allergy to pollen from one of these grasses may also indicate sensitivity to allergens from one or more of these other grasses.

Wheezy weeds

Weeds are plants, too. Many of us just don't consider them to be desirable plants. You might think that roses were weeds, for that matter, if the flowers grew unwanted in your garden. For the sake of allergies, however, when I refer to *weeds* I mean the small, wild, annual plants of no agricultural value or decorative interest to most of us. The wind-pollinated weeds that release allergenic pollen don't produce very attractive or conspicuous flowers. The most significant of these wind-pollinated weeds, in terms of allergic triggers, include

- Ragweed
- Mugwort
- Russian thistle

- ✔ Pigweed
- ✔ Sagebrush
- ✔ English plantain

The most common cause of allergic rhinitis in North America is ragweed. Ragweed is also a significant trigger of asthma. Many people who have sensitivity to ragweed may also experience cross-reactivity to cocklebur.

In the U.S., from the mid-Atlantic to northern parts of the Midwest, where ragweed is most highly concentrated, pollination usually begins around August 15 and generally lasts through October (and/or until a first frost), depending on climate conditions. Ragweeds are early risers, with most plants releasing pollen between 6 and 11 a.m. Hot and humid weather usually leads to an increased release of pollen.

Although ragweed pollen is most prevalent east of the Mississippi River, you can find related weed pollens, such as those produced by marsh elder and cocklebur, throughout most parts of North America.

Can't sneeze the forest for the trees

Of the 700 species of trees that are native to North America, only 65 produce pollen that triggers allergic rhinitis. The pollination season for most of these species usually runs from the end of winter or the beginning of spring until early summer.

Pollens from these types of trees have a much shorter range than the pollens that wind-pollinating grasses and weeds release. As a result, in most cities and towns, weed and grass pollens are far more likely to affect you than tree pollens. However, in the southeastern U.S., the spring tree season is a major problem, with high peaks of pollination over a prolonged period of time.

The trees that produce most allergenic pollen in North America include

- ✔ Elms
- ✔ Willows and poplars
- ✔ Birches
- ✔ Beeches, oaks, and chestnuts
- ✔ Maples and box elders
- ✔ Hickories
- ✔ Mountain cedars
- ✔ Ashes and olives

Ragweed to starboard, Captain!

Is that seasickness or allergies? Ragweed pollen has such a long range that it has been detected 400 miles out to sea. So if you're on the ocean during ragweed season, I suggest taking your medication with you. (Make sure it's non-drowsy, especially if you're at the helm.)

Molds

Talk about moldies and oldies: Mold spores have been suspected of being a source of respiratory allergies as far back as 1726. In fact, the fungi that produce mold spores are among the oldest forms of life on this planet. Throughout the U.S. and Canada, mold spores are some of the most common inhalant allergens, outdoors and indoors, and can be significant triggers of allergic rhinitis and other respiratory ailments.

Mold counts are usually much higher than pollen counts and usually rise to peak levels during the summer months. Outdoor mold spores are present almost year-round unless prolonged snow cover occurs, in contrast to pollens, which are released by plants, usually during distinct seasons. However, at any time, mold counts can suddenly and dramatically rise within a very short period and then drop down to previous levels just as abruptly. Because molds can also thrive indoors, you may be exposed to mold spores continuously throughout the year.

Outdoor molds grow on field crops such as corn, wheat, and soybeans and on decaying matter such as compost, hay, piles of leaves, and grass cuttings, as well as on several types of foods, including tomatoes, corn, melons, bananas, and mushrooms. (If you hunger for information on molds and food allergies, see Chapter 19.)

Spreading spores

As with grasses, weeds, and trees, only a few forms of molds produce allergens that trigger allergic rhinitis and asthma. Airborne mold spores occur almost everywhere on the planet except at the North and South poles. So unless you're a polar bear or a penguin, odds are you receive some degree of exposure to mold particles, no matter where you are. These molds include

 ✔ **Cladosporium:** These species produce some of the most abundant wind-borne spores in the world and flourish almost everywhere, except in the coldest regions.

- **Alternaria:** These outdoor molds are among the most prominent causes of allergy symptoms in sensitized people.

- **Aspergillus:** A medically important indoor mold, found in agricultural areas, crawl spaces in homes, and even outdoor air throughout North America. A variety of allergic respiratory diseases associated with exposure to aspergillus are recognized, such as allergic asthma (see Chapter 11), hypersensitvity pneumonitis ("farmer's lung"), and a serious respiratory disease known as allergic bronchopulmonary aspergillosis (ABPA).

Moldy matters

Here are some factors that can help you determine whether mold spores are triggering your allergies:

- You experience allergic rhinitis symptoms most of the year, rather than during specific seasons.

- Your symptoms worsen during summer months, even if pollen allergens aren't present to significant degree.

- Your allergies worsen near croplands, especially around grains and overgrown fields, or during or immediately following gardening.

For more information on avoiding or managing molds, see Chapter 6.

House Dust

House dust may be the most prevalent of all allergy triggers in your life. Recent studies show that the major inhalant allergens found in house dust can be the most important risk factors in triggering asthma attacks.

Let me reassure you: Dust is not dirt, and it's not an indication of poor housekeeping. I'm a clean freak, so I keep my house immaculate. However, if I go away for a week, I invariably find a coating of dust on most surfaces when I return, even though I sealed up the place and nobody has been to visit. Household dust is inescapable because it's a normal breakdown product of fibers and other materials found throughout your indoor environment.

Dust details

Common components of house dust include

- Dust-mite allergens
- Animal dander

- ✔ Insect fragments
- ✔ Fibers such as acrylic, rayon, nylon, cotton, and other materials
- ✔ Wood and paper particles
- ✔ Hair and skin flakes
- ✔ Tobacco ash
- ✔ Particles of salt, sugar, other spices, and minerals
- ✔ Plant pollen and fungal spores

Dust mites

The most potent allergen in house dust comes from the house dust mite (*Dermatophagoides pteronyssinus* and/or *Dermatophagoides farinae*, depending on where you live). A dust mite is shown in Figure 5-1. The primary food source of these eight-legged microscopic invertebrates consists of dead skin flakes that warm-blooded creatures such as humans constantly shed. (Don't worry — dust mites don't eat living skin.)

Figure 5-1: Dust mites are among the most abundant sources of allergic triggers.

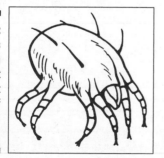

The allergenic material that dust mites produce in their waste can often cause allergy problems in humans. Because dust mites are usually as snug as bugs in a rug, we rarely come into direct contact with their bodies — just with their waste or decomposing bodies, which can also be a significant source of house dust allergens. Dust mites thrive in dark, warm, and humid environments such as mattresses, pillows, and box springs, as well as rugs, towels, upholstered furniture, drapes, and stuffed toys.

Mattresses and box springs usually provide the greatest concentration of human skin flakes for these creatures, which is why the average bed contains two million dust mites. As a result, your allergy symptoms may worsen in bed or while napping on your upholstered couch because you inhale significant amounts of dust-mite allergens while sleeping. That's why many of the avoidance and allergy-proofing steps that I recommend for your home in Chapter 6 focus on your bedroom.

If you wonder about the seriousness of dust mite infestations, consider this study: Dust mites were stained with a dye and then released on a couch in a home. (The family gave informed consent for the experiment.) By the next day, the dust mites had infested the family car, and some of the creatures were also found on the clothes of family members who had sat on the couch. Within ten days, marked dust mites were recovered from all rooms in the house.

In another experiment, dust mites in an infested rug were killed and the rug was cut into pieces and stored at different combinations of temperature and humidity. Almost two years later, the allergens from the dead mites were as potent as they had been originally.

What else is in my house dust?

Dander from household pets is another major trigger of allergic rhinitis (as well as asthma; see Chapter 11). Although you may not have pets of your own, if you're in contact with other pet-owners, dander from their animals can get on your hands or clothes, which you then introduce into your home. In addition, the urine from household pests, such as mice and rats, can be significant triggers of allergic reactions. Also, recent studies increasingly show that allergens in cockroach debris and waste can contribute to asthma attacks, especially in children.

I provide more information on all the allergens in this chapter, as well as non-allergic irritants, and ways of avoiding all of these triggers in Chapter 6 (which starts on the next page, so just keep reading).

Dust gets in your eyes . . . or nose, throat, and lungs

The following is a list of symptoms that you can use to determine whether the inhalant allergens in house dust trigger your allergies:

✔ You experience allergy symptoms as a result of dusting, making beds, or changing blankets and bed linens.

✔ Your symptoms seem to occur year-round instead of seasonally.

✔ Your symptoms are worse indoors rather than outdoors.

✔ When you awaken in bed in the morning, your symptoms are worse.

Chapter 6

Avoidance and Allergy-Proofing Your Home

*T*he three main ways of treating allergies are avoidance, pharmacotherapy (treatment with medications), and immunotherapy (treatment that modifies your immune response to allergens). Of these three methods, avoidance is the most practical and effective tool in most cases. Avoiding, or at least significantly decreasing, exposure to the substances in your environment that trigger your allergic reactions can often help relieve your symptoms, thus improving your overall health. These avoidance measures can also reduce the need for medication or shots, thereby saving you much time and money. In this chapter, I discuss the various methods of avoidance that you can use to improve your life with allergies and/or asthma.

Why Avoidance Matters

You've probably heard the joke about the patient who complains, "Doc, it hurts when I do this," to which the doctor replies, "Then stop doing that." (For more great doctor jokes, come to one of my book signings.)

Silly as that joke seems, the doctor's advice exemplifies the basic concept of avoidance, whether you're dealing with allergic rhinitis (hay fever), urticaria (hives), other allergies, or asthma. Depending on your sensitivity, avoid the substance(s) or levels of exposure to the substance(s) that trigger (that's why such substances are called *triggers*) an allergic reaction.

Avoidance seems simple enough. In real life, however, the trick is to figure out — short of living in a bubble — the practical and effective steps you can take to minimize your contact with allergy triggers.

Avoidance checklist

Environmental control measures are vital components of any allergist's treatment plan. Every practicing allergist focuses on helping you create and implement an effective avoidance strategy for yourself or your spouse, child, or other person with allergies or asthma who lives with you. The plan that you and your allergist develop will likely include these general steps:

1. **Identify allergy triggers in your environment, especially indoor allergens and irritants.**

2. **Recognize situations in which you may come into contact with those allergy triggers.**

3. **Discover how you can avoid allergens or minimize your contact with them.**

4. **Allergy-proof your home.**

Time for terminology

In case you're also allergic to jargon, the following list explains the most common technical terms that allergists use when discussing avoidance and allergy proofing:

- **Allergen load:** Your total level of exposure, at any one time, to any combination of allergens that trigger your allergies.

- **Allergic threshold:** Your level of sensitivity to an allergen. A low allergic threshold means that your sensitivity to an allergen is high — even a small exposure to the substance can trigger your symptoms. A high allergic threshold means that your body requires a higher concentration of allergens to trigger symptoms. Your threshold level, however, can decrease if you're exposed too often to large quantities of an allergen or to a combination of allergens.

- **Allergy trigger:** A normally harmless substance, such as pollen, dust, animal dander, insect stings, and certain foods and drugs, that can provoke an abnormal response by your immune system if you're sensitized to that substance. Doctors usually refer to these substances as *allergens*.

- **Cross-reactivity:** Your immune system is an expert at recognizing related allergens in seemingly unrelated sources. If you're exposed to these allergen cousins at the same time, your allergen load can exceed your allergic threshold, thereby triggering allergic symptoms.

✔ **Desensitization:** In the context of avoidance and allergy-proofing, *desensitizing* describes the active process of removing, shielding, or reducing the sources of allergens in your environment. Your allergist may advise you to desensitize your home, focusing especially on the bedroom of any person with allergies or asthma. *Desensitization* is also used to refer to a form of treatment in which an allergist injects small amounts of an allergen extract under your skin so your body can "learn" not to react to the substance (see Chapter 8).

✔ **HEPA:** High Efficiency Particulate Arrester. An air filtration process developed for hospital operating rooms and other locations that require a sterilized environment. HEPA filters absorb and contain 99.97 percent of all particles larger than 0.3 microns (one three-hundredth the width of a human hair.) If the unit truly operates at that level, only 3 out of 10,000 particles manage to sneak back into the room. Vacuum cleaners and air purifiers with ULPA (see definition later in this list) and HEPA filters are a vital tool for desensitizing and allergy-proofing your indoor environment.

✔ **HVAC:** Heating, ventilation, and air-conditioning systems — your home's lungs. The quality of air that you breathe indoors is largely dependent on the condition of these systems and the air that flows into and out of your environment through them.

✔ **ULPA:** Ultra Low Penetration Air. Even more thorough than the HEPA process, this filtration system is designed to absorb and contain 99.99 percent of all particles larger than 0.12 microns.

Knowing your limits

Avoidance measures rarely require the complete elimination of all allergy triggers and irritants in your environment. In many cases, you may only need to limit your exposure to certain triggers in order to prevent or alleviate symptoms.

Think of your allergic threshold as a cup and the allergy triggers in your environment as liquid pouring into that cup. Overflowing your small cup (low allergic threshold) may require only a small amount of liquid (allergens), thereby triggering an allergic reaction. A larger cup — a higher threshold — can accommodate more liquid without overflowing (without triggering an allergic reaction). The key to mastering your threshold is knowing your limit.

Another important concept to keep in mind when considering avoidance is to imagine a balance or scale with your allergic threshold on one side and your allergen load on the other. You won't set off your allergies unless the level of exposure to allergen triggers overloads your allergic threshold. Keep in mind, however, that your scales can tip not only from excessive exposure to a single allergen but also from exposure to small amounts of a variety of allergens.

Crossing the line

Cross-reactivity is also an important factor in causing allergic reactions, and it can contribute to overloading your allergic threshold. For example, if you have a sensitivity to ragweed, you may also have a sensitivity to allergens in melons such as honeydew, cantaloupe, and watermelon.

This phenomenon occurs because in some individuals, an allergenic cross-reactivity exists between certain food proteins and nonfood protein sources that can look similar to our immune systems. As a result, during ragweed season — in addition to ragweed allergy symptoms — you may also experience itching and swelling of your mouth and lips when eating melons, even though these fruits may not present a problem for you during the rest of the year. Some people also experience cross-reactivity reactions between latex (see Chapter 17) and — of all things — bananas, avocados, papaya, kiwi and chestnuts.

The Great Indoors

Early on, our ancestors realized that getting out of the elements and into some type of shelter was a key aspect of surviving the dangers and challenges of the prehistoric world. For the most part, we've become indoor creatures, progressing from cave and tree dwellings to suburbs, malls, and tightly sealed office buildings. In our dwellings, we're safe (for the most part) from predators (our safety from our own kind is another story), and most of us possess the means to shield ourselves from the adversities of weather and climate.

One of the downsides of modern structures is that indoor environments — at home, work, school, and even in cars and other enclosed means of transportation — can often contain far more significant sources of allergy triggers than outdoor environments. Most enclosures concentrate irritants and allergens, and because we spend so much of our time indoors, that's where we often experience the most significant exposure to allergy triggers.

Energy-conservation building codes adopted in the United States since the 1970s have worsened the concentration of allergens in structures, because airborne particles that contain allergens, as well as irritants, can often remain trapped indoors. So although I'm certainly in favor of energy efficient structures (especially when I see my utility bill), you need to insure that the air you breathe inside — especially at home — is as safe as possible.

Indoor air pollution: Every breath you take can hurt you

If you have allergic rhinitis, you may be focusing your attention solely on pollen counts, air pollution, and other elements of the outdoor environment as the prime sources for allergens and irritants that trigger your symptoms. You may have also assumed that indoor air is cleaner and safer than the air that you breathe outside. However, according to EPA studies, indoor air can actually contain as much as 70 times the pollution of outdoor air.

According to the American Lung Association, most of us spend 90 percent of our time indoors, spending 60 percent of that time at home. Therefore, indoor air pollution is a serious concern for everyone, particularly because studies show that it can cause or aggravate allergies and asthma.

Allergens on the barbie?

The issue of outdoor and indoor exposure to allergens and irritants is analogous to the difference between barbecuing outside or inside. When you cook outside, the smoke dissipates. (Yes, the smoke contributes to overall air pollution, but that issue is another story.) This backyard barbecue process is similar to the way outdoor air dilutes the effects of pollutants and allergens.

If you were crazy enough to bring your grill inside, seal all the windows and doors, turn off the ventilation, and then fire up the coals, within two minutes smoke would fill your house. Now, imagine indoor allergens and irritants as that smoke. All too frequently, many people breathe this polluted air in their indoor environments. The allergy-proofing steps that I discuss in this chapter show you how to avoid and control this type of indoor air pollution.

Allergy-Proofing Begins at Home

Allergen avoidance begins at home. While I certainly advise you to avoid or limit exposure to allergens and irritants outside — as well as at work, school, or other indoor locations — avoidance therapy can actually have the most beneficial impact in your home. Even if you're exposed to allergy triggers outside your home, reducing your exposure to those allergens and irritants at home may prevent your allergen threshold from overflowing or overloading.

On average, most of us spend one-third of our lives in the bedroom — much of that time in bed. Because we spend such a large amount of time in our bedrooms, your bedroom is the most important single area in your home. After you allergy-proof your bedroom, try to use it as much as possible to insure that you can give your allergies a rest.

In and around your home, the most common and important sources of allergens that you should focus on when allergy-proofing are

- Dust and dust mites
- Pets
- Mold
- Pollen

Controlling irritants at home is also vital to successful avoidance therapy. Although these substances don't trigger an allergic response by your body's immune system — as is the case with allergens — they often worsen existing allergy or asthma conditions.

Tobacco smoke is the most significant irritant found in the home that aggravates allergy and asthma reactions. Other important irritants, in alphabetical order, include the following:

- Aerosols, paints, and smoke from wood-burning stoves
- Glue
- Household cleaners
- Perfumes and scents
- Scented soaps

The basics of allergy-proofing are illustrated in Figure 6-1 and explained in more detail in the following sections.

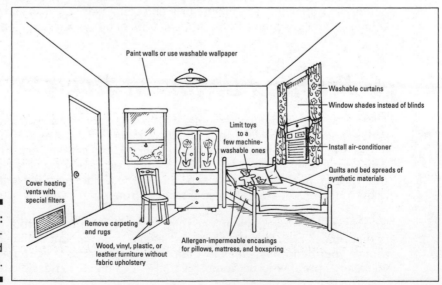

Figure 6-1:
An allergy-proofed bedroom.

Paint walls or use washable wallpaper

Washable curtains

Window shades instead of blinds

Limit toys to a few machine-washable ones

Install air-conditioner

Quilts and bed spreads of synthetic materials

Cover heating vents with special filters

Remove carpeting and rugs

Wood, vinyl, plastic, or leather furniture without fabric upholstery

Allergen-impermeable encasings for pillows, mattress, and boxspring

Controlling the dust in your house

House dust is one of the most prevalent allergy triggers in any home, and unfortunately, it's everywhere. Think of house dust as one of life's inevitabilities — along with death and taxes. House dust can trigger allergy symptoms either as an irritant to sensitized target organs (such as your eyes, nose, or lungs) or as a result of the specific allergens often contained in house dust.

Studies show that the average six-room home in the U.S. collects 40 pounds of dust each year. Please note, however, that dust is not dirt, nor is it an indication of poor housekeeping. House dust is a normal breakdown product of fibers found in pillows, drapes, clothes, linens, and other furnishings at home, work, school, or even in your car.

Ridding your house of dust mites

Allergy-proofing your bedroom and home likely involves dealing with dust mites more than with any other allergy trigger, because these microscopic creatures produce the single largest component of house dust that triggers allergies. Eighty percent of patients with allergies test positive for sensitivity to the dust mite allergen. The dust mite allergen is also the most significant allergic trigger of asthma attacks.

Although you've probably never seen them, dust mites are a fact of life — they're bound to follow almost anyplace you settle. These tiny spider relatives live in house dust where they feed on human skin scales (hence the scientific name *dermatophagoides,* meaning skin-eater), which we constantly shed (up to 1.5 grams per day — that's a lot of dust mite chow). The fecal matter (or *waste,* to put it more delicately) that they produce, at the average rate of 20 particles per day, is the most prevalent form of house dust allergens.

Controlling dust mites in the bedroom

Few of us ever go to bed alone. Dust mites thrive in dark and humid environments such as mattresses, pillows, and box springs. In fact, the average bed contains two million dust mites, which means that you may breathe in significant amounts of dust mite allergens while you sleep. Dust mites also survive well in blankets, carpets, towels, upholstered furniture, drapery, and children's stuffed toys.

Although eradication of these natural inhabitants of your home is virtually impossible — the females lay 20 to 50 eggs every three weeks — you can take practical and effective steps to minimize exposure to dust mite allergens.

In my experience, taking the following measures often results in a significant decrease in allergic symptoms and medication requirements for patients with allergies or asthma. (The appendix at the back of this book provides more information about obtaining the items I mention in this list.)

- **Beds:** Encase all pillows, mattresses, and box springs in special allergen-impermeable encasings, and mount all beds on bed frames. Wash all bed linens in hot water (at least 130 degrees) every two weeks. Only use pillows, blankets, quilts, and bedspreads made of synthetic materials. Avoid down- (feather) filled comforters and pillows.

- **Climate control:** Don't locate your bedroom in a humid area such as the basement. Likewise, use an air conditioner or dehumidifier to keep the humidity in your home below 50 percent. You may want to use a humidity gauge to monitor humidity levels.

- **Carpets and drapes:** If possible, go for the bare look in your home — remove carpeting and thick rugs. Bare surfaces such as hard wood, linoleum, or tile are inhospitable to dust mites and are also much easier to clean, thereby minimizing dust buildup. If you can't remove your carpeting and rugs, treat them with products that inactivate dust mite allergens. I also recommend washable curtains or window shades rather than heavy drapery or blinds.

- **Housekeeping:** Vacuum thoroughly, at least once a week, with a HEPA or ULPA vacuum cleaner (see "Time for terminology," earlier in this chapter). If you have allergies, wear a dust mask when you clean or engage in any activity that stirs up dust. Also, consider cleaning your furniture with a tannic acid solution.

- **Ventilation:** Use HEPA air cleaners to keep the indoor air throughout your home as pure as possible. (See "Time for terminology," earlier in this chapter.) Cover any heating vents with special vent filters to clean the air before it enters your rooms.

- **Decorations and furnishings:** Use furniture made of wood, vinyl, plastic, and leather throughout your home instead of furniture made of upholstery. Likewise, make your bedroom as uncluttered and wipeable as possible. Avoid shelves, pennants, posters, photos or pictures, heavy cushions, and other dust collectors. Limit the clothes, books, and other personal objects in your bedroom to the essentials, and make sure that you shut the ones you keep in closets or drawers when not in use.

If your child has allergies or asthma, don't make his or her bedroom a stuffed animal zoo — try to limit those types of toys to a few machine-washable ones. Keep your child's stuffed animals and toys in the closet or in a closed chest, container, or drawer when not in use.

Regulating pet dander

Pets are cherished members of many households. However, *dander* (skin flakes) from these animals is a significant source of allergy triggers for many people. All warm-blooded household pets, regardless of hair length, produce proteins in their dander and saliva that can trigger allergies. Dead skin cells in their dander can even serve as a food supply for dust mites. Cat dander residue can linger at significant exposure levels in carpets for up to 20 weeks and in mattresses for years, even after you remove the animal.

I usually advise people with allergies or asthma not to introduce a new pet into their home. If you already have a pet, I realize that removing this "member of the family" can be a very emotional issue for you and other household members, even though Fluffy or Fido's dander may be triggering your allergies or those of your children.

If finding a new home for your pet is not likely, I advise the following measures:

- ✔ Keep your pet outdoors whenever possible.
- ✔ If keeping your pet outdoors isn't possible, by all means, keep the pet out of the patient's bedroom.
- ✔ Make sure that anyone who touches your pet washes his or her hands before contacting the patient or entering the patient's bedroom.
- ✔ Washing your pet with water once a week may remove surface allergens and possibly reduce the amount of dander that can stick to other household members' clothes and body (thereby reaching the patient's bedroom). Although it may take some training (and a few scratch marks), even cats can get used to baths.

Controlling mold in your abode

Molds are some of the oldest and most common organisms on the planet, and they're widespread in most homes. Think of molds as microscopic fungi or mushrooms. You've probably encountered various forms of mold at home, from splotches on your shower door to the greenish growth on that tomato you forgot way in the back of your fridge last year (hope your mom doesn't find out).

Molds release fungal spores into the air, which settle on organic matter and grow into new mold clusters. When inhaled by sensitized individuals, these airborne spores can trigger allergic symptoms. Airborne mold spores are more numerous than pollen grains, and unlike pollen, they don't have a limited season. In many parts of the U.S. and Canada, mold spores may be present until the first snow cover.

Outdoor mold spores can enter your home through the air, by blowing in open windows and doors, and through vents. Indoor molds can grow year-round, and they thrive in dark, humid areas of the home, such as basements and bathrooms. Molds also grow under carpets, in pillows, mattresses, air conditioners, garbage containers, and refrigerators. The older your home, the larger the amount of mold that grows there.

Limiting your exposure to mold spores is a key part of allergy-proofing your home. I advise the following steps for controlling molds in and around your home:

- ✔ Avoid damp areas of your home, such as an unfinished basement or a room with a water leak. Or use a dehumidifier to lower humidity in those areas to 35 to 40 percent.

- ✔ Make sure your clothes dryer vents to the outside.

- ✔ Ventilate your bathroom well, especially after a shower or bath. Use mold-killing and mold-preventing solutions behind the toilet, around the sink, shower, bathtub, washing machine, refrigerator, and other areas of your home where water or moisture collects.

- ✔ Clean any visible mold from the walls, floors, and ceiling by using a non-chlorine bleach.

- ✔ Take out the trash and clean your garbage container regularly to prevent mold growth.

- ✔ Dry out damp footwear and clothing in which mold could breed. Don't hang clothes outside, where they can become landing areas for mold spores.

- ✔ Limit the number of indoor plants or remove them altogether, because mold may grow in potting soil. Dried flowers may also contain mold, so avoid them.

If you are have allergies or asthma, avoid exposure to outdoor molds around your home. These molds proliferate in fallen leaves, compost, cut grass, fertilizer, hay, and barns. If you need to work in your yard, wear a well-fitting face mask. Cut back any heavy vegetation around your home to allow the structure to breathe and to prevent dampness and mold growth.

Pollen-proofing

Allergic rhinitis (hay fever) is perhaps the best-known allergy of all. Many people associate this type of allergy primarily with outdoor exposure to pollen. However, you may also experience significant levels of pollen at home, and these exposures can also trigger allergic rhinitis symptoms.

Most pollens are windborne; they can often blow indoors (typically through open windows and doors) and trigger allergic symptoms such as allergic rhinitis (hay fever) within your home, not just outdoors. Wind-pollinated trees, grasses, and weeds produce pollen during various times of the year. Chapter 5 provides information on pollen counts, and the appendix includes contact information for the National Allergy Bureau so that you can obtain its reports on local pollen and mold conditions.

Take the following steps, especially during periods of high pollination, to avoid excessive exposure to pollen:

✔ Avoid intense outdoor activities, such as exercise or strenuous work, during the early morning and late afternoon hours when pollen counts are highest. If you need to work outside, wear a pollen and dust mask.

✔ Close windows and run a HEPA or ULPA air conditioner and air purifier.

✔ Make sure to clean and replace your air conditioner filters regularly.

✔ Wash your hair before going to bed to avoid getting pollen on your pillow.

✔ Use a clothes dryer instead of hanging the wash outside, where it acts as a filter trap for pollen. You may like the idea of fresh, air-dried laundry, but your target organs (see Chapter 1) won't enjoy the allergic reactions that all the fresh pollen triggers — especially if you hang sheets and pillowcases out on the line.

To find out more about the allergy-control products that I recommend in this section, turn to the appendix at the back of the book.

Chapter 7

Relieving Your Rhinitis

· ·

In This Chapter

▶ Understanding the need for rhinitis medication

▶ Winding your way through the medication maze

▶ Choosing between over-the-counter and prescription antihistamines

▶ Getting nosy with topical nasal products

▶ Combining products to manage your nasal and eye symptoms

· ·

As I mention in Chapter 6, avoidance measures and allergy-proofing can significantly improve your quality of life by decreasing your exposure to the substances that trigger your allergic reactions. However, because allergens such as pollens, molds, and dust are everywhere, complete avoidance can be difficult, if not impossible.

If you have allergic rhinitis (hay fever) and work outside, avoiding allergens is extremely challenging. Likewise, if animal dander triggers your allergies and/or asthma and your work involves contact with animals, you need to consider additional ways of dealing with your allergies. If your allergy symptoms and the underlying allergy aren't treated properly, complications such as sinusitis, asthma, and other serious respiratory ailments can also develop.

Fortunately, medications are available which, if used properly, can prevent or relieve the allergic reactions you may experience from some unforeseen exposure to allergens. In this chapter, I explain how the most common allergy medications work, what potential side effects they have, and how you can make smart choices to control your allergic reactions.

Getting Familiar with Pharmacology

The many drugs available for treating allergies have various uses and characteristics. Some allergy medications are designed for one specific purpose, while others have more flexible uses. In general, allergy medications fall into three categories of usage:

✔ **Preventive:** If used properly, these types of medications can keep your allergic reaction from developing. For people who have chronic symptoms of rhinitis, allergic or nonallergic (see Chapter 4), the most effective approach is to use antihistamines (oral or nasal — see "Dose of Prevention" later in this chapter) and topical nasal corticosteroid medications preventively (see "Topical Nasal Corticosteroids" later in this chapter).

✔ **Stabilizing:** These drugs can often stop a reaction that's already in process before your immune system can release potent chemical mediators of inflammation, such as histamine and leukotrienes (see Chapter 2) that produce noticeable symptoms.

✔ **Relief:** Most of the commonly available over-the-counter (OTC) oral antihistamines and decongestants fall into this category. These are the medications that most people use to relieve the symptoms of an allergic reaction after it's already underway. As I explain in the body of this chapter, you're usually not taking full advantage of medications, such as antihistamines and topical nasal corticosteroid sprays, if you only use them after your symptoms have been triggered.

Whether prescribed or purchased over the counter, a few basic types of drugs are used to treat allergies:

✔ Antihistamines (available in various forms OTC and by prescription)

✔ Antihistamine nasal sprays (available by prescription only)

✔ Decongestants (available OTC or by prescription in oral form or as topical nonprescription nasal sprays and drops)

✔ Topical nasal corticosteroid sprays (available only in prescription form)

✔ Topical mast cell stabilizer nasal sprays, such as cromolyn (available OTC)

✔ Anticholinergic nasal sprays (available only in prescription form)

I detail the uses and benefits of each of these types of medication in this chapter. Combinations of antihistamine (over-the-counter and prescription) and decongestant products are also used for multi-symptomatic relief, as I discuss in the section "Two for the Nose: Combination Products."

An informed patient is a healthier patient. If your doctor prescribes medication for your allergic rhinitis (or any ailment), don't hesitate to inquire about the product, why it's being prescribed, and any possilbe side effects. For further information on what you should know, see Chapter 12.

Antihistamines

As the name indicates, antihistamines are medications (available in tablet, capsule, liquid, and nasal spray forms or by injection) that counter the effects of *histamine* — a chemical substance released by the body as the result of injury or in response to an allergen. First-generation over-the-counter (OTC) antihistamines have been in use since 1942 and are frequently the first medication option for allergic rhinitis sufferers. I discuss the important differences between OTC and second-generation prescription antihistamines in the section "Newer prescription antihistamines" later in this chapter.

Both first- and second-generation antihistamines block the effects of histamine and are most effective in controlling or alleviating symptoms of sneezing, runny nose, and itchy nose, eyes, and throat. However, these medications don't usually reduce nasal congestion. As a result, they are frequently combined with a decongestant to relieve symptoms of congestion. In addition, antihistamines produce various side effects, depending on the type of product (OTC or prescription), dosage levels, and course of medication.

If you have asthma, don't be afraid to use antihistamines. In the past, product information labels advised asthma patients not to use antihistamines because these medications might theoretically dry out the airways. However, studies show that the improvement of nasal symptoms produced by antihistamines has a beneficial effect on the functioning of lower airways associated with asthma.

Histamine hints

As I explain in Chapter 1, histamine is a chemical substance produced and released by the mast cells (among the cells that line your nose and respiratory tract). You may only become aware of histamine when your immune system releases massive amounts of this chemical into nasal tissue as a reaction to injury or in the presence of an allergen. After being released from the mast cells, histamine seeks out "receptor" sites located in the tissues of the nasal lining.

Think of these receptors sites as locks. Histamine inserts itself like a key into the receptor site and triggers the familiar hay fever symptoms of allergic rhinitis. Antihistamines attach to the receptors before histamine gets to them. Because receptors only accept one chemical at a time, if histamine is blocked by antihistamines, allergic symptoms won't be triggered.

A dose of prevention

Many people tend to use antihistamines only as rescue medications. However, if you wait to take antihistamines only after your symptoms begin, the medicine can't reverse your reaction. Taking an antihistamine to relieve your symptoms is like closing the barn door after your horse has already bolted. You're not going to get that horse back (although by closing the door, you'll at least prevent any others from escaping).

Use antihistamines preventively. Take the medication two to five hours before you're exposed to the allergen. If you maintain chronic contact with allergens, take antihistamine medication on a regular basis. For example:

✔ If you're allergic to ragweed pollen, start using your medication at the beginning of August — before ragweed pollens are released in the middle of the month — and continue using the medication until after ragweed season is through. Even if you're exposed to significant amounts of allergen, you will usually experience far fewer symptoms by using this type of preventive approach.

✔ If you know that animal dander triggers your allergic rhinitis and you plan to visit someone who has pets, take your antihistamine two to five hours beforehand. Also, remember to continue with the antihistamine after you leave, because dander will probably be on your clothes.

Nonprescription antihistamines

The least costly and most common variety of antihistamine medications are first-generation nonprescription products that are available in over-the-counter (OTC) form. Hundreds of nonprescription antihistamine products line drugstore and supermarket shelves. Most of these products, however, are just different brand names for a few of the same active ingredients, such as

✔ Brompheniramine maleate — the active ingredient in Dimetapp

✔ Chlorpheniramine maleate — the active ingredient in Chlor-Trimeton

✔ Clemastine fumarate — the active ingredient in Tavist-1

✔ Diphenhydramine hydrochloride — the active ingredient in Benadryl

Although OTC antihistamines can relieve allergic rhinitis symptoms, such as sneezing, runny nose, and itchy nose, eyes, and throat, they also produce side effects that can significantly interfere with your daily life. OTC antihistamines can cross from the bloodstream into your brain, where they affect histamine receptors in the central nervous system, resulting in drowsiness — the most serious and potentially dangerous side effect of these products.

Consider these factors when taking nonprescription antihistamines:

✔ Many states in the U.S. consider people who take OTC antihistamines to be under the influence of drugs. The Federal Aviation Administration (FAA) prohibits pilots from flying if they take OTC antihistamines within

24 hours of flight time. Similar restrictions on the use of OTC antihistamines apply to truck and bus drivers and operators in other transportation industries.

✔ Operating heavy machinery or engaging in activities that require alertness, coordination, dexterity, or quick reflexes while taking OTC antihistamines is dangerous.

✔ You must avoid alcohol, sedatives, antidepressants, or other types of tranquilizers while taking OTC antihistamines.

✔ Nonprescription antihistamines can also produce other side effects including nasal stuffiness, dryness of mouth and sinus passages, dizziness, gastrointestinal irritation or distress, and urine retention (which can aggravate existing prostate problems).

✔ Recent studies show that children with allergic rhinitis who take diphenhydramine (the active ingredient in Benadryl) for their symptoms score significantly lower on learning ability tests than children who receive equivalent doses of loratadine (the second-generation antihistamine Claritin).

In my experience, many patients are unwilling to tolerate the side effects of nonprescription antihistamines. As a result, they are less willing to take a long-term or even mid-term preventive course of a nonprescription antihistamine medication. Instead, patients may resort to OTC antihistamines as quick, short-term fixes after allergens trigger their allergic rhinitis symptoms. This approach often leads to a pattern of debilitating, recurring symptoms that can diminish the patient's quality of life and increase their chances of developing other serious respiratory ailments.

Newer prescription antihistamines

Many people assume that OTC medications are somehow safer than prescription products. In the case of antihistamines, however, the reverse may be true. Due to significant advances in research since the development of first-generation antihistamines over 50 years ago, several of the newer prescription antihistamines have fewer side effects. (However, the majority of the existing prescription antihistamines are still of the older, first-generation type, and just like all the OTC antihistamines, they can potentially cause drowsiness.) Some of the benefits of these newer second-generation medications include:

✔ Not crossing the blood-brain barrier. This means that second-generation products are non-sedating, such as loratadine (Claritin) and fexofenadine (Allegra), or only cause mild sedative effects, as in the case of cetirizine (Zyrtec).

✔ Side effects other than drowsiness, such as dry mouth, constipation, urine retention, or blurred vision occur less frequently or are much less noticeable with second-generation antihistamines.

✔ Although second-generation antihistamines cost more than nonprescription antihistamine products, the prescription products work longer and require only one or two doses per day to prevent or relieve allergic rhinitis symptoms.

✔ In some cases, second-generation products work as rapidly as the first-generation drugs. For example, loratadine (Claritin) and cetirizine (Zyrtec) usually start functioning within 30 minutes.

✔ Overall, patients who use second-generation antihistamines usually experience much less disruption or impairment in their daily lives.

Because of these factors, second-generation antihistamines, such as those listed in Table 7-1, can greatly improve the treatment of allergic rhinitis. In my experience, patients are far more likely to stick with second-generation antihistamines for the prescribed course, which often results in a more effective prevention of allergic rhinitis symptoms and a significant improvement of their overall condition.

When used in combination with certain systemic antifungals (such as ketoconazole), antibiotics (such as erythromycin), or any medical condition that might affect liver function, Seldane and Hismanal (no longer available in the U.S. but still sold in Canada and other countries) can — in rare cases — produce abnormal and potentially fatal heart rhythms. Make sure that you inform your doctor about any and all medications you already take — including OTC products — when you receive a prescription for another drug.

A.m./p.m. dosing

As part of their cost-cutting efforts, some managed care organizations experiment with a dosing schedule that consists of prescribing a non-sedating prescription antihistamine during the day and a less expensive, sedating OTC antihistamine at night. Although the concept may seem logical in theory, the reality of this practice can actually cause many problems. Because antihistamines continue to act in the body for a long time, the sedative side effects of the first-generation product may persist during the day. Studies show that using a first-generation product at night leads to sedation, performance impairment, and decreased alertness the next day.

Antihistamines and children

Treating children with any type of illness can be quite a challenge, and allergic rhinitis is certainly no exception. Besides the difficulty of getting children to actually take medications, parents also need to be concerned about side effects. In this regard, some of the second-generation antihistamines, such as the following, can be especially useful when treating children with allergic rhinitis:

Table 7-1 **Prescription Antihistamines**

Active Ingredient	Formulation	Brand Name	Total Usual Daily Dose for Children under 12 Years (See Formulation Details)	Total Usual Daily Adult Dose
Cetirizine	5 mg, 10 mg tablet (ages 12 years and older) syrup, 5 mg per teaspoon (2-5 years)	Zyrtec	Syrup, ½ teaspoon (2.5 mg) once per day for ages 2-5 years; 1-2 teaspoons (5-10 mg) once per day for ages 6-11 years	1 tablet once per day
Fexofenadine	30 mg tablet (6-11 years)	Allegra-Pediatric	1 tablet twice per day	Not applicable
Fexofenadine	60 mg capsule, 60 mg tablet (12 years and older)	Allegra	Not approved for children under 12 years of age	1 capsule twice per day 1 tablet twice per day
Fexofenadine	180 mg tablet (12 years and older)	Allegra-24 Hour	Not approved for children under 12 years of age	1 tablet once per day
Fexofenadine (with 120 mg pseudoephedrine)	60 mg tablet (12 years and older)	Allegra-D	Not approved for children under 12 years of age	1 tablet twice per day
Loratadine	10 mg tablet (6 years and older)	Claritin	1 tablet once per day (6-11 years)	1 tablet once per day
Loratadine	10 mg tablet (rapidly disintegrating) (6 years and older)	Claritin RediTabs	1 tablet once per day (6-11 years)	1 tablet once per day
Loratadine (with 120 mg pseudoephedrine)	5 mg tablet (12 years and older)	Claritin-D 12 Hour	Not approved for children under 12 years of age	1 tablet twice per day

mg = milligram

(continued)

Table 7-1 (continued)

Active Ingredient	Formulation	Brand Name	Total Usual Daily Dose for Children under 12 Years (See Formulation Details)	Total Usual Daily Adult Dose
Loratadine (with 240 mg pseudoephedrine)	10 mg tablet (12 years and older)	Claritin-D 24 Hour	Not approved for children under 12 years of age	1 tablet once per day
Loratadine	Syrup, 5 mg per teaspoon (for ages 6-11 years; approval pending for ages 2-5 years)	Claritin Syrup	2 teaspoons (10 mg) once per day for ages 6-11 years; 1 teaspoon (5 mg) once per day for ages 2-5 years*	2 teaspoons (10 mg) once per day

The following drugs are no longer available in the U.S.

Astemizole	10 mg tablet (12 years and older)	Hismanal	Not approved for children under 12 years of age	1 tablet once per day
Terfenadine	60 mg tablet (12 years and older)	Seldane	Not approved for children under 12 years of age	1 tablet twice per day
Terfenadine (with 120 mg pseudoephedrine)	60 mg tablet (12 years and older)	Seldane-D	Not approved for children under 12 years of age	1 tablet twice per day

*Soon to be approved in the U.S. for this age group

mg = milligram

✔ **Loratadine (Claritin):** Your doctor can prescribe this medication in a once-a-day kid-friendly syrup or rapidly disintegrating tablet form (Claritin RediTabs) for children as young as 6 years.

✔ **Cetirizine (Zyrtec):** Your doctor can prescribe this medicine for children as young as 2 years in a once-a-day syrup form.

Antihistamine nasal sprays

On the front lines of allergic rhinitis treatment, the most recent addition to the antihistamine arsenal in the U.S. is *azelastine hydrochloride*. The FDA has approved azelastine for use as a nasal spray under the product name Astelin. Here are some basic facts you need to know about this nasal spray:

✔ Azelastine hydrochloride is highly effective for the treatment of seasonal allergic rhinitis symptoms, such as sneezing, runny nose, and itchy nose, eyes, and throat.

✔ In contrast to most oral antihistamines, studies show that azelastine often helps reduce nasal congestion (stuffy nose), which may make it particularly useful in dealing with the congestion that often accompanies allergic rhinitis due to late-phase reactions (see Chapter 2).

✔ You can use azelastine nasal spray in combination therapy with topical nasal corticosteroid sprays or oral antihistamines in cases that require greater prevention or relief.

✔ The recommended dosage for azelastine is two sprays in each nostril twice a day for patients over 12 years of age and one spray in each nostril twice a day for children ages 5 to 11 years.

✔ The spray usually starts to take effect within three hours.

✔ Side effects may include a bitter taste and drowsiness in cases of prolonged use.

Decongestants

People commonly use decongestants for the relief of stuffy nose symptoms associated with allergic rhinitis. You can find decongestants in two forms: systemic decongestants in tablet, capsule, or liquid forms, and topical decongestants in the form of nasal sprays or nose drops. Unlike antihistamines, no second-generation decongestants have yet been developed.

Decongestants shrink swollen and irritated mucosal membranes by constricting blood vessels through action on the sympathetic nervous system. That's why these drugs are medically classified as *sympathomimetics*.

Systemic decongestants

Nonprescription oral decongestants are among the most widely used OTC products in the world, and you can find them in various tablet, capsule, and liquid forms. These medications work by shrinking blood vessels, thus reducing the amount of fluid that leaks into tissues lining the nose, thereby decreasing nasal congestion. The three most commonly used decongestants are pseudoephedrine, phenylephrine, and phenylpropanolamine. Pseudoephedrine is the most frequently used active ingredient in OTC oral decongestants, such as Sudafed, and in antihistamine-decongestant combinations such as Actifed and Dimetapp.

Here is some basic information you need to know before using this type of decongestant:

✔ Systemic decongestants are often combined with other drugs, such as antihistamines, antipyretics (fever reducers), analgesics (pain relievers), antitussives (cough suppressants), or expectorants to provide multi-symptom relief for headaches, fever, cough, sleeplessness, and other symptoms of the common cold, flu, allergic rhinitis, and other ailments.

✔ Oral forms of systemic decongestants can cause side effects, such as sleeplessness, nervous agitation, loss of appetite, dryness of mouth and sinuses, high blood pressure, and heart palpitations if used consistently over a long period of time.

If you have a medical condition such as arrhythmia, coronary heart disease, hypertension, hyperthyroidism, glaucoma, diabetes, and urinary dysfunction, you should not take any product containing a decongestant (even OTC), without first checking with your doctor.

✔ Because of the stimulant effect of oral decongestants, use them cautiously with children. (Believe it or not, most of the parents in my practice are not interested in unduly stimulating their kids.)

Topical nasal decongestants

Nonprescription decongestant nasal sprays and nose drops can provide quick and effective short-term relief of nasal congestion. However, you should only use them occasionally, and not for more than three to five days in a row, because long-term or consistent use can result in adverse effects such as *nasal rebound* (described in the nearby sidebar of the same name).

Never use topical decongestant nasal sprays and drops with children under the age of 6 without a doctor's supervision. If you use them properly, OTC topical decongestants generally produce few side effects other than occasional sneezing and dry nasal passages. The most common OTC topical decongestant drugs and brand-name medications include:

✔ Naphazoline, found in Privine

✔ Oxymetazoline, found in Afrin, Allerest, Dristan Long Lasting, and Sinex Long Lasting

✔ Phenylephrine, found in Neo-Synephrine, Sinex

✔ Xylometazoline, found in Otrivin

The dosage levels and usage frequency of these medications vary depending on each product's formulation and method of application. As always, you need to carefully read all product instructions and warnings before using any medication.

The long-lasting products require no more than two doses a day to remain effective, but other short-acting products may work for only one to four hours. Therefore, you may need to apply short-acting products several times a day, as long as you don't exceed safe dosage levels and don't use the product continuously without checking first with your physician.

Two for the Nose: Combination Products

Antihistamines and decongestants can often be more effective in treating the full range of allergic rhinitis symptoms if you combine them in one preparation. You can find numerous oral OTC combination products in tablet, capsule, and liquid forms on store shelves.

An antihistamine, such as chlorpheniramine or brompheniramine, is often combined with a decongestant, such as phenylpropanolamine or pseudo-ephedrine. These products are also frequently combined with other active ingredients — analgesics (pain relievers), antitussives (cough suppressants), and antipyretics (fever relievers), for example — to provide relief for a variety of ailments, such as cold and flu symptoms.

The onset of action and dosage frequency vary with different products. Tablets and capsules generally come in two varieties:

✔ **Rapid release:** These medications start working quickly but usually lose effectiveness within four hours.

✔ **Sustained release:** As you may expect, these products work the opposite way; they act slower but last longer than rapid release medications — usually six to eight hours or longer.

Non-drowsy OTC formulas may contain pain relievers, fever reducers, cough suppressants, or other active ingredients for multi-symptom relief but do not contain first-generation antihistamines, which cause drowsiness. Therefore, these formulas don't usually provide relief from the sneezing, runny nose, and itchy nose, eyes, and throat that are significant symptoms of allergic rhinitis.

Nasal rebound

No, nasal rebound is not a new basketball technique. This condition, more formally known as *rhinitis medicamentosa,* results from prolonged overuse of OTC decongestant nasal sprays and drops. Overusing such medications can irritate and inflame the mucous membranes in your nose more than before you used the spray, leading to more serious nasal congestion.

Unfortunately, some people increase their use of the topical product as their congestion worsens, leading to a vicious cycle in which more use produces more congestion. When this happens, higher doses do not clear the congestion — they only make it worse.

To break this vicious cycle, you must stop using your topical OTC decongestant. Your doctor may also need to prescribe a short course of oral and/or topical nasal corticosteroids to clear your nasal congestion and allow you to tolerate the discontinuation of the topical OTC decongestant.

Remember, the warning on the label that directs you not to use the nasal decongestant spray or drops longer than three to five days really means three to five days and no more. If your stuffy nose persists beyond this point, consider using an oral decongestant.

The decongestant in combination products can still cause sleeplessness, nervous agitation, loss of appetite (in fact, the decongestant phenylpropanolamine is the active ingredient in several popular diet pills, such as Dexatrim), dryness of mouth and sinuses, high blood pressure, and heart palpitations, especially in older patients. Likewise, the antihistamine in combination products can still cause drowsiness. For example, the antihistamine diphenhyramine (Benadryl) is the active ingredient in many popular sleep aids, such as Nytol. See the following section for more details.

The upside and downside

Because of their sedative effects, OTC antihistamines are generally thought of as *downers.* Likewise, because decongestants act as stimulants, they are considered *uppers.* You may think that combining these two types of drugs in a single OTC product cancels out both the sedative and stimulant side effects. However, a person may experience both the upper and downer effects at the same time, resulting in an agitated, jittery form of drowsiness.

If a patient's condition warrants a combination product, I usually prescribe a non-sedating antihistamine formulated with a decongestant, such as Claritin D, Claritin D 24-hour, or Allegra D. The decongestant (pseudoephedrine) in these products usually doesn't produce as great a stimulant effect as other decongestants, such as phenylephrine and phenylpropanolamine. As a result, the patient gets the benefits of both a nonsedating antihistamine and a less stimulating decongestant action, minimizing the adverse downer or upper side effects.

Most OTC liquid forms are short-acting, which means that they usually require up to four doses a day. However, you may prefer to use liquids, especially syrup forms that often contain flavorings (and sometimes sweeteners), to treat children as well as adults who have trouble swallowing tablets and capsules. Another option in these cases is to use prescription chewable formulations of these products, such as AH-Chew Chewable Tablets.

One size fits all

Although combination antihistamine and decongestant products may work well for short-term treatment of allergic rhinitis when you need quick relief from symptoms, the products are less viable for long-term use because you can't adjust the dosage levels of the individual active ingredients. Each dose, whether in tablet, capsule, or liquid form, delivers the same amount of antihistamine and decongestant (as well as other active ingredients) to your system whether you need relief from one symptom or the full range of ailments.

If you're considering switching combination products because the one you use doesn't seem effective, check the active ingredients on other medications to make sure that you don't buy the same antihistamine and decongestant combination under a different brand name.

Topical Nasal Corticosteroids

The most effective medication currently available for controlling the four major symptoms of allergic rhinitis — sneezing, itching, runny nose, and nasal congestion — is *topical nasal corticosteroid spray*. Patients and the general public commonly refer to these corticosteroid products as *steroids* or *cortisone*. However, my colleagues and I use the proper term *corticosteroid* for these types of nasal sprays so as to avoid confusion.

The spray is available by prescription only, administered by aqueous (non-CFC propellant) mechanical pump or metered-dose spray forms. The following information can help you and your doctor decide whether topical nasal corticosteroids will work for you:

- ✔ Topical nasal corticosteroid sprays suppress the inflammation of nasal passages, thereby clearing your nose for easier breathing.
- ✔ Topical nasal corticosteroid sprays are most effective if you use them daily as preventive medications. For a guide to safe dosage levels, see Table 7-2.

Never exceed dosage levels with these products to minimize the possibility of the medication causing systemic side effects, such as those associated with oral corticosteroids, as I explain in the "Steroids to avoid" sidebar.

✔ Topical nasal corticosteroid sprays provide gradual relief at the outset of allergic rhinitis symptoms. Initially, you may need to use the medication for several days before the spray suppresses the inflammation. Full effectiveness may require two to three weeks of daily application.

✔ Only use topical nasal corticosteroids if your nose is clear enough for the spray to penetrate. If your nose is seriously congested, you may need to use a topical nasal decongestant for only the first three to five days just prior to administering the topical nasal corticosteroid spray.

✔ In order to prevent injuring your septum (the bone that divides the nose into two nostrils), direct the spray away from the septum and slightly in the direction of your ears. Think of the Fifth Dimension hit "Up, Up and Away" . . . from the septum (perhaps I'm dating myself) as a reminder of how to aim the spray. You may even want to spray the product once in the air to judge the force of the spray before using it in your nose.

✔ You can often minimize the adverse side effects of nasal irritation, burning, drying, and nosebleeds by using an aqueous (AQ) formulation of a topical nasal corticosteroid because of its gentler action on the nasal lining.

Although evidence indicates that topical nasal corticosteroid sprays are highly effective and safe for children, some concern exists about the possible effects the sprays may temporarily have on the rate of growth in children who use these products. If your child uses a topical nasal corticosteroid spray, make sure that your child's physician knows about your concerns so he or she can accurately monitor your youngster's growth.

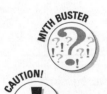

The negative perception that some people have of steroids is mostly due to attempts by some athletes to build up muscle mass by abusing anabolic steroids. In fact, the type of steroids used in topical corticosteroid nasal sprays are a completely different type of drug than anabolic steroids (which are actually male hormones).

Steroids to avoid

Although topical nasal corticosteroid sprays are highly effective and safe, using other forms of steroids is less advisable and potentially unsafe. The following steroids are potentially harmful to you:

✔ **Oral corticosteroids:** I advise using quick bursts of short-acting oral steroids (such as prednisone or methylprednisolone) only in cases of severe nasal rebound or nasal polyps, where a topical decongestant nasal spray can't penetrate sufficiently to decongest your nose. In such cases, you may require a short course of oral corticosteroids to sufficiently clear your congestion so you can use a topical nasal corticosteroid spray.

✔ **Intranasal injections:** Cortisone shots into the nose are not appropriate treatment for allergic rhinitis because of their potential for serious side effects, including vision disturbances and possibly even blindness.

Table 7-2   **Topical Nasal Corticosteroid Sprays**

Active Ingredient	Formulation	Brand Name	Total Usual Daily Dose for Children under 12 Years (See Formulation Details)	Total Usual Daily Adult Dose
Beclomethasone	42 mcg per inhalation	Beconase, Vancenase Pockethaler	1 spray each nostril three times per day (6-11 years)	1 spray each nostril 2-4 times per day
Beclomethasone	42 mcg per inhalation	Beconase AQ, Vancenase AQ	1-2 sprays each nostril twice per day (6-11 years)	1-2 sprays each nostril twice per day
Beclomethasone	84 mcg per inhalation	Vancenase AQ Double Strength	1-2 sprays each nostril once per day (6-11 years)	1-2 sprays each nostril once per day
Budesonide	32 mcg per inhalation	Rhinocort, Rhinocort Aqua	Rhinocort 2 sprays each nostril, twice per day or 4 sprays each nostril once per day (6-11 years) Rhinocort Aqua 1-2 sprays each nostril once per day (6-11 years)	Rhinocort 2 sprays each nostril twice per day or 4 sprays each nostril once per day Rhinocort Aqua 1-4 sprays each nostril once per day
Flunisolide	25 mcg per inhalation	Nasarel, Nasalide	1 spray each nostril three times per day or 2 sprays each nostril twice per day (6-11 years)	2 sprays each nostril twice per day
Fluticasone	50 mcg per inhalation	Flonase	1 spray each nostril once per day; may be increased to 2 sprays each nostril once per day (4-11 years)	2 sprays each nostril once per day or 1 spray each nostril twice per day; may be decreased to maintenance dose of 1 spray each nostril once per day

(continued)

mcg = microgram

Table 7-2 (continued)

Active Ingredient	Formulation	Brand Name	Total Usual Daily Dose for Children under 12 Years (See Formulation Details)	Total Usual Daily Adult Dose
Mometasone	50 mcg per inhalation	Nasonex	1 spray each nostril once per day; may be increased to 2 sprays each nostril once per day (3-11 years)	2 sprays each nostril once per day
Triamcinolone	55 mcg per inhalation	Nasacort, Nasacort AQ	2 sprays each nostril once per day (6-11 years)	2 sprays each nostril once per day

mcg = microgram

Cromolyn Sodium

Cromolyn sodium, an anti-inflammatory OTC nasal spray, may be highly effective in controlling symptoms of allergic rhinitis when you use it properly. (You can find this medicine under the brand name Nasalcrom.) Cromolyn sodium stabilizes mast cells, thereby preventing the release of histamine and other chemical mediators that can cause nasal inflammation.

As I explain more extensively in Chapter 1, mast cells are important players in the process of an allergic reaction. These cells are present in large numbers in the nose and lungs. When the body's immune system detects the presence of an allergen, mast cells activate and release several substances, including histamine, that produce allergic rhinitis symptoms.

To help determine whether cromolyn sodium nasal spray might work for you, here are some facts about its recommended use and effectiveness:

- ✔ Cromolyn sodium is most effective if you start using it two to four weeks before exposure to allergens. In cases of occupational allergic rhinitis or of limited exposure to allergens, using the spray immediately prior to allergen exposure, if your nasal passages aren't already congested, may also provide some relief.

- ✔ If allergic rhinitis symptoms are already present, you may need a short course of a combination antihistamine-decongestant for the first few days that you use cromolyn sodium.

- ✔ Because cromolyn sodium has an excellent safety profile and produces no significant side effects, doctors may often prescribe it for children and pregnant women.

- ✔ You can purchase cromolyn sodium in a metered spray form. The recommended dosage for adults and children over 6 years is one spray in each nostril, three to six times per day at regular intervals. Only administer cromolyn sodium to children between 2 and 6 years under the supervision of a doctor.

Anticholinergic Sprays

Ipratropium bromide is the active ingredient in the anticholinergic products (drying agents) that sell under the brand name Atrovent Nasal Spray. As the name of this drug class indicates, anticholinergics counter cholinergic activity by blocking *acetylcholine* — a neurotransmitter that stimulates mucus production — from attaching to chemical receptors in the nose. Therefore, these sprays reduce the amount of mucus in your nose.

Here are some basic facts about anticholinergic sprays:

- ✔ Ipratropium bromide effectively reduces symptoms of runny nose, as seen in conditions such as vasomotor (nonallergic) rhinitis (see the nearby "Skier's nose" sidebar) or the common cold.

- ✔ Ipratropium bromide has little effect on other allergic rhinitis symptoms, such as stuffy nose, sneezing, or itchy nose.

- ✔ Your doctor can prescribe Atrovent Nasal Spray in two strengths — 0.03 percent for relief of runny nose associated with allergic and nonallergic rhinitis in adults and children over 6 years, and 0.06 percent for relief of runny nose associated with the common cold in adults and children over 12.

- ✔ Spray two sprays per nostril two to three times per day (0.03 percent) or three or four times per day (0.06 percent) at regular intervals for the recommended dosage.

Leukotriene Modifiers

Leukotrienes play a significant role in asthma attacks. These chemicals, found in the mast cells that line the airways of the lungs and nose, enhance mucus production, constrict the bronchial passages, and promote further inflammation of the respiratory lining by attracting additional inflammatory cells into the airways. Leukotriene modifiers, such as montelukast (Singulair) and zafirlukast (Accolate), are relatively newer drugs that inhibit or stabilize leukotriene activity, thus decreasing the amount of mucus generated by exposure to allergens.

A few isolated studies show that leukotriene modifiers may effectively treat patients whose allergic rhinitis symptoms don't respond solely to antihistamines. If you're in that category, ask your doctor whether leukotriene modifiers may work for you. One of these drugs, Singulair, shows promise in treating symptoms of allergic conjunctivitis.

Remedies for Sore Eyes: Allergic Conjunctivitis

Allergic conjunctivitis often coexists with allergic rhinitis. In fact, most of the same allergens as those involved in allergic rhinitis can trigger allergic conjunctivitis. Characteristic symptoms of this ailment include redness on the eyeballs and the underside of the eyelids and swollen, itchy, and watery eyes.

Skier's nose

Ever notice how often skiers blow their noses? When I was training at National Jewish Hospital in Denver, I managed to get to the ski slopes occasionally. When I did, I noticed many boxes of tissues at the bottom of the ski lifts. As I discovered, the tissue boxes were there because of what people call *skier's nose,* which is triggered by cold air and is symptomatic of vasomotor rhinitis (see Chapter 4).

I've since found that Atrovent Nasal Spray works well to prevent skier's nose, if you use it before going up the slope, and also for treatment once symptoms appear. However, doctors also use anticholinergic eye drops similar to ipratropium bromide (the active ingredient) to dilate patients' eyes, so make sure that you keep the spray away from your eyes or you won't see that mogul coming right at you.

Because the mechanisms of allergic rhinitis and allergic conjunctivitis are similar, conjunctivitis is often treated with some of the same types of drugs used to control rhinitis in ophthalmic solutions specifically formulated for safe use in the eye. Treatment can include

✔ **Prescription antihistamines:** Two newer second-generation prescription antihistamines, *levocabastine* (Livostin) and *emedastine* (Emadine), appear to be more effective than conventional OTC antihistamines for the treatment of allergic conjunctivitis. Normal recommended dosage for both of these products is one drop per eye up to four times a day for up to two weeks.

✔ **Over-the-counter decongestants:** Products include Clear Eyes, Clear Eyes ACR, Visine A.C., Visine L.R., Visine Moisturizing, and Visine Original.

✔ **Combinations of OTC antihistamines and decongestants:** Product names include Naphcon-A, Vasocon-A, Ocuhist, Prefrin, and VasoClear.

✔ **Mast cell stabilizers:** This group of medications inhibit mast cells from releasing chemical mediators of inflammation, thus potentially preventing allergic symptoms from developing. These types of eyedrop products include

• **Cromolyn sodium (Crolom, Opticrom — not available in the U.S.):** As I mention earlier in the chapter, cromolyn sodium works best if you use it preventively, prior to allergen exposure. Likewise, it's more effective if you administer it on a regular basis, four times a day. For infrequent allergen exposure (when visiting someone with pets, for example) use cromolyn sodium immediately before you visit. This product has also demonstrated some effectiveness in treating forms of *vernal conjunctivitis* (a chronic eye condition that can cause severe burning and intense itching of the eyes and marked sensitivity to bright light).

- **Nedocromil sodium (Alocril):** This medication, already available in a metered-dose inhaler (MDI) formulation for the treatment of asthma (Tilade), has recently been approved in the U.S. as an ophthalmic solution. Alocril is indicated for treatment of itching of the eyes associated with allergic conjunctivitis and can be prescribed for children as young as 3 years of age. This product provides effective relief of both the early and late-phase allergic response (see Chapter 2). The normal dosage for Alocril is one to two drops in each eye twice per day.

- **Lodoxamide (Alomide):** This drug isn't approved for use specifically in the U.S. for allergic conjunctivitis, but it has shown some effectiveness in clinical trials as a treatment for vernal conjunctivitis. Normal dosage is one to two drops per eye, four times per day, for up to three months.

✔ **Nonsteroidal anti-inflammatory drugs (NSAIDs):** Ketorolac (Acular) is a type of NSAID that is indicated for the relief of the itching, redness, and tearing of seasonal allergic conjunctivitis. Normal dosage is one drop per eye, four times per day.

✔ **Combination antihistamine and mast cell stabilizer:** The most recent additions to allergic conjunctivitis eye products are olopatandine (Patanol), and ketotifen (Zaditor), which are available by prescription in the U.S. The normal recommended dosage for Patanol is one to two drops twice per day, six to eight hours apart. For Zadator, the recommended dosage is one drop in each eye every eight to 12 hours.

Doctors prescribe topical corticosteroid eye drops for severe cases of allergic conjunctivitis that are unresponsive to the medications I describe in the preceding section. However, you should monitor the use of topical corticosteroid eye drops closely because using these products improperly can lead to very serious adverse side effects. You should never use topical corticosteroid eye drops in cases where a viral infection of the eyes, such as herpes, may be suspected, because the use of these products may result in prolonging the course of and increasing the severity of this type of viral infection. In addition, prolonged use of these topical corticosteroid eye drops may result in glaucoma, vision disturbances, and cataract formations. You should consider consulting a qualified ophthalmologist before routinely using topical corticosteroid eye products.

I commonly recommend that patients with allergic conjunctivitis use eye drops during peak pollination seasons in addition to their other prescribed medication for allergic rhinitis to minimize eye discomfort. Try not to rub your eyes. Even though they may itch, rubbing them usually only makes matters worse. Instead, gently rinsing your eyes with clean water or a soothing OTC sterile irrigating solution can often wash away pollen and help relieve your symptoms.

If you experience severe allergic conjunctivitis, your doctor may prescribe an oral antihistamine, eye drops, and/or a combination of two different eye drop products for maximum relief of your symptoms.

Chapter 8

Allergy Testing and Allergy Shots

● ●

● ●

Depending on the severity and nature of your allergies and the degree of exposure that you receive to triggering allergens, avoidance measures and *pharmacotherapy* (treatment with medications) alone may not effectively manage your symptoms. You may need to identify and address the root causes of your condition instead of simply treating your symptoms. Your doctor may refer you to an allergist for the following specialized diagnostic and treatment procedures:

✔ **Skin tests:** Doctors use these tests to confirm that your symptoms result from allergies instead of some other cause. Doctors also use skin tests to identify, if possible, the specific allergens that trigger your allergy symptoms. Later in this chapter, I explain the two most common types of allergy skin testing that doctors use.

✔ **Immunotherapy:** Also known as *allergy shots, desensitization, hyposensitization,* or *allergy vaccination,* the advisability of this treatment depends on whether skin testing provides clear evidence that you are allergic to specific allergens, what those allergens are, and how they correlate with your medical history. (I go into more immunotherapy details later in this chapter.)

Skin Tests

Allergists consider skin tests the most reliable and precise method for diagnosing allergies. Doctors use skin tests to determine whether a minute dose of a suspected allergen — which an allergist or clinic staff member administers in solution form on or just below your skin — produces a small-scale, localized positive reaction — a *wheal and erythema (flare) reaction.* A wheal and erythema reaction is a reddening and small-scale swelling of your skin, resembling a mosquito bite, hive, or bump at the site of the allergen test. A positive reaction can confirm that you have sensitivity to the administered allergen and may also indicate your specific sensitivity level to that allergen.

You should remain under observation for at least 30 minutes after your skin tests. If the tests do produce a positive reaction, your allergist or test administrator will examine and measure the resulting wheal and erythema. Clinicians use these measurements to help determine your level of sensitivity to the allergen that they have administered. If your physician concludes that you need immunotherapy, knowing your level of sensitivity to the allergen is often important in determining a safe starting dosage for your first series of allergy shots.

Pins and needles

Most allergists use two types of skin tests to evaluate allergic ailments:

- **Prick-puncture:** Sometimes referred to as a *scratch test,* clinicians perform this test on the surface of your back or on your forearm.

- **Intracutaneous:** Allergists perform this test, also known as *intradermal testing,* only if the prick-puncture test fails to produce a significant positive result. The intracutaneous test involves a series of small injections of allergen solution in rows just below the surface of the skin on your arm or forearm.

A positive reaction usually appears within 20 minutes for both prick-puncture and intracutaneous tests. With either test, don't worry about someone turning you into a pincushion or sticking you with a giant syringe. The intracutaneous test uses only very fine needles just beneath the surface of the skin and, like the prick-puncture test (on the surface of the skin), produces minimal discomfort.

Skin tests and antihistamines: Not a good mix

After carefully reviewing your condition and history, if your doctor advises skin testing, you probably will need to discontinue using your antihistamine medications (and other products in certain cases) for several days prior to the test. The presence of these drugs in your body can interfere with the skin test results. However, it's unlikely that you will need to stop most of your other medications.

Never abruptly stop taking your asthma medications without first checking with your doctor. Fortunately, most asthma medications won't interfere with allergy skin testing.

The following list offers some general guidelines about discontinuing various common products; however, your allergist can provide you with more exact instructions, based on the specific medications that you take.

✔ Discontinue first-generation, over-the-counter (OTC) antihistamines such as Benadryl, Chlor-Trimeton, Dimetapp, Tavist-1, and similar products for 48 to 72 hours before your skin test.

✔ You may need to stop using prescription non-sedating antihistamines, such as Allegra, Claritin, Zyrtec, or Seldane, for as long as two to four days prior to testing. Likewise, studies show that Hismanal can interfere with skin tests for as long as three months. Therefore, you and your physician need to plan accordingly if you take Hismanal and anticipate taking a skin test. (Seldane and Hismanal are no longer available in the U.S. but are still sold in Canada and other countries; see Chapter 7.)

✔ If you take beta-blockers (Inderal, Tenormin) or monoamine oxidase inhibitors (Nardil, Parnate), make sure your allergist knows, because he or she must take special precautions when administering skin tests to patients who take these types of medications. These drugs can sometimes prevent the effectiveness of *epinephrine,* a rescue medication that doctors use for emergency treatment in case a rare, severe allergic reaction occurs after skin testing. Therefore, if your doctor advises you not to stop taking beta-blockers or monoaminoxidase inhibitors, your allergist may decide to use a RAST blood test rather than proceed with allergy skin testing (see "Blood testing for allergies" later in this chapter.)

✔ Because of their antihistamine effects, some antidepressants can also interfere with skin tests. If you're taking antidepressants, such as trycyclic antidepressants (Elavil or Sinequan), check with the doctor who prescribed these medications to see whether it's safe to briefly stop taking those products or possibly substitute another antidepressant (such as Prozac or Paxil) that doesn't have antihistaminic properties. If discontinuing these drugs to undergo skin testing is permitted, you may need to stop taking these medications for three to five days prior to your test.

You should never stop taking any prescribed medication (for any medical condition) without first checking with your physician.

✔ Skin conditions such as contact dermatitis, eczema, psoriasis, or *lesions* (irritations) in the skin test area can also interfere with your test results. Make sure that your doctor knows about any such conditions before he or she performs your skin test.

Starting from scratch: Prick-puncture procedures

Allergists consider prick-puncture tests the most convenient, least expensive, and most precise screening method for detecting specific IgE antibodies produced by your immune system (see Chapter 2) in response to a wide variety of inhalant and food allergens.

Antibodies are the agents that our immune systems normally produce to attack the harmful viruses and bacteria that constantly invade our bodies. However, with allergies, your immune system develops sensitivities to otherwise harmless substances — such as ragweed pollen or animal dander — and produces antibodies to defend against these substances, known as *allergens*.

When your immune system detects the presence of allergens to which it has previously produced IgE antibodies, these antibodies bind to mast cells in the area (such as your respiratory tract) where the allergen has been detected. This binding causes the release of chemicals such as histamines and leukotrienes as part of your body's mistaken defense against allergens. These chemicals then trigger allergy symptoms. (See Chapter 2 for more information on this process.)

To perform a prick-puncture test, an allergist or other qualified medical professional first places a drop of a suspected allergen (in solution form) on your back or on your forearm. The test administrator then uses a device that pricks, punctures, or scratches the area to see whether the allergen produces a reaction. The device only scrapes the skin, without drawing blood.

Alternatively, multiple prick-puncture tests can be administered simultaneously with a Multi-Test — a sterile, disposable multiple skin test applicator with eight heads. In this procedure, the applicator, with a specific allergen extract on each of its eight applicator heads, is applied directly to the patient's skin, as shown in Figure 8-1.

Figure 8-1:
A multiple skin test applicator can be used to administer prick-puncture skin tests.

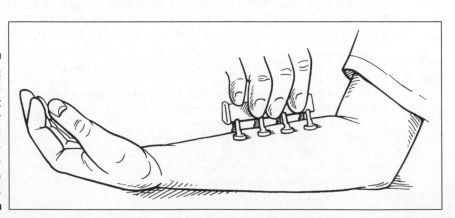

To conclusively identify inhalant allergens, you may have to undergo as many as 70 prick-puncture tests. The number of tests you receive varies according to factors such as the area where you live, work, or go to school and the types of allergen exposure that you receive. In many cases, your doctor requires fewer tests.

The number of prick-puncture tests that your doctor may need to administer to determine your specific food allergies may vary from 20 to 80. However, only a few selected foods (peanuts, shellfish, fish, tree nuts, eggs, milk, soy, and wheat) account for the vast majority of cases of allergic food reactions. By first taking a detailed medical history, in many cases your doctor may only need to perform a few carefully chosen food allergen skin tests to help confirm a very likely diagnosis of food hypersensitivity ("food allergy" — see Chapter 19).

Some food allergies, such as peanut hypersensitivity, can trigger serious reactions. If a patient tells me, "Doctor, anytime I eat anything that has peanuts in it, I nearly die," I take his or her word for it. If you suffer from specific severe food allergy reactions, I strongly advise against skin tests — and never intracutaneous tests — because the resulting positive reaction can produce serious or even life-threatening results. (See Chapter 19 for more information on food allergies.) Always tell your doctor — before he or she performs a skin test — about any serious food reactions that you may have experienced in the past.

Getting under your skin

If your prick-puncture tests are inconclusive, your doctor may need to perform up to 40 intracutaneous tests (but rarely in the case of suspected food allergies) to produce a significant positive reaction and confirm the diagnosis of an allergy.

Because intracutaneous tests involve the injection of an allergen extract just below the surface of your skin, the risk — although small — exists of a wide-spread systemic reaction. Never take an intracutaneous test for a particular allergen without first undergoing a prick-puncture test for that same allergen. The type of adverse reaction that may result from administering a particular allergen is usually far less serious with a prick-puncture test and alerts your allergist to the danger of performing an intracutaneous test with that allergen.

Because of a variety of factors, including the types of allergen extracts that your allergist administers, delayed reactions can occur with prick-puncture tests but occur more often following intracutaneous tests. The characteristic signs of these reactions include swollen, reddened, numb bumps at the skin test site.

Delayed reactions can develop 3 to 10 hours after your test and may continue for up to 12 hours thereafter. The bumps usually disappear 24 to 48 hours later. In some cases, these delayed reactions (known as *late-phase skin reactions*) can provide further evidence of your sensitivity level to the allergen (which I explain in Chapter 2).

Skin-test side effects

Skin testing occasionally produces adverse side effects in very sensitive individuals, but only rarely. As you would expect, adverse reactions occur far less frequently with prick-puncture tests than with more invasive intracutaneous tests. These side effects can range from large local reactions on the skin to systemic reactions, such as sneezing, coughing, tightness of the chest, swelling of the throat, itchy eyes, and postnasal drip.

In very rare cases, death from *anaphylaxis* (a life-threatening reaction that affects many organs simultaneously) has occurred following a skin test. For this reason, the medical facility where doctors perform your skin test needs to have appropriate emergency equipment and drugs on hand in the unlikely event that using these items becomes necessary.

Blood testing for allergies

Although most allergists consider skin tests the gold standard for diagnosing allergies, they may not work for all patients. Your allergist may advise diagnosing your allergic condition with a blood test known as *radioallergensorbent testing* (RAST). (Try saying that a few times, and you'll know why doctors use the acronym.) Your doctor may advise a RAST test instead of a skin test for the following reasons:

✔ Your prescribing physician may advise you not to discontinue medications such as antihistamines and antidepressants, which can interfere with skin test results, or beta-blockers and monoamine oxidase (MAO) inhibitors, which can cause complications when medications such as epinephrine are needed to treat serious allergic reactions.

✔ If you suffer from a severe skin condition such as widespread eczema or psoriasis (over a large part of your body), your doctor may not find a suitable skin site for testing.

✔ If your sensitivity level to suspected allergens is so high that any administration of those allergens may result in potentially serious side effects, you should avoid allergy skin testing.

✔ Another reason why RAST may be advisable is when problematic behavioral, physical, or mental conditions prevent a person from cooperating with the skin testing process. In those types of cases, RAST may serve as the next best alternative for diagnosing that patient's allergic condition.

Because RAST may require only one blood sample to analyze many allergens, this method may seem more convenient than skin testing. However, except for the cases that I list previously in this section, most allergists rarely use RAST because it isn't as accurate as skin testing and may result in an incomplete profile of your allergies. In addition, the RAST process is more expensive and time-consuming, because a laboratory must analyze blood samples and report test results, which often takes at least two days. If your results return inconclusive, your allergist must perform the test again and wait for new results. In contrast, skin testing usually provides results on the spot in 15 to 30 minutes.

Immunotherapy

Immunotherapy is currently the most effective form of treating the underlying immunologic mechanism (see Chapter 2) that causes allergic conditions such as allergic rhinitis (hay fever), allergic conjunctivitis, allergic asthma, and allergies to insect stings. (Chapter 21 provides details on how allergists treat stinging insect hypersensitivity with venom immunotherapy, or VIT.) However, at the present time, immunotherapy doesn't provide a safe and effective treatment for food allergies.

How immunotherapy works

The main goals of immunotherapy include

- Decreasing production of IgE antibodies, which are the agents that cross-link with allergens at receptor sites on the surfaces of mast cells, thus initiating the release of potent chemical mediators of inflammation such as histamine and leukotrienes. These chemicals trigger allergic reaction symptoms. (See Chapter 2 for an extensive explanation of the complex immune system responses involved in allergy and asthma symptoms.)

- Initiating the production of other allergen-specific IgG antibodies, also known as *blocking* antibodies. Immunotherapy can stimulate your body to produce these blocking antibodies, which compete with IgE for allergen binding on the surface of mast cells, thus preventing the initial sensitization, activation, and subsequent release of potent chemical mediators of inflammation from these cells. To find out more about the cast of Ig (immunoglobulin) antibodies and other characters involved in the complex immune system responses that result in allergy and asthma symptoms, turn to Chapter 2 (especially if you're a budding immunologist).

- Stabilizing the actual mast cells (and basophils) themselves. This means that even if IgE antibodies and allergens cross-link on the surface of these cells, your potential allergic reaction is usually less severe, since the release of potent chemical mediators of inflammation is reduced. In addition, immunotherapy can result in decreasing the actual number of mast cells (and basophils) in the affected areas. This reduction in activation and numbers of these cells also results in suppressing the inflammatory late-phase allergic response following allergen exposure (see Chapter 2).

Does immunotherapy make sense for you?

Immunotherapy may be appropriate for treating your allergies, depending on the following factors:

✔ Effectively avoiding allergens that trigger your allergies is impractical, or even impossible, because the life you lead inevitably results in allergen exposure.

✔ Your allergy symptoms are consistently severe or debilitating.

✔ Managing your allergy symptoms requires prohibitively expensive courses of medication, which produce side effects that adversely affect your overall health and quality of life. If the health and financial costs of allergy drugs outweigh their benefits, immunotherapy may make more sense for you.

✔ Allergy testing provides conclusive evidence of specific IgE antibodies, thus allowing your allergist to identify the particular allergens triggering your symptoms.

✔ You haven't experienced serious adverse side effects, as a result of skin testing, to the allergens that your doctor will use in your subsequent course of immunotherapy.

✔ You can make the commitment to see the therapy process through. Immunotherapy isn't a quick fix, and it requires a significant investment of your time.

✔ If you suffer from an unstable heart condition and you take beta-blockers such as Inderal or if you take monoamine oxidase (MAO) inhibitors, don't consider immunotherapy unless your physician advises you that the benefits of starting immunotherapy outweigh the risks of discontinuing those medications.

Getting shots

Injections (shots) are the most effective and reliable method of administering the specially prepared, diluted allergen extracts that allergists use when providing immunotherapy treatment. If needles give you nightmares, relax. Immunotherapy injections ("allergy shots") are much less painful or traumatic than the deep intramuscular shots often needed to effectively administer immunizations or certain medications (such as cortisone or penicillin). That's because doctors usually administer allergy shots with the same type of fine needle used in intracutaneous testing, thus causing minimal discomfort.

I'm often amazed at how well kids handle allergy shots after getting over their initial fear of the first shot. After the first shot, allergy shots aren't usually a problem for most children, especially after they notice that their symptoms are starting to improve. I'm not claiming that kids love getting allergy shots (or going to the doctor for anything besides a lollipop), but they usually quickly learn that receiving these injections beats not being able to breathe properly.

The allergens that doctors most commonly use in immunotherapy treatments for allergic rhinitis, allergic conjunctivitis, and allergic asthma include extracts of inhalant allergens from tree, grass, and weed pollens; mold spores; dust mites; and sometimes animal danders.

In preparing your allergen extract (serum or vaccine), your doctor includes only those allergens to which you have previously demonstrated sensitivity in your skin testing results. If your skin tests show sensitivity to multiple allergens (you're sensitive to many grass and weed pollens, for example), your allergist may mix all the different grass extracts into one vial and all the different weed extracts into another vial. Preparing the vials in such a combination ensures that you receive only one shot for each group of extracts, thus reducing the number of injections you need for effective therapy.

Your allergist may even determine that mixing the doses of all your allergens into a single shot on a particular visit is an option for you based on your allergic sensitivity, the volume of extract that needs to be administered, and the types of allergen extracts he or she uses for your therapy. In some cases, for your comfort, it may be preferable to split the required dose of your allergy shot into two or more separate injections.

Although this treatment can greatly reduce your allergy symptoms, immunotherapy isn't considered a guaranteed permanent cure for genetically predetermined allergies (see Chapters 1 and 2). You should still continue practicing avoidance measures while receiving immunotherapy; doing so can significantly enhance the effectiveness of your treatment.

Immunotherapy can significantly improve your allergy symptoms, thus reducing your need for allergy medication, making this treatment the closest thing to a "cure" for allergies currently available. However, always tell your allergist if you're considering taking medications — including over-the-counter (OTC) drugs — for allergies or nonallergic conditions. Also, always report any changes in your medical condition to your allergist, even if the changes may not seem directly connected to your allergies. Pregnancy, which I mention in the nearby sidebar, is an example of a change in medical condition that you need to report to your allergist.

Your adherence is key for an effective immunotherapy program. You should follow and maintain the injection schedule (see next section) that your allergist prescribes as closely as possible. However, you should avoid shots under the following circumstances:

Pregnancy and immunotherapy

If you become pregnant while receiving immunotherapy, you will be glad to know that your allergy shots are safe during pregnancy. In fact, your allergist may advise you to continue receiving immunotherapy, possibly at a reduced dose to minimize any risks of reactions to allergy shots, but also at a dose that continues to provide relief from your allergy symptoms.

If you stop treatment, you can run the risk of experiencing worsening symptoms. This worsening can lead in turn to increased needs for medication that may not be desirable during your pregnancy. However, if you're already pregnant and are considering whether or not to start a course of immunotherapy, your allergist may advise you to delay beginning this form of treatment until after delivery.

✔ **Exercise:** Make sure that you don't engage in strenuous physical activity for at least one hour before and two hours after your allergy shots. Exercising at these times can increase your risk of experiencing a serious adverse reaction because exercise increases your blood circulation, potentially resulting in a rapid absorption of the allergen from the shot and possibly even causing a severe reaction.

✔ **Illness:** If you run a fever, tell your allergist. Receiving an allergy shot while ill isn't a good idea because your fever symptoms can make detecting an adverse reaction to the shots difficult.

✔ **Immunizations:** Try to avoid scheduling any immunization injections on the same day as your allergy shots because potential adverse effects from the immunization can make a reaction from an allergy shot difficult to identify. If you do get an immunization shot on the day of your scheduled allergy shots, let your allergist know — he or she may advise you to not get your allergy shots that same day.

Shot schedules

The most effective way of administering immunotherapy is by providing *perennial therapy,* which involves receiving shots of allergen extracts year-round. Studies show that perennial therapy provides the longest and most successful reduction of your level of sensitivity to specific allergens.

Here's how a typical course of perennial immunotherapy may work:

1. Your allergist begins your therapy by administering shots once or twice a week, starting with a very small amount of a diluted dose of allergen extracts.

2. Your allergist gradually increases your allergen dose by increasing the amount and concentration of the extract week by week until you reach the maintenance dose in about three to six months. The *maintenance dose* refers to the predetermined amount of maximal concentration or the highest strength that you can tolerate that doesn't produce adverse reactions.

3. After you reach your maintenance dose, allergy symptom relief usually starts to occur. When relief begins, you can continue receiving injections at the maintenance dose level. Likewise, your allergist may extend the interval between your shots from one week to as many as four, depending on your response to the treatment and the levels of exposure that you receive in your environment to the allergens in question.

Every time you receive your allergy shots, expect to wait at least 20 minutes afterwards in your allergist's office so that a medical staff member can inspect and evaluate the areas of skin (sites) around your injections. Another benefit to staying in your allergist's office after your injection is that, in the rare event that you experience a severe reaction, qualified medical personnel can immediately provide emergency assistance.

A long-term relationship

For inhalant allergens, an effective immunotherapy program usually requires injections for at least three to five years. In many cases, if your sensitivity to allergens improves over this immunotherapy period, you can maintain your allergy improvement for several years even after discontinuing the shots.

However, in some cases, the withdrawal of immunotherapy results in the reappearance of allergic symptoms. Therefore, your allergist will need to evaluate the specifics of your individual case when he or she considers the possibility of discontinuing immunotherapy.

Side effects

The possibility — however small — of anaphylactic reactions exists any time your allergist injects allergenic proteins into your body. In some unfortunate cases, people have died after receiving an allergy shot. Therefore, although the odds of a serious reaction to allergy shots are far less than those of getting into a bad car crash on the way to your allergist's office, I strongly advise taking as many precautions as possible. After receiving an allergy shot, immediately tell your doctor or nurse if you experience any of the following signs of serious adverse side effects:

✔ Itchiness of the feet, hands, groin area, and underarms

✔ Large-scale skin reactions such as hives or flushing

- ✔ Upper and lower respiratory symptoms, such as sneezing, coughing, tightness of the chest, a swollen or itchy throat, itchy eyes, postnasal drip, difficulty swallowing, and a hoarse voice

- ✔ Nausea, diarrhea, and stomach cramps

- ✔ Dizziness, fainting, or a severe drop in blood pressure

Because the threat of severe adverse reactions exists, I strongly advise against giving yourself allergy shots at home. Although practices vary in different areas, the vast majority of my colleagues insist that patients receive their allergy shots only in an appropriate medical facility because of the small chance of adverse, life-threatening reactions.

On the Horizon

New forms of immunotherapy treatment are just around the corner. The most promising therapies include

- ✔ **Sprays:** Nasal sprays that are under development may provide a less needle-dependent form of administering allergen extracts to patients.

- ✔ **Anti-IgE antibodies:** The agent in this medication named Xolair (still undergoing clinical trials) is a high-tech antibody known as *recombinant human monoclonal antibody* (rhuMab-E25). Researchers have designed this drug to bind to the part of the IgE antibody that otherwise would bind with the IgE receptor site on mast cells, thus preventing the activation of these cells and subsequent allergic reaction. In my opinion, this drug not only shows the potential to improve asthma and allergic rhinitis treatment, but it may also include the potential to block many types of allergic reactions that science hasn't had much success in controlling adequately — for example, severe allergic food reactions.

Chapter 9

Avoiding Allergy Complications

● ●

In This Chapter

▶ Knowing the complications of untreated allergies

▶ Diagnosing sinus and ear infections

▶ Clearing the nosy road to your ears and sinuses

▶ Preventing infections

● ●

*B*ecause many people refer to allergic rhinitis as *hay fever,* they often think that this allergic condition is just a nuisance rather than a serious disease. However, as I explain in Chapter 4, allergic rhinitis isn't a simple problem. Allergic rhinitis is an ailment that often requires serious attention and management, not only because the symptoms can severely affect your quality of life, but also because a lack of treatment or poor management of allergic rhinitis can lead to serious complications, such as *sinusitis* — an inflammation of the sinuses — and *otitis media* — an inflammation of the middle ear. In this chapter, I explain the causes and symptoms of these two common types of infections, and I describe appropriate methods of preventing and treating them.

Sinusitis

If you've ever had a cold or nasal symptoms that didn't seem to go away, you may have actually been suffering from a form of sinusitis. This often painful condition develops as a result of swollen nasal and sinus passages that frequently result from allergic rhinitis. Many patients often confuse sinusitis symptoms with the symptoms of a cold, flu, or allergy.

Sinusitis is one of the most common health problems in the United States. Current estimates are that sinusitis affects 35 million people in this country each year. Because of the pain and discomfort that sinusitis causes, it's one of the most common reasons for doctor visits in the U.S.

Consult a doctor as soon as you suspect you may have sinusitis. Complications such as recurrent bronchitis, otitis media, nasal polyps, and aggravation of asthma can occur if you manage your sinusitis poorly. Chronic sinus infections can result in swollen adenoids that may require surgery to remove. On a more positive note, studies show that asthma patients who effectively manage their sinusitis can significantly improve their respiratory symptoms.

Common causes

In a significant number of sinusitis cases, allergic rhinitis precedes the start of a sinus infection. Research shows that over half of all children in the U.S. who receive treatment for sinusitis also have allergic rhinitis.

Vasomotor rhinitis, a nonallergic form of rhinitis that results from sudden temperature changes or exposure to tobacco smoke, pollutants, and other irritants (see Chapter 4), can also contribute to sinusitis. Swimmers, divers, fliers (passengers, as well as flight crews), and other people with this form of rhinitis who frequently experience pressure and weather changes may be particularly prone to developing sinusitis if they don't effectively manage their rhinitis symptoms.

Other factors (you may have one or more of these) that can also increase your chances of developing sinusitis include

- **Upper respiratory viral infections:** Viruses such as those associated with the common cold are the most frequent causes of sinusitis.

- **Bacteria:** The same family of germs that can cause acute otitis media (*Streptococcus pneumonia, Haemophilus influenza, Moraxella catarrhalis*) can cause acute bacterial sinusitis. Unlike viral infections, this type of sinusitis responds to antibiotic therapy.

- **Fungal:** This type of sinusitis infection can develop in otherwise healthy patients who have been on long-term antibiotic treatment or have been taking oral corticosteroids on a chronic basis. *Aspergillus* is the most common fungus that causes these types of cases and is also frequently implicated in cases of *allergic fungal sinusitis.* Characteristic signs and symptoms of this form of recurring fungal infection, which can often affect individuals with allergic rhinitis and/or asthma, are sinus infections and *nasal polyps* (growths in the nose).

- **Nasal rebound:** Overuse of over-the-counter topical nasal decongestants can also predispose you to sinusitis. (See Chapter 7 for more information.)

- **Anatomical obstructions:** Nasal polyps, other growths, enlarged adenoids (particularly in children), and a deviated nasal septum (the great divide between the nostrils — see Chapter 4 for more details) can increase your chances of developing sinusitis.

✔ **Other diseases:** Patients with cystic fibrosis, in which abnormally thick mucus is produced and the function of the *cilia* (tiny hair-like cells that sweep debris-laden mucus through the airways) is impaired, frequently suffer from sinus infections. In addition, AIDS and other immune deficiency diseases often weaken the body's defenses to the point where bacteria and viruses can cause many types of infections, including sinusitis. These patients with compromised immune systems may be particularly vulnerable to various forms of fungal sinus infections.

Sinus science

Allergists refer to the sinuses that surround your nose — called *paranasal sinuses* — when they discuss sinusitis. *Para* is Greek for around or near. *Nasal,* of course, refers to the nose, and *sinus* is Latin for a hollow place. Your sinuses are hollow cavities in the bones that surround your nasal cavity (see Figure 9-1), hence *sinusitis,* which means inflammation *(itis)* of the sinuses.

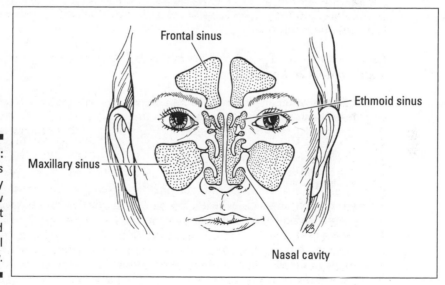

Figure 9-1: Your sinuses are actually hollow cavities that surround your nasal cavity.

The three types of paranasal sinuses come in pairs (one on each side of the nose) and are named for the bones that house them:

✔ **Maxillary sinuses:** The largest of the sinuses, located in your cheekbones.

✔ **Frontal sinuses:** These sinuses reside in your forehead above your eyes.

✔ **Ethmoid sinuses:** These sinuses are immediately behind your eyes and nose.

The other sinus affected by sinusitis is the *sphenoid* sinus, located behind your nose near the base of your brain.

Sinus infections most often affect the maxillary, frontal, and ethmoid sinuses. The most commonly seen complication affects the orbit around the eye, causing *cellulitis* and possibly forming an *abscess* (a localized collection of pus surrounded by inflamed tissue). Patients with this type of infection may look as though they've been severely punched in the eye. Because the sphenoid sinus is near the brain, an infection in this area, although rare, is usually associated with infections in all the other sinuses *(pansinusitis)* and can have very serious consequences if infected fluids spread to the central nervous system. Untreated sinusitis has the potential to lead to life-threatening conditions, such as *meningitis* (an infection of the membranes that envelop the brain and spinal cord) and brain abscesses.

Your maxillary sinuses are present at birth, along with immature ethmoid sinuses, which begin to fully develop when you're between 3 and 7 years old. Therefore, contrary to previous medical opinion, children under 5 can experience sinus infections that require appropriate therapy. If your young child has allergic rhinitis, effectively treating his or her condition is vital in reducing the risk of developing sinusitis.

Practical sinus

Sinuses are a vital part of your body's defense against the airborne bacteria, viruses, irritants, and allergens that you constantly inhale. Under normal circumstances, the mucus in your sinuses traps most of these intruders. Cilia, which are tiny, hair-like projections of certain types of cells that line the sinuses (and other parts of the respiratory tract), sweep the particle-laden mucus through connecting *ostia* (sinus drainage openings) into your nasal passages, which then drains into your throat. From your throat, the mucus moves into your stomach, where your digestive system can neutralize and eventually eliminate the offending substances.

In addition to keeping your respiratory system clear, your sinuses serve other important roles. For example, your sinuses act as:

- Air pockets that lighten your skull — otherwise, your head would be too heavy for your neck. Calling someone an airhead is actually an anatomically correct statement.
- Resonance chambers that provide space for your voice to resonate.
- Climate adjusters, warming and humidifying the air that you inhale.
- Insulators, which also warm the base of your brain, located directly behind your nose.
- Shock absorbers, protecting the inside of your skull from injury.

Allergic rhinitis irritates the nasal and sinus lining, causing the linings to swell, which narrows the ostia (sinus drainage openings) into the nasal cavity. At the same time, your immune system's allergic response to allergic rhinitis increases mucus production. This combination of increased mucus flow and a swollen sinus lining overwhelms the cilia's abilities to sweep out the mucus, which then becomes infected.

Think of a swiftly flowing stream. If the stream dams up, the water usually stagnates and turns into a breeding ground for all sorts of organisms. The same process applies to your sinuses, which is why it's crucial to avoid letting them turn into swamps.

How long has this been goin' on?

Although no universal definition exists for the various presentations of sinusitis, most doctors base their sinusitis classifications on the duration and types of symptoms involved. Therefore, doctors often use the following terms to classify cases of sinusitis:

✔ **Acute sinusitis:** Symptoms of acute sinusitis persist for up to three to four weeks, although some doctors may diagnose symptoms that continue for up to eight weeks as acute. Typical symptoms of acute sinusitis include:

• Upper-respiratory infection.

• Runny nose with infected mucus that often appears as cloudy, thick, yellowish or greenish nasal discharge.

• Cloudy, yellowish, or greenish postnasal drip (often of such a quantity that you may need to swallow frequently).

• Facial pain or pressure around cheeks, eyes, and lower nose, especially while bending over or moving vigorously (for example, during exercise).

• Nasal congestion, headache, fever, and cough.

• In some cases, a reduction or loss of the sense of smell, pain in upper teeth or the upper jawbone, and bad breath.

• In some children, nausea and vomiting due to gagging on infected mucus.

✔ **Chronic sinusitis:** When your condition lasts longer than four weeks, doctors usually consider you a chronic sufferer. In many cases, chronic sinusitis can last for months with combinations of the same symptoms as acute sinusitis, although you may not have a fever. For this reason, many people with chronic sinusitis think that they suffer from frequent or constant colds.

✔ **Recurrent sinusitis:** Doctors usually define recurrent sinusitis as three or more episodes of acute sinusitis per year. The recurring episodes may occur as a result of different causes. If you have recurrent sinusitis, your doctor may refer you to an allergist to determine whether allergies are the underlying cause of your condition. (See Chapter 8 for more details on allergy testing.)

Diagnosis

Often, your doctor can diagnose sinusitis based on your symptoms and medical history. Your doctor may ask questions like the following:

✔ When did you first notice the symptoms?

✔ What hurts? Where do you feel the pain?

✔ Do you have a history of allergies and sinus problems in your family?

✔ What have you done to treat your symptoms? What sorts of medications have you taken, and what has been their effect?

Your doctor also conducts a physical exam of your nose and sinuses in order to confirm diagnosis. This exam may include

✔ Taking your temperature to check for fever and listening to your chest to see whether the infection has spread to your lungs.

✔ Lightly tapping your forehead and cheekbones to check for sensitivity in your frontal and maxillary sinuses.

✔ Looking for infected mucus in your nose and the back of your throat. This exam may require insertion of a flexible fiberoptic device, known as an *endoscope,* so your doctor can clearly view potentially infected areas.

Your doctor may need to use sophisticated imaging techniques to confirm the diagnosis of sinusitis. *Computed tomography (CT)* is currently the gold standard for these purposes and, in many cases, is replacing the use of less-accurate sinus X-rays. A CT scan, also known as a *CAT scan,* is a diagnostic test that combines the use of X-rays with state-of-the-art computer technology. This test uses a series of X-ray beams from many different angles to create cross-sectional images of your body — in this case, of your head and sinuses. These images are assembled in a computer into a three-dimensional picture that can display organs, bones, and tissues in great detail.

Treatment

To effectively treat your sinusitis, you need to effectively manage your allergic rhinitis. In many cases, appropriately treating your allergic rhinitis also improves your sinusitis. As I explain in Chapter 6, avoidance and allergy-proofing are crucial tools you can use to effectively treat your allergies. Chapter 7 provides you with an in-depth explanation of allergy medications that you may find appropriate for your condition.

In addition to addressing your allergic rhinitis, doctors can also prescribe a variety of treatments for sinusitis, ranging from medication to irrigation to surgery.

Antibiotics

Antibiotics are the most common medications that doctors prescribe to clear up the bacterial infection in your sinuses. When taking antibiotics, keep the following in mind:

- ✔ Because the blood flow to your sinuses is poor, you may need to take your prescribed antibiotics for a while before you notice a beneficial effect. However, most cases of acute sinusitis respond to antibiotic treatment within two weeks.

- ✔ In cases of chronic sinusitis, don't be surprised if your doctor prescribes a six- to eight-week course of antibiotic therapy to eliminate your bacterial infection.

- ✔ In some cases of acute or chronic sinusitis, you may notice a sudden improvement in your symptoms soon after you start a course of antibiotics, and you may consider stopping the medication at that point. However, you must take the complete course of antibiotics to ensure that all the bacteria have been completely eliminated.

Other medications

In addition to prescribing antibiotics to clear up the bacterial infection in your sinuses, your doctor may also prescribe medications to treat symptoms of allergic rhinitis, which I describe extensively in Chapter 7.

Irrigation

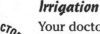

Your doctor may advise you to use a nasal douche cup, nasal bulb syringe, Water Pik with nasal attachment, or some other type of nasal wash device to irrigate your nostrils with warm saline solution. You can use these devices at home to relieve pressure and congestion in your nasal passages. Ask your doctor for specific instructions on how to use nasal wash devices.

Get steamed

Your doctor may also advise a simple home remedy to help clear your sinuses and relieve discomfort. This remedy consists of inhaling steam to liquefy and soften crusty mucus while moisturizing your inflamed passages.

I suggest using the following method for inhaling steam:

1. Boil water in a kettle on the stove.

2. Carefully pour the boiling water in a pan or basin on a low table.

3. Sit at the table and drape a towel over your head, leaning over the pan or basin to form a kind of human tent with your head as the pole.

4. Hold your face a few inches above the steaming water and breathe the steam through your nose for approximately ten minutes.

Two steam treatments a day may provide relief of your sinusitis symptoms. However, you still need to deal with the underlying cause of the sinus infection, so I don't advise relying solely on this home remedy as the only therapy for your infectious sinusitis.

Sinus surgery

If other treatment methods don't provide effective relief of your sinusitis, you may need surgery, especially if physical obstructions such as a deviated septum or nasal polyps contribute to your condition. However, if allergic rhinitis is the underlying cause of your sinusitis, surgery alone won't resolve your sinus problems. You must continue managing your allergic rhinitis to avoid further complications. By the same token, treating your allergies alone won't reverse the damage that sinusitis may have already caused.

If your doctor thinks that surgery is advisable, he or she will refer you to an ear, nose, and throat specialist, or ENT, otherwise known as an *otolaryngologist* (remember that word for your next Scrabble game — you could score big). Surgery should be recommended only after thoroughly examining your condition and reviewing your medical history.

Never hesitate to ask your surgeon for further information concerning your planned surgical procedure, such as how long the procedure takes, where and when it will be performed, any possible complications that may occur, and how soon you can get back to work or school.

The good news about surgery for your sinuses is that the two most common procedures are minimally invasive and can usually be performed on an outpatient basis with local anesthesia, although a doctor may use general anesthesia in certain cases. The two procedures most often used are

- **Antral puncture and irrigation:** This procedure opens up your sinuses so they can drain and irrigate properly.

- **Functional endoscopic sinus surgery:** This procedure is more complex than antral puncture and irrigation. Functional endoscopic sinus surgery often involves enlarging the openings from the ethmoid and maxillary sinuses into the nasal cavity and removing and cleaning the infected sinus membranes, resulting in improved drainage. This procedure reestablishes the ventilation of your ethmoid, maxillary, and frontal sinuses. Otolaryngologists perform this type of surgery with high-tech computer-assisted instruments and navigation devices to ensure pinpoint accuracy.

Prevention

If you have allergic rhinitis, consider taking the following preventive measures to keep your sinuses clear in the event that you come down with an upper respiratory infection (such as the common cold) or experience an allergy attack:

✔ Take appropriate medications, such as the ones that I list in Chapter 7, which your doctor can prescribe.

✔ Drink plenty of water to keep your mucus thin and fluid so your sinuses can drain more easily.

✔ Be nice to your nose — blow it gently, preferably one nostril at a time.

✔ Avoid flying. If you have to travel by air while you have a cold or an allergy attack, use a topical nasal decongestant spray prior to takeoff. The spray prevents the sudden pressure changes from blocking your sinuses and ears.

✔ Avoid swimming. You probably won't feel like going to the beach or the pool if you have a cold or allergy attack, and your sinuses won't enjoy the pressure changes that swimming and diving involve.

Otitis Media

Otitis media is an inflammation of the middle ear, as well as a condition in which fluid accumulates in your ear. This condition is in contrast to *otitis externa,* which affects the external auditory canal, known commonly as *swimmer's ear.* Based on the definitions I've provided of sinusitis and rhinitis (see Chapter 4), you can probably already guess what *otitis* means: an inflammation *(itis)* of the ear *(otikos* in Greek.) *Media* means middle, by the way. The middle ear is the part of the ear that is affected most by inflammatory disease processes, as I explain later in this section. Otitis media can often develop as a result of allergic rhinitis and from complications of sinusitis.

Middle ear infections and fluid in the ear are especially common in young children and infants. In fact, otitis media is the most common reason in the U.S. for pediatric visits, with doctors treating at least 10 million children annually for ear infections. Otitis media can have serious consequences for youngsters, in particular by adversely affecting a child's development and learning ability due to potential hearing loss.

The most common forms of otitis media are

- ✔ **Acute otitis media (AOM):** This condition involves inflammation and infection of the middle ear and Eustachian tube. The peak incidence is between six months and one year of age, decreasing with age and with fewer episodes after 7 years of age.

- ✔ **Otitis media with effusion (OME):** Doctors also refer to this condition as *serous otitis media* — fluid in the middle ear. This condition, which occurs commonly in children ages 2 to 7 years, can lead to hearing loss if not treated properly.

Common causes

In a significant number of cases, allergic rhinitis precedes an ear infection. A long-term study of 2,000 children found that 50 percent of the patients with chronic and recurrent ear infections who were 3 years and older had allergic rhinitis.

Other conditions that can increase your chances of developing ear infections include

- ✔ Sinusitis. The same factors that can lead to sinus infections, such as exposure to allergens, tobacco smoke, pollutants, and other irritants, can also contribute to ear infections.

- ✔ Enlarged adenoids.

- ✔ Unrepaired cleft palate.

- ✔ Nasal polyps.

- ✔ Excessive buildup of earwax.

- ✔ Poorly functioning thyroid gland, resulting in frequent nasal congestion.

- ✔ Benign or malignant tumors.

- ✔ Teething. Some physicians believe that teething in young children can also contribute to ear infections, but a direct connection has not yet been clearly established.

Many of the conditions in the previous list affect infants and young children. Always ask your physician to check your child's ear for infection and fluid in the middle ear anytime he or she is ill.

Getting an earful

The visible part of your ear — that funny-looking protrusion on the side of your head — is only the tip of the iceberg. Much of your ears' functions take place inside your skull in chambers, tubes, and passages that register and conduct sound and also provide your sense of balance.

The ear is made up of the following parts, as shown in Figure 9-2:

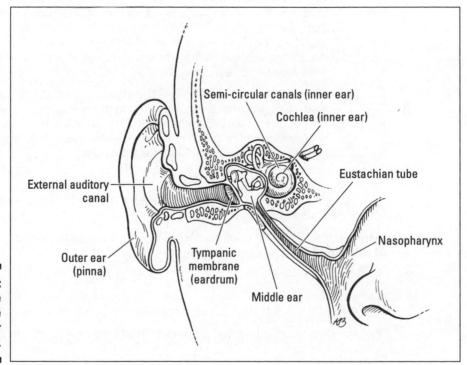

Semi-circular canals (inner ear)

Cochlea (inner ear)

Eustachian tube

External auditory canal

Nasopharynx

Outer ear (pinna)

Tympanic membrane (eardrum)

Middle ear

Figure 9-2: See how the less visible part of your ear appears.

- ✔ **Outer ear:** Also known as the *pinna,* this structure is what many of us think of as the ear. The primary function of this skin-covered flap of elastic cartilage is to funnel sound into the middle ear.

- ✔ **Middle ear:** This air-filled chamber contains the *tympanic membrane* (commonly known as the *eardrum*) and small bones that enable your eardrum to function. Through its connection (the Eustachian tube) to the *nasopharynx* (back of the nose), your middle ear also equalizes the air pressure on both sides of your eardrum.

- ✔ **Inner ear:** Your inner ear contains sensory receptors that provide your hearing and balance. The hearing receptors are enclosed in the *cochlea,* a fluid-filled chamber, while the balance receptors are in the semi-circular canals (refer to Figure 9-2).

✔ **Eustachian tube (ET):** Your Eustachian tube is an extension of the middle ear that connects to the back of your nose. The ET, which is often the origin of ear infections, serves three important functions:

- The ET provides ventilation for your middle ear.

- The ET helps equalize air pressure inside your ear, buffering the eardrum from the force of external air, and helps dissipate the energy of sound waves from your inner ear into your throat.

- Because it's closed most of the time, your ET serves as an important barrier to viruses, bacteria, irritants, and allergens that enter your middle ear. Similar to the function of your sinuses, cilia (tiny hair-like projections of certain cells) in the middle ear sweep debris-laden mucus from your middle ear through the ET into the back of your nasal cavity. The cilia prepare the mucus for drainage into your throat and eventually into your stomach.

The ET briefly opens to allow the cilia to sweep mucus away when you swallow, yawn, sniff, or strain. In many children, however, the ET doesn't fully develop until age 6, causing the ET to ineffectively ventilate, clear, or protect the middle ear. Therefore, large numbers of young children get middle ear infections.

Acute otitis media (AOM)

Many of us suffer *acute otitis media (AOM)* — an inflammation and infection of the middle ear and Eustachian tube — in early childhood. The main symptoms include

✔ Earache — sometimes with intense, stabbing pains — and fever. Occasionally this symptom is accompanied by vomiting and diarrhea.

✔ Possible hearing loss and occasional dizziness and ringing in the affected ear.

✔ With infants, high fever, irritability, and a tendency to pull on the affected ear.

✔ In some cases, discharge of infected fluid from the middle ear (if your eardrum has been perforated).

An AOM infection generally develops as a result of an allergic, bacterial, or viral ailment that inflames your nose, sinuses, middle ear, and Eustachian tube. Your ET may swell shut, trapping infected fluid, which then presses on your eardrum, causing the pain you associate with an earache. If you don't rectify this situation, infected fluids can eventually reach the membranes that cover your brain, leading to meningitis and even possibly death.

Because sinusitis and otitis media often coexist, doctors usually treat these conditions with the same medications. Treatment of AOM usually includes a course of antibiotics (available by prescription only) to rid your middle ear of infection. The antibiotic drugs that doctors commonly prescribe include

- ✔ Amoxicillin (Amoxil). If this drug isn't effective, your doctor may prescribe amoxicillin/potassium clavulanate (Augmentin).
- ✔ Clarithromycin (Biaxin) or azithromycin (Zithromax).
- ✔ Trimethoprim-sulfamethoxazole (Bactrim or Septra).
- ✔ A third-generation cephalosporin antibiotic, such as cefuroxime (Ceftin), cefpodoxime (Vantin), cefprozil (Cefzil), and cefixime (Suprax).

If you're allergic to penicillin, make sure your doctor knows. Some people who have penicillin allergies may also have adverse reactions to cephalosporin medications (see Chapter 20 for information on adverse drug reactions).

Otitis media with effusion (OME)

When you have otitis media with effusion (OME, also known as *serous otitis media*), your middle ear traps either infected or sterile fluid. The most common symptoms of OME are

- ✔ Plugged-up ears (similar to the discomfort that you may experience when descending in an airplane)
- ✔ Some hearing loss

Children with OME may not show obvious symptoms of the ailment. However, if your child acts inattentive, doesn't seem to hear well (for example, he or she always wants the television volume turned up loud), and/or talks loudly, make sure your doctor examines your child's ears. Undetected or poorly treated OME can result in hearing loss, poor language development, learning disorders, and eventual behavioral problems.

OME treatments can also include non-prescription oral decongestants and nasal decongestant sprays, as well as topical nasal corticosteroid sprays. (For more information on these types of medicines, see Chapter 7.)

For children with chronic OME that lasts more than six to eight weeks, your pediatrician may refer your child to an ear, nose, and throat (ENT) specialist for surgery. The most common OME treatment procedures are

- ✔ **Myringotomy:** The ENT surgeon makes a small incision in the eardrum that permits drainage of the trapped fluid. This procedure is helpful both for diagnostic purposes (to identify infecting organisms) and to relieve the severe pain, pressure, and fever associated with an acute middle ear infection.

✔ **Tympanostomy:** This procedure includes surgically inserting small plastic tubes (known as *pressure equalization* or *PE tubes*) in the eardrum to equalize air pressure in the ear and to drain fluid from the middle ear and Eustachian tube. ENT surgeons usually perform tympanostomies with a general anesthetic, and occasionally with local anesthetic (for older children or adults), as an outpatient procedure. In most cases, doctors recommend that PE tubes remain in place for 6 to 18 months or until they fall out. Children often don't notice the tubes once they've been in place for a while. Generally, children with tubes shouldn't go swimming. However, in some cases, an ENT surgeon may fit your child with earplugs, making water activities a possibility.

✔ **Adenoidectomy:** If your child's Eustachian tube is chronically blocked and your child is more than 3 years old, your doctor may recommend removing your child's adenoids. (Removing the tonsils is no longer an effective or appropriate procedure for treatment of ear problems.)

Diagnosis

The first step in diagnosing suspected ear infections usually involves examining your middle ear. Your doctor usually uses an *otoscope* (a metal instrument you've probably seen before) to look for an obvious sign of infection. AOM often appears as a swollen, red, inflamed bulging of the tympanic membrane (eardurm) with poor or no movement. Otitis media with effusion (OME) can appears as a pink or white opaque, withdrawn tympanic membrane with poor or no movement.

Other diagnostic procedures for both AOM and OME may include

✔ **Tympanometry:** This procedure measures the eardrum's response at various pressure levels and helps to diagnose middle ear effusions and Eustachian tube dysfunction.

✔ **Audiometry:** This procedure evaluates the effect of chronic middle ear effusions on a person's hearing. Audiometry is especially important for children because hearing loss can cause delayed speech and language development.

Prevention

As with sinusitis, one of the most important steps you can take to prevent ear infections, if you also have allergic rhinitis, is to effectively treat your allergies. Effectively treating your allergies includes using the avoidance measures that I describe in Chapter 6 and also the appropriate medications, if necessary, to manage allergic rhinitis symptoms, as I explain in Chapter 7. You also need to take the preventive measures that I describe in the "Sinusitis" section of this chapter to keep your sinuses clear if you have an allergy attack or a cold or other upper respiratory infection.

Part III

Asthma: A Disease in Search of Good Management

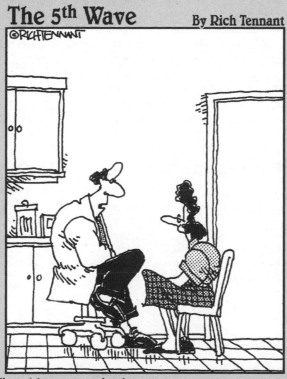

The 5th Wave   By Rich Tennant

"Sudden perspiration, shallow breathing, and a rapid heart rate are all signs of an asthma attack. The fact that these symptoms only occur when the pool boy is working in your backyard, however, raises some questions."

In this part . . .

Asthma is not a recurring chest cold, a psychological disorder, a minor annoyance, or a condition that you usually outgrow. It's a multifaceted, chronic, inflammatory airway disease of the lungs that causes breathing problems and that requires proper diagnosis, early and aggressive treatment, and effective long-term management.

In this part, you find an extensive discussion of the underlying inflammatory response that characterizes asthma, what you should know about diagnosing your condition and avoiding triggers of the disease, the range of long-term and quick-relief medications that your doctor may prescribe for you, and essential information about developing an effective long-term asthma management plan.

In addition, I also include chapters that focus on taking care of a child with asthma and vital information on continuing your asthma treatment during pregnancy.

Chapter 10

The Basics of Managing Asthma

hrough the ages, asthma has affected people from all walks of life, in all parts of the world. The Roman emperor Caesar Augustus was only one of many historical figures who suffered from this serious respiratory disease (see Chapter 23). As far back as 2,500 B.C., Chinese doctors documented cases of asthma, as did chroniclers in many subsequent civilizations, including those of ancient Greece. In fact, *asthma* is the ancient Greek word for a classic symptom of this disease: *panting* or *breathlessness*.

Unfortunately, although asthma is chronicled in ancient history, the disease is still very much a part of the modern world. According to many experts, asthma is a global epidemic, and the prevalence and severity of the disease continue to grow in many parts of the world, including the United States. As I explain in Chapter 11, an increase of indoor air pollution may be one of the most important factors in this rising incidence of asthma.

More than 17 million people in the U.S. have some form of asthma. That equals three times the number of asthma cases diagnosed in 1960, despite major medical breakthroughs during the last 40 years in diagnosing and treating airway obstruction — the basis of this disease.

Here are more highlights of the state of asthma today:

✔ Asthma is the most common chronic disease of childhood. At least five million children in the U.S. suffer from this illness, which accounts for 20 percent of missed school days — second only to viral upper respiratory infections such as the common cold. Acute asthma attacks are the most common reason for emergency treatment of children in this country.

✔ In the U.S., people with asthma account for more than two million emergency room visits and over nine million doctors' appointments per year. Asthma and related respiratory problems are responsible for more than

500,000 hospitalizations and over 100 million days of restricted activity annually. Costs associated with asthma, including treatment, medications, and lost productivity, exceed $11 billion each year.

✔ Occupational asthma is an increasingly serious problem in the U.S. More than 15 percent of newly diagnosed asthma cases in this country have been linked to workplace irritant and allergen exposure. Doctors recognize more than 250 chemicals as asthma triggers.

✔ The prevalence and severity of asthma continues to rise for poorer Americans, particularly inner-city residents. Among African-Americans, asthma rates are 22 percent higher than among whites. African-Americans between the ages of 15 and 24 have the highest death rates from asthma. The undertreatment of poorer patients, resulting from inadequate access to effective medical care, may be a major cause of this troubling discrepancy between ethnic groups. A lack of coordinated and comprehensive public health policy that could help more Americans recognize asthma symptoms and seek effective treatment may also play a part in the asthma-rate discrepancies between different groups.

✔ Although the mortality rates of other serious illnesses are declining, deaths due to asthma continue to rise. More than 5,000 Americans — many between the ages of 5 and 34 — die each year because of asthma. Most of these deaths, however, are clearly preventable. With proper diagnosis, effective and timely treatment, and an asthma management plan that empowers a person with asthma (and the patient's family) to control symptoms of the disease, the vast majority of asthma patients can lead fulfilling and productive lives, free from the worry of life-threatening asthma attacks.

Defining Asthma

Asthma is a chronic, inflammatory lung disease that causes breathing problems. It is also a complex, multifaceted condition that many people — asthmatics themselves, family members, and even some doctors — may not recognize or may improperly diagnose, often as a chest cold or bronchitis.

Here are some other important points to keep in mind about asthma:

✔ Inflammation of the airways (bronchial tubes) is the single most important underlying factor in asthma. If you have asthma, your symptoms may come and go, but the underlying inflammation usually persists. Episodes of asthma symptoms can vary in length from minutes to hours and even from days to weeks, depending on your medical treatment (see Chapter 12), the severity of your symptoms (see Chapter 13), and the character of the triggering mechanism (see Chapter 11).

✔ Although no cure exists for asthma, in most cases the effects of the disease are manageable and reversible — unlike, for example, emphysema, in which the destruction of *alveoli* (tiny air sacs in the lungs that perform oxygen exchange) is irreversible. However, poorly managed or undertreated asthma may lead to loss of airway functions and, in some cases, irreversible lung damage as a result of airway remodeling. (I explain airway remodeling in "How airway obstruction develops," later in this chapter.)

✔ Early, aggressive treatment with appropriate medication is vital to effectively managing your asthma.

✔ Asthma often begins in childhood and affects boys more commonly than girls. In child-onset asthma, *atopy* (the genetic susceptibility for the immune system to produce antibodies to common allergens, leading to allergy symptoms) and/or a family history of allergies are the strongest identifiable predisposing factors for developing the disease. Atopic dermatitis (eczema) and allergic rhinitis (hay fever) may serve as key indicators of atopy in infants and young children.

✔ Important symptoms of asthma in infancy and early childhood include persistent coughing, wheezing, and recurring or lingering chest colds.

✔ Heredity can play a role in asthma. For example, two-thirds of asthma patients have a close relative with asthma. However, asthma in your family doesn't guarantee that you'll definitely develop asthma. You inherit the tendency to the disease, not the disease itself.

✔ Not all asthma is allergic, and not all allergies lead to asthma. In some cases of adult-onset asthma (which often develops in people over 40 and is less common than child-onset asthma), atopy may not be present. Instead, sinusitis, gastroesophageal reflux (GER), nasal polyps, and sensitivities to aspirin and related over-the-counter (OTC) nonsteroidal anti-inflammatory drugs (NSAIDs), such as ibuprofen (Advil), ketoprofen (Actron, Orudis), or naproxen (Aleve), and newer prescription NSAIDs, known as COX-2 inhibitors — including celecoxib (Celebrex) and rofecoxib (Vioxx) — can more commonly trigger symptoms of adult-onset asthma, as I explain in greater detail in Chapter 11.

Triggers, attacks, episodes, and symptoms

A wide variety of allergens, irritants, and other factors such as colds, flu, exercise, and drug sensitivities can trigger asthma symptoms — what you may refer to as *asthma attacks* or *asthma episodes*. Asthma symptoms can range from decreased tolerance to exercise to feeling completely out of breath and from persistent coughing to wheezing, chest tightness, or life-threatening respiratory distress. In many cases, a bothersome cough may be the only symptom of asthma that you even notice.

Why aren't these antibiotics curing my bronchitis?

Bronchitis is a general term for inflammation of the *bronchi,* or airways. (*Itis* is Greek for swelling or inflammation, as in *tonsillitis,* an inflammation of the tonsils; *appendicitis,* an inflammation of the appendix; or *rhinitis,* an inflamed nose.) The most frequent causes of bronchial or airway inflammation are viral or bacterial infections, smoking, or asthma.

Because the coughing symptoms in different types of airway inflammation can appear similar and because bacterial infections of the airway are common, many patients who actually have asthma often are mistakenly treated with antibiotics. Although these drugs can often clear bacterial infections of the airways, they don't relieve or control asthma symptoms.

If you experience lingering coughs, recurring colds, or similar symptoms that could indicate bronchitis, make sure — as I explain in "Testing your lungs," later in this chapter — that your doctor performs appropriate lung function tests to check for reversible airflow obstruction, a hallmark of asthma. Performing such tests gives doctors the information they need to prescribe appropriate and effective treatment for your condition.

Experiencing asthma symptoms, whatever the intensity, means that your asthma is temporarily not well controlled. Such symptoms may indicate that your asthma needs more effective management, as I explain in "Managing Your Asthma: Essential Steps" later in this chapter.

It's not in your head

Until recently, asthma was often considered a nervous disorder, thought to be caused by anxiety and psychological stress. We now know that this misconception has no basis in fact.

Asthma occurs in the airways of your lungs, not in your head. Although anxiety and stress can aggravate your asthma (as well as other illnesses), psychological factors are not the underlying cause of your condition.

The many faces of asthma

Asthma can show up in various ways. The core mechanism underlying asthma's many manifestations, however, is a complex interaction in the lungs between inflammatory cells, as well as other types of cells, and tissues that reside in your airway. I explain this process further in "Asthma and Your Airways," later in this chapter.

Allergies and asthma all over the world

According to numerous samples of populations in many countries, large numbers of people have allergic sensitivities that frequently increase their risk of developing symptoms associated with asthma. Here's a sampling of allergy and asthma surveys from the around the globe:

✔ Almost half of the U.S. population has some sensitivity to allergens, and a third of homes in the U.S. contain conditions such as elevated humidity levels that frequently lead to the proliferation of significant sources of household allergens like molds and dust mites. (See Chapter 11 for practical and important tips on allergy-proofing your home.)

✔ Based on allergy skin testing (see Chapter 8), at least half of all children in Hong Kong and other Chinese cities demonstrate allergic sensitivities, especially to cockroach and dust mite allergens. Likewise, as many as one-quarter of schoolchildren in Costa Rica may have asthma.

✔ Studies in Germany found that at least one-third of Germans have sensitivities to pollens, dust mites, and other common inhalant allergens, while as many as a quarter of that country's population experiences symptoms of asthma and allergic rhinitis.

✔ Indian research shows that as many as one-fifth of Bombay residents have hyper-responsive airways, a significant indicator of asthma (see Chapter 10), and equivalent numbers also experience sensitivities to dust mites.

✔ Australia and New Zealand consistently report two of the highest incidences of childhood asthma of any nations in the world. In Australia, the prevalence of childhood asthma has been reported as high as over 20 percent in certain childhood age groups, while in New Zealand, comparable studies reveal a prevalence of asthma of more than 16 percent in similar childhood age groups.

✔ If you're thinking of moving to the desert to escape your allergies, consider the significant numbers of allergists in the telephone directories of cities such as Phoenix or Tucson, and also consider this: Studies in Kuwait show that as many as a quarter of Kuwaitis experience some sensitivity to dust mites.

Because such a wide range of factors can precipitate asthma symptoms, and because certain triggers can cause stronger reactions in some asthma patients than in others, doctors often classify asthma according to the triggers that instigate your symptoms. Classifying asthma in this way can help you and your doctor understand the cause of your symptoms.

Although a certain precipitating factor may predominate in many asthma cases, multiple triggers affect the majority of people with asthma. For example, most asthmatics have exercise-induced asthma (EIA), sometimes known as exercise-induced bronchospasm (EIB) — which I explain in the next section — in addition to asthma that manifests as a result of other types of triggers or precipitating factors. The next sections list the main asthma classifications that many doctors use.

Allergic asthma

Throughout the world, triggers of this common form of asthma include inhalant allergens such as dust mites, animal dander, fungal spores, and pollens from trees, grasses, and weeds (see the nearby sidebar "Asthma and allergies all over the world"). If you suffer from allergic asthma, you may be sensitive to a combination of many of these allergens and probably suffer from allergic rhinitis (hay fever) and/or allergic conjunctivitis, which I explain in detail in Chapter 4.

I advise you to develop and implement — in consultation with your doctor — effective allergy-proofing and avoidance measures to limit your exposure to allergy triggers as part of your overall asthma management plan. (Chapter 11 explains how to avoid the many forms of asthma triggers and precipitating factors.)

Depending on your degree of sensitivity and levels of exposure to inhalant allergens, your doctor may also recommend allergy testing (which an allergist usually performs) to determine what triggers your allergic asthma and whether immunotherapy (allergy shots) may provide an appropriate and effective treatment for your condition.

Immunotherapy can, in certain cases, reduce your level of sensitivity to the allergens that affect you, thus decreasing your allergy and asthma symptoms. (To find out more about immunotherapy, turn to Chapter 8.)

Nonallergic asthma

Irritants such as tobacco smoke; household cleaners; soaps; perfumes and scents; glue; aerosols; smoke from wood-burning appliances or fireplaces; fumes from unvented gas, oil, or kerosene stoves; and indoor and outdoor air pollutants can also trigger asthma.

Aspirin triad

The syndrome consisting of 1) asthma, 2) nasal polyps, and 3) aspirin-intolerance is commonly referred to as the *aspirin triad*. Many patients with this syndrome also have a history of recurrent sinusitis. For these people, aspirin, other related OTC NSAIDs, and newer prescription NSAIDs known as COX-2 inhibitors can trigger adverse reactions that can result in severe or potentially life-threatening asthma attacks — including some of the worst I've treated in my many years of practice.

If you suffer from this type of sensitivity, I strongly advise you to wear a MedicAlert bracelet or pendant. This device alerts medical personnel not to administer any medication to which you're sensitive in the event that you're unconscious or unable to communicate during an emergency. See the appendix at the back of this book for more information on MedicAlert bracelets and pendants.

Upper respiratory tract infections, such as the common cold and flu, as well as sinusitis, nasal polyps, gastroesophageal reflux (GER), and aspirin sensitivity (see "Aspirin-induced asthma" later in this chapter), may also aggravate airway inflammation and trigger asthma symptoms in some people.

Occupational asthma

Current estimates are that occupational asthma, which can be triggered by a wide range of allergens and irritants, affects as many as 15 percent of asthma patients in the U.S. The precipitating factors in occupational asthma cases often include exposure to fumes, chemicals, gases, resins, metals, dust, insecticides, vapors, and other substances in the workplace that can induce or aggravate airway inflammation.

Exercise-induced asthma (EIA)

Symptoms of *exercise-induced asthma* (EIA) — also known as *exercise-induced bronchospasm* (EIB) — occur to varying degrees in a majority of asthmatics. Exercising that involves breathing cold, dry air — such as running outdoors in winter — may trigger EIA symptoms more often than activities that involve breathing warmer, humidified air, such as swimming in a heated pool.

Certain medications can help you prevent and control EIA symptoms so that you can enjoy many types of exercise and sports activities, in spite of your condition. Chapter 12 provides information on these medical products, which you should take only according to your doctor's advice.

Aspirin-induced (and food-additive-induced) asthma

A significant number of people who have both asthma and nasal polyps may experience intensified asthma symptoms if they take aspirin and related medications, such as OTC nonsteroidal anti-inflammatory drugs (NSAIDs) and newer prescription NSAIDs, known as COX-2 inhibitors, such as celecoxib (Celebrex) and rofecoxib (Vioxx). Some asthma sufferers may also experience intensified symptoms if they ingest *sulfites* (preservatives found in beer, wine, and many processed foods) or *tartrazine* (FDC yellow dye No. 5), which is used in many medications, foods, and vitamin products.

Because approximately 10 percent of asthma patients have some level of sensitivity to aspirin and the other substances that I mention, if you have a history of nasal polyps and sinusitis in addition to asthma, I strongly recommend using acetaminophen-based products, such as Tylenol, instead of aspirin or NSAIDs for the relief of your common aches and pains.

If you are sensitive to food additives, I advise checking labels on liquid medications, such as cough syrups and other liquid cold and flu remedies, to see whether they contain tartrazine. When in doubt, ask your pharmacist. If you have a sulfite sensitivity, you should also be careful about consuming beer, wine, and processed foods and also carry rescue medication, such as an EpiPen kit and/or a short-acting inhaled bronchodilator, with you in the event that you experience respiratory symptoms after unintentionally consuming food or liquids that contain these sulfites.

Asthma and Your Airways

Your airways are vital to your health. This network of bronchial tubes enables your lungs to absorb oxygen into the bloodstream and eliminate carbon dioxide — the process that we call *respiration,* or breathing. Most people take breathing for granted — you usually don't need to think about it, unless something interferes with this process by obstructing your airways.

The inflammatory response

In asthma, airway obstruction is most often the result of an underlying airway inflammation that leads to one or more of the following conditions (which I explain in "How airway obstruction develops" later in this chapter):

- Airway hyperresponsiveness
- Airway constriction
- Airway congestion

These airway conditions can become part of an overall, ongoing process known as the *inflammatory response.* This complex response can develop into a vicious cycle of worsening inflammation, hyperresponsiveness, constriction, and congestion, in which your airways become more and more sensitive and inflamed as a result of reacting to allergens, irritants, and other precipitating factors.

Burning your lungs

You need to realize that the ongoing, underlying airway inflammation is often so subtle that it can go unnoticed. Asthma symptoms are often just the tip of the iceberg. If you have the disease, the inflammation smolders away in your airways, whether or not you're actually experiencing asthma symptoms.

Imagine if you had a rash or sunburn and only took pain relievers to deal with the discomfort, rather than staying out of the sun or treating the cause of the problem. The underlying airway inflammation in asthma is similar to having a sunburn in your bronchial tubes, as my good friend Nancy Sander, founder of the Allergy and Asthma Network • Mothers of Asthmatics, Inc. (AANMA), likes to explain. If you suffer from asthma, the insides of your airways are often red and inflamed, and, as with a bad rash or sunburn, the top layer of airway tissue may peel.

Breathing basics: How your lungs function

To better understand how asthma adversely affects your airways, consider what happens in normal breathing:

1. The air you inhale flows through your nose or mouth into your *trachea,* or windpipe.

2. Your trachea then divides into right and left main *bronchi* (or branches), splitting and funneling the air into each of your lungs.

3. The main bronchi continue branching, like tree branches, within your lungs, dividing into a network of airways called *bronchial tubes.* The outside of your bronchial tubes consists of layers of smooth, involuntary muscles that relax and tighten your airways as you inhale and exhale. Doctors refer to the process of airway relaxation as *bronchodilation.* Likewise, doctors refer to the tightening, which helps your lungs push out air when you exhale, as *bronchoconstriction.*

4. Your network of airways ultimately leads to *alveoli,* tiny air sacs that look like small clusters of grapes. The alveoli contain blood vessels and provide the means for vital respiratory exchange: Oxygen from the air you inhale is absorbed into the bloodstream, while carbon dioxide gas from your blood exits as you exhale.

What you can't see can hurt you

If your lungs were external organs — like gills — or if your body were transparent so that you could see what happens internally, I think that asthma would be treated earlier and more aggressively because you and your doctor could easily see how the underlying disease affects you.

As I explain in "Testing your lungs" later in the chapter, you need to make sure that your doctor performs appropriate pulmonary (lung) function tests if you have bouts of wheezing, recurring coughs, lingering colds, or other symptoms that could indicate an underlying respiratory ailment.

How airway obstruction develops

Here's an overview of how the mechanisms of asthma interact. Although I've itemized these processes to explain them, keep in mind that these processes are often ongoing events that can occur simultaneously in your lungs. As you read these descriptions, take a look at Figure 10-1, which compares a normal airway with an asthmatic airway.

✔ **Airway constriction:** When a trigger or precipitating factor irritates your airways, causing the release of chemical mediators such as histamine and leukotrienes from the mast cells of the *epithelium* (the lining of the airway), the muscles around your bronchial tubes can tighten, leading to *airway constriction*. This process results in narrowing airways and breathing difficulty. Airway constriction can also occur in people who don't have asthma or allergies if they are exposed to substances that can harm their respiratory systems, such as poisonous gases or smoke from a burning building.

✔ **Airway hyperresponsiveness:** The underlying airway inflammation in asthma can cause *airway hyperresponsiveness* as the muscles around your bronchial tubes twitch or feel ticklish. This twitchy or ticklish feeling indicates that your muscles overreact and tighten, causing acute bronchoconstriction or bronchospasms even if you're exposed only to otherwise harmless substances, such as allergens and irritants, that rarely provoke reactions in people without asthma and allergies (see "The many faces of asthma" earlier in the chapter).

✔ **Airway congestion:** Mucus and fluids are released as part of the inflammatory process and can accumulate in your airways, overwhelming the *cilia* (tiny hair-like projections from certain cells that sweep debris-laden mucus through your airways) and leading to *airway congestion*. This accumulation of mucus and fluids may make you feel the urge to cough up phlegm to relieve your chest congestion.

✔ **Airway edema:** The long-term release of inflammatory fluids in constricted, hyperresponsive, and congested airways can lead to *airway edema* (swelling of the airway), causing bronchial tubes to become more rigid and further interfering with airflow. In severe cases of airway congestion and edema, a chronic buildup of mucus secretion leads to the formation of mucus plugs in the airway, which limit airflow.

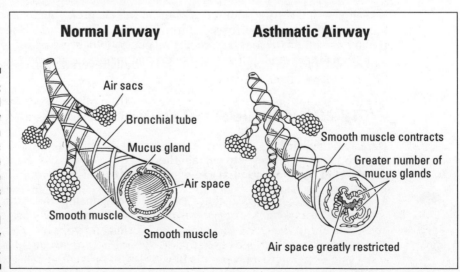

Figure 10-1: A normal airway and an asthmatic airway. Note the muscle contractions (bronchospasms) and airway constriction.

Normal Airway

Air sacs
Bronchial tube
Mucus gland
Air space
Smooth muscle
Smooth muscle

Asthmatic Airway

Smooth muscle contracts
Greater number of mucus glands
Air space greatly restricted

✔ **Airway remodeling:** If airway inflammation is left untreated or poorly managed for many years, the constant injury to your bronchial tubes due to ongoing airway constriction, airway hyperresponsiveness, and airway congestion can lead to *airway remodeling,* as scar tissue permanently replaces your normal airway tissue. As a result of airway remodeling, airway obstruction can persist and may not respond to treatment, leading to the eventual loss of your airway function as well as potentially irreversible lung damage.

This vicious cycle of asthma mechanisms can develop gradually, over hours or even days following exposure to triggers or precipitating factors. After this cycle is set in motion, you can suffer severe and long-lasting consequences.

Diagnosing Asthma

Effectively managing your asthma begins with your doctor correctly diagnosing your condition. In order to determine whether asthma causes your respiratory symptoms, your doctor should take your medical history, perform a physical exam, test your lung functions, and perform other tests, as I explain in the following sections.

The diagnostic processes that your doctor uses are crucial because, as my friend Nancy Sander notes, asthma is not a neat little package of symptoms that you or your doctor can easily identify and eliminate. Asthma symptoms vary widely from patient to patient. In fact, your own symptoms may change over time.

The key points that your doctor should establish in diagnosing your asthma include the following:

✔ You experience episodes of airway obstruction.

✔ Your airway obstruction is at least partially reversible (and can be improved through treatment).

✔ Your symptoms result from asthma, not from other conditions that I describe in "Considering other possible diagnoses" later in this chapter.

Taking your medical history

A careful, thorough medical history is vital in diagnosing the correct cause of your respiratory symptoms. For this reason, your doctor may ask a lot of questions about many aspects of your condition and your life. Keeping track of symptoms in a diary may help provide your doctor with details that can assist him or her with a proper diagnosis. Try to provide your doctor with as much information as possible about the following subjects:

✔ The type of symptoms you experience, which may include coughing, wheezing, shortness of breath, chest tightness, and productive coughs (coughs that bring up mucus).

✔ The pattern of your symptoms:

  • Perennial (year-round), seasonal, or perennial with seasonal worsening

  • Constant, episodic, or constant with episodic worsening

✔ The onset of your symptoms: At what rate do your symptoms develop — rapidly or slowly? And does that rate vary?

✔ The duration and frequency of your symptoms and whether the type and intensity of symptoms vary at different times of day and night. Especially note if your episodes are more severe when you wake up in the morning.

✔ The impact that exercise or other physical exertion has on your symptoms.

✔ Your exposure to potential asthma triggers. In addition to the allergens, irritants, and precipitating factors that I list in "The many faces of asthma" earlier in this chapter, your doctor also needs to know about endocrine factors, such as adrenal or thyroid disease. Special considerations for women are pregnancy or changes in the character or duration of their menstrual cycles.

✔ The development of your disease, including any prior treatment and medication you've received or taken and their effectiveness. Your doctor particularly wants to know whether you presently take or have previously taken oral corticosteroids and, if so, the dosage and frequency of use.

✔ Your family history, especially whether parents, siblings, or close relatives suffer from asthma, allergic or nonallergic rhinitis, other types of allergies, sinusitis, or nasal polyps.

✔ Your social history, including

  • The characteristics of your home, such as its age and location, type of cooling and heating system, condition of the basement, whether you have a wood-burning stove, humidifier, carpet over concrete, mold and mildew, and the types of bedding, carpeting, and furniture coverings that you use.

  • Whether anyone smokes in your home or the other locations where you spend time, such as work or school.

  • Any history of substance abuse.

✔ The impact of the disease on you and your family, such as

  • Any life-threatening symptoms, emergency or urgent care treatments, or hospitalizations.

- The number of days you (or your child with asthma) tend to miss from school or work, the economic impact of the disease, and its effect on your recreational activities.

- If your child has asthma, your doctor may ask you about the effects of the illness on your youngster's growth, development, behavior, and extent of participation in sports.

✔ Your knowledge, perception, and beliefs about asthma and long-term management of the disease, as well as your ability to cope with the illness.

✔ The level of support you receive from your family and their abilities to recognize and assist you in case your symptoms suddenly worsen.

Examining your condition

A physical exam for suspected asthma usually focuses not just on your breathing passageways, but also on other characteristics and symptoms of atopic disease. The significant physical signs of asthma or allergy that your doctor looks for primarily include

✔ Chest deformity, such as an expanded or over-inflated chest, as well as hunched shoulders

✔ Coughing, wheezing, shortness of breath, and other respiratory symptoms

✔ Increased nasal discharge, swelling, and the presence of nasal polyps

✔ Signs of sinus disease, such as thick or discolored nasal discharge

✔ Any allergic skin conditions, such as atopic dermatitis (eczema — see Chapter 16)

Testing your lungs

As a society, we're used to routinely taking our temperature or regularly having our doctor check our pulse and blood pressure, in addition to monitoring our blood sugar and cholesterol levels on a consistent basis. However, we're not yet in the habit of having routine pulmonary (lung) function tests, which may be why asthma is so frequently not diagnosed at an early stage but rather after a severe episode.

Objective pulmonary-function tests are the most reliable means of assessing the extent to which your lung function is limited or affected. The following sections explain the most important tests that doctors use to diagnose asthma.

Spirometry

In order to determine whether you have airway obstruction and whether your condition is reversible (can improve with appropriate treatment), doctors often use a *spirometer* to measure the volume of air you exhale from your large and small airways before and 15 minutes after inhaling a short-acting inhaled beta$_2$-adrenergic bronchodilator. Figure 10-2 shows a patient using a spirometer.

Spirometry provides many types of airflow measurements, including:

- **Forced vital capacity (FVC):** The maximum volume (in liters) of air that you can exhale after the maximum point of inhaling.

- **Forced expiratory volume (FEV$_1$):** The volume (in liters) of air that you exhale in the first second, as forcefully as possible. A reduction in FEV$_1$ is the most common indicator of airway obstruction used by physicians and is often seen in patients with symptoms of asthma. This test, the most important measurement in the diagnosis and management of asthma, generally measures obstruction of the large airways, although FEV$_1$ can also reveal severe obstruction, if present, of the small airways. A baseline FEV$_1$ (before using a bronchodilator) that is lower than normal but that increases by at least 12 percent 15 minutes after inhaling a short-acting bronchodilator (post-bronchodilator) allows your doctor to more conclusively establish the diagnosis of asthma.

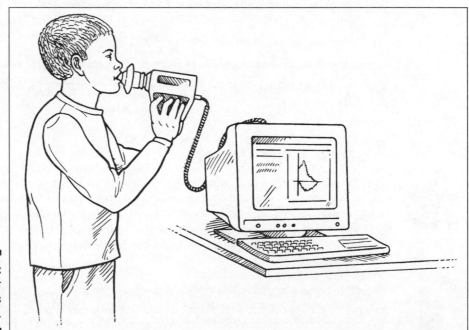

Figure 10-2:
A spirometer measures airflow.

BERGER BIT

The jaws of asthma

Picture one of those scary shark movies: People swim about peacefully on the ocean surface until suddenly, a fin breaks the waves (ominous music) and a shark attacks a hapless swimmer. The shark doesn't just materialize out of nowhere; it's been lurking around underwater, probably for a long time. But the swimmers on the surface don't notice it until it's too late.

Your asthma episodes are similar to that shark attack (without the bite marks). If you rely only on short-acting inhaled beta$_2$-adrenergic bronchodilators — known as rescue medications — to treat your asthma

symptoms when they flare up, that's the equivalent of swimming in shark-infested waters, hoping that someone rescues you if the creature comes after you.

I constantly advise my patients (and you, throughout this book) to manage their asthma on a consistent, long-term preventive basis and to avoid a crisis management approach. (The section "Managing Your Asthma: Essential Steps" later in this chapter provides you with more details.) You can control your asthma — don't let your asthma control you!

✔ **Maximum midexpiratory flow rate (MMEF):** The middle part of your forced exhalation (in liters per second). This measurement is also referred to as the *forced expiratory flow rate between 25 and 75 percent* (FEF 25-75%) of the forced vital capacity (FVC). A reduction in this measurement can indicate obstruction of the small airways of the lungs.

Your doctor compares the values obtained from spirometry (lung function tests) to the predicted normal reference values, based on your age, height, sex, and race, as established by the American Thoracic Society. The percent of predicted normal of your measured FEV$_1$ is one of major criteria your doctor uses to classify your level of asthma severity (see Chapter 13 for information on the four levels of asthma severity).

TIP

Doctors consider spirometry a valuable diagnostic tool for diagnosing childhood cases of asthma in children over 4 years of age. However, for children under that age, the test can be difficult, if not impossible, to perform. In those cases, your child's physician may decide that trying a peak flow meter or other less complicated assessment process is more suitable (see Chapter 14 for information on diagnosing asthma in infants and children).

Peak flow meters

Just as diabetics check their blood sugar levels with a monitoring device and people with hypertension take their own blood pressure, you can also keep an eye on your lung functions at home with a peak flow meter. Peak flow meters, which are available in a variety of shapes and sizes from different manufacturers (see the appendix), are convenient, portable, and easy-to-use devices for monitoring *peak expiratory flow rate* (PEFR), the maximum rate of air (in liters per minute) that you can force out of your large airways, as a measurement of lung function.

This measurement isn't as accurate as spirometry, but you can easily perform it at home. Measurements of PEFR are also a vital part of long-term management of your asthma, as I explain in "Periodic assessment and monitoring" later in this chapter.

Bronchoprovocation

If spirometry indicates normal or near-normal lung functions but asthma continues to seem the most likely cause of your symptoms, your doctor may decide that a form of challenge test is necessary for a more conclusive diagnosis.

Challenge tests usually involve your doctor administering small doses of inhaled methacholine or histamine to you or making you exercise under his or her observation. The goal of such tests is to see whether these challenges cause obstructive changes in your airways, thus provoking mild asthma symptoms. Your doctor usually measures your lung functions before and after each test.

Considering other possible diagnoses

Although asthma causes most recurring episodes of coughing, wheezing, and shortness of breath, other disorders can cause these symptoms in some cases. With infants and children, underlying problems may include

- An upper respiratory disease, such as allergic rhinitis or sinusitis
- A swallowing mechanism problem or the effects of gastroesophageal reflux (GER)
- Congenital heart disease, often leading to congestive heart failure
- An obstruction of large airways, possibly caused by
  - A foreign object in the trachea or main bronchi, such as a small piece of popcorn that your child may have accidentally inhaled
  - Problems of the *larynx* (the cartilaginous portion of the upper respiratory tract that contains the vocal cords) or with the vocal cords themselves
  - Benign or malignant tumors or enlarged lymph nodes
- An obstruction of the small airways, as a result of
  - Cystic fibrosis
  - Abnormal development of the bronchi and lungs
  - Viral infection of the *bronchioles* (small bronchi)

With adult cases, underlying problems may include

- Chronic bronchitis and/or emphysema, collectively referred to as *chronic obstructive pulmonary disease* (COPD)

- Pulmonary embolism (a blood clot, air bubble, bacteria mass, or other mass that can clog a blood vessel)

- Heart disease

- Problems of the vocal cords or the larynx

- Benign or malignant tumors in the airways

- A cough reaction due to drugs such as ACE inhibitors that you may be using to treat other conditions, such as hypertension

Classifying asthma severity

If your doctor diagnoses you with asthma based on the results of your medical history, the physical exam, and appropriate tests, studies, and assessments, he or she also needs to define the severity of your condition. Physicians classify asthma — whether allergic or nonallergic — according to four levels of severity.

Experts from different fields of medicine have developed these severity classifications, which provide the basis for "stepwise" management of asthma. I explain stepwise management and asthma severity levels in detail in Chapter 13.

Referring to a specialist for diagnosis

In order to diagnose your condition, you or your physician should consider consulting an asthma specialist such as an allergist or pulmonologist (lung doctor) when

- Your diagnosis is difficult to establish.

- Your diagnosis requires specialized testing, such as allergy testing (see Chapter 8), bronchoprovocation (see "Testing your lungs" earlier in this chapter), or *bronchoscopy* (an exam of the interior of your bronchi using a slender, flexible fiber-optic bronchoscope).

- Your doctor advises you to consider immunotherapy (allergy shots).

- Other conditions such as sinusitis, nasal polyps, severe rhinitis, gastro-esophageal reflux (GER), chronic bronchitis and/or emphysema (COPD), vocal cord problems, or *aspergillosis* (a fungal infection that can affect the lungs) complicate your condition or diagnosis.

Managing Your Asthma: Essential Steps

If you're diagnosed with asthma, you and your doctor need to develop and implement appropriate long-term and emergency-management plans to effectively treat your condition. In my experience, motivated patients (with family members) who address their conditions through this type of thorough, individualized process almost always lead fulfilling and productive lives.

Management basics

Your asthma management plan requires your full participation in order to work most effectively. One of the most important ways for you to actively participate in your asthma treatment is to learn not just about the complexities of the disease, but also about medications, self-monitoring, allergies, triggers, and precipitating factors.

Your asthma management plan should address the following key areas:

- ✔ Objective assessments and monitoring of your lung functions. In addition to helping diagnose asthma, these tests and assessments are vital in tracking how your condition develops and responds to prescribed treatment.

- ✔ Long-term pharmacotherapy, which involves using medications to prevent symptoms by treating the underlying airway inflammation, congestion, constriction, and hyperresponsiveness.

- ✔ Short-term pharmacotherapy, which involves using fast-acting rescue medications when your condition suddenly deteriorates.

- ✔ Ways of avoiding and controlling your exposure to asthma triggers and precipitating factors.

- ✔ Using appropriate medication to prevent symptoms if you're exposed to allergens, irritants, and other asthma triggers.

- ✔ An ongoing process of education for you and your family about asthma. This process can involve information and resources that your doctor, clinic staff, and patient support groups provide or recommend, as well as relevant books, newsletters, videos, and other helpful materials that you and your family gather.

Your asthma therapy goals

Your asthma management plan should be results-oriented. I advise developing an overall goal, in consultation with your doctor, that aims for the highest attainable improvement of lung functions and enables you to maintain near-normal levels of exercise and other physical activities.

Other results that you should expect from asthma therapy include

- Preventing chronic and troublesome symptoms of asthma, such as coughing, shortness of breath, wheezing (especially upon awakening in the morning), and episodes that disturb your sleep at night
- Preventing recurring aggravation of symptoms
- Minimizing the need for emergency care and hospitalization
- Providing the most effective medication therapy that results in minimal or no adverse side effects

Based on the previous goals, if you feel that your doctor isn't providing adequate and effective treatment for your condition, I recommend consulting an asthma specialist, such as an allergist or pulmonologist. Too often, referrals are made only after a patient's symptoms have gotten out of control.

In my experience, after patients receive appropriate care for their asthma and understand that, in most cases, their asthma management goals are clearly achievable, they usually lead normal lives and will *never* tolerate going back to being frequently ill with asthma attacks.

In addition, you or your physician may also want to consider consulting an asthma specialist if

- You've suffered a life-threatening asthma attack.
- You're not meeting the goals of your asthma therapy.
- You require more education and guidance on possible treatment complications, the avoidance and control of triggers and precipitating factors, and following your asthma management program.
- You have severe persistent asthma that requires constant daily use of preventive medications and frequent use of short-acting inhaled beta$_2$-adrenergic (beta$_2$-agonist) bronchodilators.
- Your condition requires continuous use of oral corticosteroids, high-dose inhaled topical corticosteroids, or more than two bursts of oral corticosteroids within one year.
- You have a child under age 3 who has moderate persistent or severe persistent asthma (see Chapter 13) and requires constant use of preventive medication and frequent use of short-acting inhaled beta$_2$-adrenergic bronchodilators.
- You care for a person with asthma who experiences significant psychological, emotional, or family problems that interfere with or prevent that person from following an appropriate asthma management plan. Such experiences can lead to worsening asthma symptoms, which pose a threat to the patient's health. In this event, it may also be advisable for him or her to undergo evaluation by a mental health professional.

Periodic assessment and monitoring

Ongoing monitoring of your condition is a key component of your long-term asthma management plan. This section summarizes recommended assessment measures, which I explain more fully in Chapter 13.

Asthma assessment measures should cover the following areas:

- **Signs and symptoms of asthma:** Your doctor should instruct you on how to recognize patterns of worsening symptoms. Your doctor also needs to assess your symptom history during each office visit. Make sure that you let your doctor know about any episodes of severe asthma symptoms, because they can indicate that some aspect of your asthma management plan is inadequate, and your doctor needs to reevaluate your condition and modify your treatment plan.

- **Lung functions:** Your doctor will use spirometry to monitor your lung functions at least every one to two years, depending on how severe your asthma is and how you respond to treatment. Using a peak flow meter to self-monitor your lung functions should also be an essential element of your asthma management plan, as I explain in the next section.

- **Quality of life:** Evaluating the extent to which asthma may adversely affect your physical fitness, your ability to work or attend school, your emotional state, and your mental condition is an important aspect of determining whether you're meeting your goals of asthma treatment.

- **Medication therapy:** Your doctor should assess the effectiveness of the medication prescribed as part of your asthma management plan, including any side effects you may experience as a result of the drugs.

- **Communication:** Effective communication between you (and your family) and your physician about your asthma management plan is also vital in treating your condition.

Peak flow monitoring: Try this at home!

If you have persistent asthma, learn how to monitor your peak expiratory flow rate (PEFR) and make sure that you have a peak flow meter at home. By tracking your PEFR, you can objectively assess your lung functions and detect changes in your airflow that can provide an early signal of a worsening of your condition. Chapter 13 provides detailed information on your PEFR.

"Dear asthma" diary

In addition to tracking your PEFR, keeping a daily symptom diary can also provide your physician with valuable information to use when assessing your condition. A typical daily symptom diary is usually in the format of a table with columns and rows where you can record daily information about your asthma.

That information usually includes any symptoms you may experience, your PEFR readings, all the medications you've taken (including OTC products), your exposures to possible triggers, suspected early warning signs of asthma symptoms, questions you may have for your doctor, and any unscheduled office visits, after-hours treatments, emergency care, or hospitalizations that may have occurred within the dates of a diary page. See Chapter 13 for more details about tracking your asthma symptoms.

Handling emergencies

In addition to teaching you how to monitor your symptoms to recognize early warning signs of a worsening condition, your doctor should also

- ✔ Give you a written action plan that you can follow in case your condition deteriorates. Children with asthma need a plan that they can use at school, day care, or summer camp. Your written action plan must clearly instruct you how to adjust your medications in response to particular signs, symptoms, and PEFR levels, as well as tell you when to call for medical help.

- ✔ Teach you to seek medical help early if your episode is severe, if medication doesn't provide rapid, sustained improvement, or if your condition continues to deteriorate.

- ✔ Advise you to keep on hand appropriate medications, peak flow meters, and inhalant devices, such as nebulizers, to treat severe episodes at home if you suffer from moderate-to-severe persistent asthma or have a history of severe asthma attacks.

- ✔ Warn you against trying to manage severe episodes with home remedies, such as drinking large amounts of water, breathing steam or moist air (from a hot shower), taking over-the-counter (OTC) medications such as antihistamines, cold and flu remedies, pain relievers, or using OTC bronchodilators. Although these types of inhalers can sometimes provide temporary relief of airway constriction, they certainly aren't the preferable approach when appropriate medical care is required for treating acute asthma emergencies. (See Chapter 12 for information on asthma medications.)

Managing asthma at school

If your child has asthma, you should inform teachers, administrators, and the school nurse. I advise taking the following steps to ensure that your child's school days are as healthy, safe, and fulfilling as possible:

✔ Meet with school staff to inform them about any medications that your child may need to take while on campus, as well as any physical activity restrictions that your doctor may advise. (With proper management of their conditions, most children with asthma can participate in sports and physical education classes.)

✔ File treatment authorization forms with the school office and discuss what school personnel need to do in case of an asthma emergency. You also need to provide phone numbers and other avenues for school personnel to reach you and your child's physician in the event of an emergency.

✔ Inform school personnel of allergens and irritants that can trigger your child's asthma symptoms and request that the school remove the sources of those triggers if possible.

For more information on managing childhood asthma, turn to Chapter 14.

Chapter 11

Pulling Asthma Triggers

● ●

In This Chapter

▶ Identifying what's triggering your asthma symptoms

▶ Avoiding inhalant allergens

▶ Controlling triggers in your home

▶ Recognizing triggers in your workplace

▶ Keeping clear of food and drug triggers

▶ Dealing with other conditions that can aggravate your asthma

● ●

*W*ater covers two-thirds of the world's surface. If you have asthma, it may seem at times that the rest of the planet consists of nothing but asthma triggers. Throughout the world and in virtually every aspect of our everyday lives, countless precipitating factors — allergens, irritants, or other medical conditions — can induce asthma symptoms.

Avoiding or limiting your exposure to these precipitating factors is vital for effective management of your condition. Avoiding asthma triggers can help you experience fewer respiratory symptoms and potentially allow you to reduce your need for medication, especially rescue drugs such as short-acting beta$_2$-adrenergic (beta$_2$-agonist) bronchodilators (see Chapter 12 for details on asthma medications).

Although certain triggers frequently dominate each individual's asthma, controlling your condition often requires dealing with a host of precipitating factors — an especially common situation if you have allergic asthma, one of the most frequent types of asthma. Allergic asthma is usually associated with allergic rhinitis (hay fever) and/or allergic conjunctivitis (see Chapter 10 for details of allergic asthma).

If the prospect of dealing with a world full of asthma triggers seems daunting, don't despair. Throughout this chapter, I provide information and tips, based on extensive experience and the latest research findings, that can help you — in consultation with your doctor — implement practical and effective measures for avoiding or reducing exposure to your asthma triggers.

What Triggers Your Asthma?

One of the most important steps you need to take to effectively manage your asthma is to identify the triggers and precipitating factors that may affect your condition. These triggers, shown in Figure 11-1, include

- ✔ Inhalant allergens, including animal danders, dust mite and cockroach allergens, some mold spores, and certain airborne pollens of grasses, weeds, and trees (see Chapter 5).

- ✔ Occupational irritants and allergens, found primarily in the workplace, that induce occupational asthma (see "Working Out Workplace Exposures," later in this chapter) or aggravate an already existing form of the disease.

- ✔ Other irritants that you inhale, such as tobacco smoke, household products, and indoor and outdoor air pollution.

- ✔ Nonallergic triggers, including exercise and physical stimuli such as variations in air temperature and humidity levels.

- ✔ Other medical conditions, including rhinitis, sinusitis, gastroesophageal reflux (GER), and viral infections; sensitivities to aspirin, beta-blockers, and other drugs; and sensitivities to food additives — particularly sulfites.

- ✔ Emotional activities, such as crying, laughing, or even yelling. Although emotions themselves are not the direct triggers of asthma symptoms, activities associated with emotions (happy or sad) can induce coughing or wheezing in people with pre-existing hyperreactive airways (see Chapter 10), as well as in individuals who don't have asthma but who may suffer from other respiratory disorders. For example, your friend with a bad cold may say, "Please don't make me laugh; if I do, I'll start coughing."

Evaluating triggers

In order to determine what triggers your asthma symptoms and your sensitivity levels to those triggers, your doctor should take a thorough medical history.

Keeping an asthma diary (see Chapter 10) can assist in your doctor's assessment, by providing details of your symptoms and your exposures to potential triggers. You should also prepare to give your doctor specific information about the respiratory symptoms you experience, as I explain in Chapter 10.

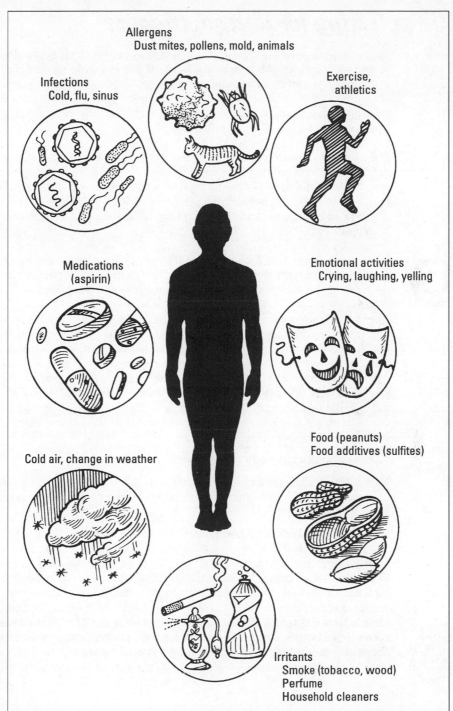

Allergens
Dust mites, pollens, mold, animals

Infections
Cold, flu, sinus

Exercise,
athletics

Medications
(aspirin)

Emotional activities
Crying, laughing, yelling

Cold air, change in weather

Food (peanuts)
Food additives (sulfites)

Irritants
Smoke (tobacco, wood)
Perfume
Household cleaners

Figure 11-1:
Common
triggers of
asthma.

Testing for allergic triggers

Many asthma patients experience *perennial* (year-round) symptoms that worsen during particular seasons. Because such a wide range of triggers can contribute to perennial asthma episodes, you should provide your doctor with a record of the seasonal patterns of your symptoms. Your record contains valuable clues to help your doctor narrow down the factors that affect your condition.

For example, if your asthma consistently worsens during late summer and fall in the eastern parts of the United States, your physician may suspect ragweed as a prime cause of the allergic reactions that aggravate your condition. However, doctors usually advise allergy testing (see Chapter 8) to investigate other possible causes and to confirm the diagnosis and determine appropriate treatment.

If you have persistent asthma (see Chapter 10) with perennial symptoms that occur primarily indoors, allergy testing can help your doctor identify several of the triggers, such as dust mites, that may be affecting you.

Nocturnal or *nighttime asthma,* which often shows up as a nighttime cough, wheezing, and/or shortness of breath, that disturbs your sleep and may require you to use your short-acting adrenergic bronchodilator (see Chapter 12) can often be severe. This condition is often triggered by allergens in the bedroom, postnasal drip from allergic rhinitis (see Chapter 4), or chronic sinus problems (such as sinusitis; see Chapter 9). Other factors that can trigger nocturnal asthma include

- Gastroesophageal reflux (GER)
- A drop in your body temperature
- Low circulation of *adrenal gland* (glands above your kidneys) *hormones,* such as *cortisol,* a hormone produced by the *cortex* (outer layer) of the adrenal gland
- A delayed reaction (known as a *late-phase reaction;* see Chapter 2) to allergens that you've been exposed to previously during the day

The *circadian rhythm* (also known as *diurnal variation*), which is your body's internal clock, may also affect your asthma, making you more susceptible to symptoms in the early morning hours (around 3 to 5 a.m.). Studies have shown that asthmatic airways are more *hyperreactive* (or *twitchy*) at these times. If you work at night and sleep during the day, you may experience these symptoms while sleeping during daytime hours.

Controlling Inhalant Allergens

Inhalant allergen triggers, also known as *areoallergens,* are probably the most familiar asthma precipitants because they're also associated with allergic rhinitis and similar conditions (see Chapter 4). If you have allergic asthma, reducing your exposure to inhalant allergens is the first and most important step you should take — in consultation with your doctor — to manage your condition.

Effectively avoiding inhalant allergen triggers usually begins at home, with a primary focus on the bedroom because most of us spend, on average, one-third of our lives there. Even if you're exposed to triggers in other aspects of your life, reducing your exposure at home to inhalant allergens (and irritants) through allergy-proofing (see Chapter 6) can significantly help prevent the onset of asthma symptoms.

Avoiding animal allergens

Pet dander, which contains traces of animal urine, feces, and saliva, is a potent trigger of symptoms for many people with asthma. Although household dogs and cats are the most common sources of these allergens, all warm-blooded animals, such as horses, rabbits, small rodents, and birds, produce dander — regardless of hair length — that can cause allergic reactions and aggravate your asthma. Urine from these animals is also a source of allergens. Animal dander also serves as a food supply (along with dead human skin scales) for dust mites, as I explain in Chapter 5.

I advise people with allergies or asthma not to introduce new pets into their homes. If you already have a pet, limiting your exposure to the animal can often improve your condition and can eventually result in substantially reducing your medication requirements. Bear in mind that even if you find a new home for your dog or cat, the animal's dander can linger at levels that can trigger allergic responses for up to six months. If you can't bear parting with Fluffy or Fido, see the measures I advise in Chapter 6 for more pet relief. At the very least, I advise making the asthma patient's bedroom a "pet-free" zone.

Dealing with dust mites

Dust mites abound almost everywhere humans settle, and they thrive especially well in mattresses, carpets, upholstered furniture, bed covers, linens, clothes, and soft toys. The main diet of these microscopic spider relatives consists of the dead skin scales that humans constantly shed. Dust mite fecal matter is one of the most allergenic components of house dust allergens.

Although eradicating these dusty denizens is virtually impossible — the females lay 20 to 50 eggs every three weeks — you can take practical and effective steps to minimize exposure to the allergens that dust mites produce. See Chapter 5 for more dirt on dust mites, and Chapter 6 for details on measures to control these creatures.

Controlling your exposure to cockroaches

As if you need another reason to avoid cockroaches, exposure to allergens from cockroach droppings (yuck!) in house dust can trigger and aggravate your asthma symptoms. Studies show that inner-city children who unfortunately receive high levels of exposure to cockroach allergens, especially in the bedroom, can develop increasingly severe asthma.

Cockroach allergens are particularly common in inner-city apartments. Many asthmatic patients of inner-city clinics have been found to test positive for cockroach allergens (through allergy skin testing) but have improved after immunotherapy (allergy shots) with cockroach allergen extract. (See Chapter 8 for more information on allergy skin testing and immunotherapy.)

Controlling cockroach allergens in your home should include these key measures:

- ✔ Exterminate cockroach infestations. During the fumigation process, stay out of your home, and allow it to air out for several hours before re-entering. (This advice applies to anyone, regardless of whether or not you have asthma.)

- ✔ Clean your entire home thoroughly after extermination.

- ✔ Set roach traps.

- ✔ Seal any cracks or other conduits into your home to prevent reinfestation.

- ✔ Keep your kitchen clean by washing dishes and cookware promptly and by emptying garbage and recycling containers (including old newspapers) often, and avoid leaving food out.

Managing mold triggers

The airborne spores that molds (fungi) release in typically damp areas of many homes, particularly from basements, bathrooms, air conditioners, garbage containers, and under carpeting, can trigger allergy and asthma symptoms when you inhale them. Fungi can also thrive in leaf piles, compost heaps, cut grass, fertilizer, hay, and barns around your home. Airborne mold spores are more numerous than pollen grains and don't have a limited season (as I explain in Chapter 5). Depending on where you live, you may receive exposure to airborne spores during many parts of the year, based on levels of humidity.

See Chapter 5 for more moldy matters, including tips on translating mold counts. Chapter 6 explains what you can do to reduce mold exposures.

Avoiding pollen problems

From spring through fall, many varieties of trees, grasses, and weeds release pollens that can trigger symptoms of allergic rhinitis and/or allergic conjunctivitis. These reactions can also affect your asthma, aggravating the underlying airway inflammation.

Many people primarily associate pollens with outdoor exposure. However, because most pollens are wind-borne, they can often make their way indoors and trigger allergy and asthma symptoms in your home.

See Chapter 6 for steps you can take to avoid excessive exposure to pollen, especially during periods of high pollination, and see Chapter 5 for more pollen particulars, including tips on pollen counts.

Clearing the Air at Home

Our indoor environments at home, work, school, and cars as well as other enclosed means of transportation can often provide far more significant sources of asthma triggers than the outdoors, because most enclosures concentrate irritants and allergens. According to the American Lung Association, many of us spend 90 percent of our time indoors — 60 percent of that time within our own homes. Therefore, you should seriously consider the effects of indoor air pollution because it can induce or aggravate allergies and asthma.

Household irritants

The most significant irritant triggers of asthma in many households are

- Tobacco smoke (see the next section)
- Fumes and scents from household cleaners, strongly scented soaps, perfumes, glues, and aerosols
- Smoke from wood-burning appliances or fireplaces
- Fumes from unvented gas, oil, or kerosene stoves

Other sources of indoor air pollution include pollens and mold spores that get inside, especially on windy days when windows and doors are open. These allergenic materials can also infiltrate your home via your clothing and hair. In fact, if you have allergic asthma, you may wake up congested and wheezing in the morning because allergenic materials find their way into your house so easily. (The pollen or mold spores in your hair probably wound up on your pillow, so you spent the night breathing those allergens into your lungs.)

No smoking, please

As far as truly irritating irritants go, here's a no-brainer: Tobacco smoke is the number one indoor air pollutant. Secondhand smoke has been associated with an increase in the following adverse effects: persistent wheezing associated with asthma, hospital admissions for respiratory infections, earlier onset of respiratory allergies, decreased lung function, and even increased incidence of *otitis media with effusion* (inflammation of the middle ear; see Chapter 9).

Tobacco smoke frequently precipitates asthma symptoms in children. In fact, numerous studies show that parental smoking, especially by the mother, is a major risk factor in the development of asthma in infants, who are exposed to the smoke during the first few months of life. Therefore, don't smoke and make sure that those around you don't smoke, especially if you have children.

Filters and air-cleaning devices

The quality of the air you breathe indoors largely depends on the condition of your heating, ventilation, and air-conditioning (HVAC) system, as well as the air and particles that circulate throughout it.

If you're exposed to airborne allergens and irritants such as animal dander, mold spores, pollen, and tobacco smoke, you may want to consider using air filters on your HVAC ducts to reduce the level of allergy and asthma triggers circulating through your home. Keep in mind, however, that these filters won't remove substances that have already settled in bedding, carpeting, and furniture — especially dust mite allergens. Dust mite allergens are generally larger than other airborne allergens and irritants, and they usually fall from the air within a few minutes of being stirred up in dust or air currents.

The two types of air filtration systems often recommended by doctors for reducing indoor levels of airborne allergen and irritants are

 ✔ **High Efficiency Particulate Matter (HEPA):** These filters are designed to absorb and contain 99.97 percent of all particles larger than 0.3 microns (one-three hundredth the width of a human hair). If the unit truly operates at that level, only 3 out of 10,000 particles get into your indoor environment. Vacuum cleaners and air purifiers with HEPA and ULPA filters (see the next section for more information) can play a vital part in allergy-proofing your home.

✔ **Ultra Low Penetration Air (ULPA):** This system filters more thoroughly than the HEPA process and is designed to absorb and contain 99.99 percent of all particles larger than 0.12 microns.

If your home doesn't have a central HVAC system, you can purchase stand-alone HEPA and ULPA air cleaners for use in individual rooms. The appendix at the back of this book provides information on finding and purchasing these items.

Vacuum cleaning is also vital for reducing your exposure to allergens and irritants at home. However, many standard vacuum cleaners only absorb larger particles, and they allow many allergens to escape in the exhaust. This is often why you may experience asthma symptoms after housework: The vacuuming may actually have made matters worse for you by simply stirring up triggering substances that you then inhaled.

In order to avoid stirring up asthma triggers when you vacuum, ask your doctor whether he or she thinks investing in a vacuum cleaner that uses a HEPA or ULPA filtration process may work for you. You can find more information on HEPA- or ULPA-filtered vacuums in the appendix.

Working Out Workplace Exposures

Exposures to many types of chemicals and dust in workplace environments can induce different forms of occupational asthma. In many cases, people who have asthma but haven't yet developed obvious symptoms of the disease may experience asthma episodes for the first time as a result of exposure to occupational triggers. Allergic and nonallergic triggers may both play a part in occupational asthma, which may account for as many as 15 percent of all new asthma cases each year in the U.S.

Targeting workplace triggers

Doctors and other health care professionals typically associate occupational asthma with exposure to the following workplace triggers:

✔ **Industrial irritants:** These irritants can include chemicals, fumes, gases, aerosols, paints, smoke, and other substances you primarily find in the workplace. Tobacco smoke in the workplace can cause many asthma symptoms. Likewise, other irritants in the workplace can include perfumes, food odors, and even other workers who use heavily scented perfumes and colognes.

✔ **Physical stimuli:** These stimuli include conditions in your workplace, especially variations in temperature and humidity, such as heat and cold extremes or air that's especially dry or humid.

✔ **Occupational allergens:** Many occupations involve exposure to or contact with substances made of plant materials, food products, and other items that contain allergenic extracts that can trigger allergic reactions, thus inducing occupational asthma in sensitized people. For example, "Baker's asthma" can occur in workers who receive constant respiratory exposure to the allergens contained in flour. (Eating the resulting baked food usually doesn't produce symptoms in these workers, however.) Latex is another common occupational allergen, as I explain in the sidebar "Latex and your lungs."

Diagnosing and treating workplace triggers

Your physician should distinguish between asthma that results from exposure to certain substances in the workplace, school, or other frequented locations (other than your home) and a pre-existing condition that is aggravated by occupational allergens and irritants. This determination is vital to developing appropriate and effective methods of avoiding or reducing your exposure to occupational substances that may affect your asthma.

Diagnosing your occupational asthma is important for your long-term health and the effective management of your disease. The sooner you can effectively avoid or reduce your exposure to triggers at work, the better you can control your asthma.

In diagnosing a case of occupational asthma, your doctor may first need to assess the following factors:

✔ The pattern of your symptoms. Symptoms that improve when you're away from work strongly suggest that your problem is indeed work-related.

✔ Whether your co-workers suffer from similar symptoms.

✔ Whether your first noticeable asthma episode at work occurred after a particularly significant exposure, such as a spill of chemicals or other industrial substances.

Depending on the severity of your condition, your doctor may prescribe medications that control your asthma symptoms at work. In most cases, however, for this treatment to be effective, your doctor will probably advise you to find ways of avoiding or at least reducing your exposure to workplace triggers.

Latex and your lungs

Latex is increasingly a part of the environment in most medical facilities, due to the need during recent years for more aggressive infection control measures. This rubber compound is found particularly in medical gloves and other medical equipment, such as latex ports in intravenous tubing for administration of fluids and medications.

Because many surgical gloves contain corn starch powder that's coated with latex allergen, health care workers often inhale airborne allergen latex particles. These exposures can result in allergens from the rubber compounds sensitizing medical personnel. Thus, latex has become one of the most frequent causes of occupational allergy and asthma in the health care industry. In addition, patients being treated in medical facilities can also receive exposures and be sensitized to latex.

These exposures can lead to serious symptoms of allergic rhinitis, asthma, urticaria (hives) angioedema (deep swellings), and in, extreme cases, anaphylaxis (a potentially life-threatening reaction that affects many organs simultaneously).

It's the allergens in natural rubber contained in many latex products (including condoms) that mainly cause Type I immediate hypersensitivity IgE-mediated reactions. (I explain this mechanism in Chapter 2.) For this reason, the FDA now requires labeling of all medical devices or packaging containing natural rubber latex.

If you're at risk for allergic reactions to latex exposure, you should make sure that any physician who treats you knows this fact so that you can, ideally, receive medical/dental care in a latex-free environment — a setting in which no latex gloves are used and no latex accessories (such as catheters, adhesives, tourniquets, and anesthesia equipment) come into contact with you. Similarly, if your occupation involves contact with latex, you should find out what you can do to avoid or minimize your exposure to this allergen. In health care settings, powder-free latex gloves and non-latex gloves and other medical articles are increasingly becoming available. Using these alternative products can often substantially reduce the risk that you may suffer an allergic reaction to latex.

Additionally, I advise you to wear a MedicAlert bracelet or pendant to alert medical personnel not to use latex articles in the event that you're unconscious or unable to communicate during a medical emergency. (The appendix provides information on obtaining these bracelets and pendants.) If you've experienced a serious allergic reaction to latex, you should also ask your doctor whether an emergency epinephrine kit, such as an EpiPen or AnaKit, with an injectable dose of epinephrine, is advisable for you.

Avoiding Food and Drug Triggers

Some people with asthma also suffer from sensitivities to certain foods and medications containing substances that can trigger severe and, in some cases, potentially life-threatening asthma episodes. In the following sections, I explain the most significant sensitivities that can adversely affect your asthma and what you can do to avoid them.

Aspirin sensitivities

Approximately 10 percent of asthma patients experience some level of sensitivity to aspirin, aspirin-containing compounds (such as Alka-Seltzer, Anacin, and Exedrin) and nonsteroidal anti-inflammatory drugs (NSAIDs). If your medical history includes nasal polyps and sinusitis in addition to asthma, I strongly recommend using acetaminophen-based products such as Tylenol instead of aspirin or NSAIDs for the relief of common aches and pains.

A more serious form of aspirin sensitivity is the *aspirin triad*. This condition affects aspirin-intolerant patients who have asthma and chronic nasal polyps as well as a history of sinusitis. If you suffer from the aspirin triad, adverse reactions to aspirin, aspirin-containing compounds, NSAIDs, and newer prescription NSAIDs, known as COX-2 inhibitors, including celecoxib (Celebrex) and refecoxib (Vioxx), can result in severe or potentially life-threatening asthma attacks.

I strongly advise anyone with this level of sensitivity to wear a MedicAlert bracelet or pendant. This device alerts medical personnel not to administer any medication to which you are sensitive if you're unconscious or unable to communicate during a medical emergency. See the appendix for more information on MedicAlert bracelets and pendants.

Beta-blockers

Doctors frequently prescribe beta-blocker medications, including Inderal, Lopressor, and Corgard, to treat conditions such as migraine headache, high blood pressure, glaucoma, angina, or hyperthyroidism. If you have one of these disorders and you also have asthma, you should know that taking beta-blockers can worsen your asthma symptoms by blocking the $beta_2$-adrenergic receptor sites in your airways that cause bronchodilation, thus making your asthma less responsive to $beta_2$-adrenergic ($beta_2$-agonist) bronchodilators.

Occasionally, taking beta-blockers can trigger asthma episodes in susceptible individuals who have not previously experienced any respiratory symptoms.

Because beta-blockers may possibly trigger asthma symptoms, make sure that any doctor you consult for any of the conditions I mention in this section knows that you have asthma and/or has your complete medical history. If beta-blockers aren't advisable, your doctor may prescribe alternative forms of medication therapy, such as other families of anti-hypertensives or other types of anti-migraine drugs.

Sensitivities to sulfites and other additives

Sulfites are often used as antioxidants to preserve beverages such as beer and wine and foods such as dried fruit, shrimp, and potatoes. These antioxidants are also often used in salad bars and in guacamole. Exposure to these food additives can trigger severe asthma symptoms — including potentially life-threatening bronchospasm (constriction of the airways) — in as many as 10 percent of people who have severe persistent asthma when these individuals inhale sulfite fumes from treated foods. Severe asthmatics who require long-term treatment with oral corticosteroids (see Chapter 12) are more likely to be sulfite-sensitive and may be especially at risk for severe adverse reactions to these additives.

If you're sensitive to sulfites, avoid consuming beer, wine, and processed foods. Also, carry rescue medication, such as an EpiPen and/or a short-acting inhaled bronchodilator, with you in the event that you unintentionally ingest food or liquids that contain sulfites. Eating more fresh foods, instead of processed foods, particularly fruits and vegetables, is a good idea anyway, regardless of whether or not you have asthma.

Tartrazine (FDC yellow dye No. 5), used in many medications, foods, and vitamin products, may also cause adverse reactions in asthmatics. If you're sensitive to this food additive, check the labels on liquid medications, such as cough syrups and other liquid cold and flu remedies, to see whether they contain tartrazine or sulfites. When in doubt, ask your pharmacist.

Food allergies

Many people with asthma develop hypersensitivities to certain foods. However, although certain foods have the potential to cause anaphylaxis, they don't appear to significantly increase the underlying airway inflammation that's characteristic of asthma in most patients.

If your infant or young child has food allergies, it may indicate a tendency to develop other allergy-related problems. In this case, your doctor should evaluate your child for possible signs of asthma and other atopic diseases, such as allergic rhinitis and atopic dermatitis.

If you've experienced an episode of anaphylaxis, ask your doctor whether an emergency epinephrine kit, such as an EpiPen (or EpiPen Jr. for children under 66 pounds) or AnaKit, with an injectable dose of epinephrine, is advisable for you. I also strongly advise that you wear a MedicAlert bracelet or necklace in case you're unable to speak during a reaction. The appendix at the back of this book provides more information on obtaining these items.

If you're hungering for details on food allergies, turn to Chapter 19.

Other Medical Conditions and Asthma

In addition to the triggers that I discuss previously in this chapter, certain activities, illnesses, and syndromes can also induce your asthma symptoms or make them worse. Managing these precipitating factors is as vital to effectively controlling your asthma as is avoiding allergens and irritants.

Exercise-induced asthma (EIA)

Symptoms of exercise-induced asthma (EIA — also known as *exercise-induced bronchospasm* or EIB) occur to varying degrees in a majority of asthmatics. For certain individuals, physical activity may be the only trigger that precipitates asthma symptoms such as coughing, wheezing, and shortness of breath. Occasionally, patients mistakenly attribute their EIA symptoms to just "being out of shape." Typically, EIA begins minutes after you begin vigorous activity, when the airways in your lungs become narrow and constricted. These asthma symptoms usually reach their peak of severity between five and ten minutes after you stop exercising. In many cases, the symptoms can spontaneously resolve (without the use of a short-acting inhaled bronchodilator) within 30 minutes.

Exercises that involve breathing cold, dry air — such as running outdoors — are more likely to trigger EIA than activities that involve breathing warmer, humidified air, such as swimming in a heated pool.

Although EIA usually relates to outside activities, using home exercise equipment or simply running up the stairs can precipitate an asthma episode in some people. If you have an increased sensitivity for EIA, make sure that your doctor knows so that he or she can evaluate and treat your condition appropriately.

Asthma and athletics

Unless your condition is properly diagnosed and treated, EIA might prevent you from participating in the activities that you truly enjoy. Although the symptoms usually last for only a few minutes, the episode can still be a frightening experience for many people and may even unnecessarily limit your activities. Fortunately, your doctor can prescribe medications that you can use to preventively control your EIA symptoms, thus allowing you to enjoy many types of exercise and sports activities in spite of your asthma.

Keeping a record of your activities, noting when you experience asthma symptoms and what steps you normally take to relieve your symptoms, can assist your doctor in developing the most effective treatment program for managing your EIA. Because certain drugs are more effective in preventing and controlling EIA if taken according to your exercise schedule, *when* you take your prescribed medication is just as important as *what* medications you take. Therefore, working with your doctor to determine the best time to take your medication provides maximum relief from EIA. Chapter 12 presents information on these drugs, which you should take only according to your doctor's advice.

In many cases, competitive athletes with asthma or EIA use inhaled topical corticosteroids daily to control their airway inflammation. Many competitive athletes also add a long-acting inhaled beta$_2$-adrenergic bronchodilator daily, such as salmeterol (Serevent), twice a day and/or a short-acting inhaled beta$_2$-adrenergic bronchodilator, such as albuterol (Proventil, Ventolin), prior to exercise or athletic events. These medications help prevent asthma episodes when athletes exert themselves.

Contrary to popular myth, sports federations such as the NCAA or the U.S. Olympic Committee haven't banned the use of inhaled topical corticosteroids that athletes take to control asthma symptoms. (The steroids that various sports committees ban are actually male hormones, taken by tablet or injection, that some athletes use to build muscle mass.)

Warming up and cooling down to prevent EIA

Many doctors advise some type of warm-up and cool-down routine (even if you don't have asthma) when engaging in exercise or sports-related activity. Consult with your physician to determine the type of pre- and post-exercise routine that's most beneficial for you. After you've determined the warm-up and cool-down plan that works best for you, incorporate that routine into your asthma management plan.

As long as you stick to your asthma management plan, asthma shouldn't prevent you from enjoying or even excelling at a wide range of physical activities. Consider the examples of Jackie Joyner-Kersee and other Olympic champions who also suffer from asthma. (See Chapter 24 for more famous folks with asthma — the list may surprise you!)

Rhinitis and sinusitis

Poorly managing allergic and nonallergic forms of rhinitis can lead to *sinusitis*. This infection of the sinuses can also cause aggravation of your asthma symptoms, especially if it isn't responsive to repeated courses of antibiotic treatment. If so, sinus surgery may be necessary to treat sinusitis and reestablish control over asthma symptoms. Studies show that asthma patients who effectively manage their rhinitis and/or sinusitis can significantly improve their asthma symptoms.

Because your respiratory tract is essentially a continuum, treating your nose and sinuses can actually help treat the underlying inflammation that characterizes asthma. In fact, when dealing with serious respiratory diseases such as asthma, doctors increasingly consider it vital to treat the whole patient — not just the patient's lungs. For more information on dealing with sinusitis and other rhinitis complications, turn to Chapter 9.

Gastroesophageal reflux (GER)

The digestive disorder *gastroesophageal reflux* (GER, also known as *gastroesophageal reflux disease,* or *GERD*), occurs when the valve that connects the esophagus to the stomach doesn't function properly. As a result, stomach acid and undigested food can wash up into the esophagus (and occasionally, through inhalation, into the respiratory tract) from the stomach in individuals who suffer from GER. You can see a cross-section of the organs involved in GER in Figure 11-2.

Patients who suffer from GER often burp during and after meals, complain of an acid taste in their mouth, and feel a burning sensation in their throat or chest, symptoms that they typically describe as heartburn or indigestion.

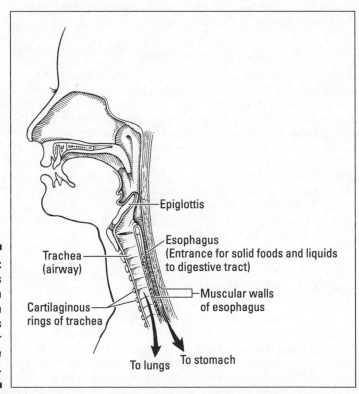

Figure 11-2: GER occurs when stomach contents spill over into the trachea.

Epiglottis

Esophagus (Entrance for solid foods and liquids to digestive tract)

Trachea (airway)

Muscular walls of esophagus

Cartilaginous rings of trachea

To lungs   To stomach

GER is a trigger of asthma symptoms in a large number of asthmatics and is, in particular, a major trigger of adult-onset asthma (see Chapter 10) in patients whose asthma symptoms (coughing, wheezing, shortness of breath) are not usually associated with allergic triggers. If you're asthmatic, the flow of acidic digestive contents into your respiratory airways can make your underlying airway inflammation worse. GER, with or without inhalation of stomach contents, has also been associated with increased bronchospasm due to irritation of the esophagus.

If you have frequent heartburn and poorly controlled asthma, particularly with episodes that occur at night and disturb your sleep, your doctor should investigate the possibility that GER contributes to your asthma symptoms.

To help alleviate the effects of GER, your doctor may advise the following:

- ✔ Avoid eating or drinking within three hours of going to bed.

- ✔ Avoid heavy meals and minimize dietary fat. Also, try to eat several small meals over the course of the day instead of fewer, larger meals.

- ✔ Eliminate or cut down on the consumption of chocolate, alcoholic beverages, coffee, tea, and colas, and carbonated beverages in general.

- ✔ Avoid or reduce smoking and the use of any tobacco products.

- ✔ Try elevating the head of your bed, by using 6- to 8-inch blocks, so that your stomach contents are less likely to rise to the point that you can inhale them while sleeping. Adding pillows under your head can also be of some benefit.

- ✔ To control the digestive problems that result from your GER symptoms, use appropriate over-the-counter (OTC) products, including Zantac, Tagamet, Axid, and Pepcid AC. Your physician may also prescribe other medications, such as Prilosec and Prevacid, that decrease *gastric* (stomach) acid secretion.

Viral infections

Viral respiratory infections such as the common cold or flu can aggravate airway inflammation and trigger asthma symptoms. Asthmatic children under 10 are particularly prone to asthma symptoms precipitated by *rhinovirus infections* (upper respiratory infections, usually referred to as the common cold).

Rhinovirus infections cause bronchial hyperreactivity and promote allergic inflammation, leading to increased asthma symptoms. For infants and toddlers, viral infections of all types are the most frequent cause of severe asthma episodes. That's because infants and younger children have smaller airways that are often more susceptible to bronchial obstruction.

Inform your doctor whenever you experience flu or cold symptoms. As comforting as you may find chicken soup when you're sniffly and sneezy, you may require early and aggressive medication therapy to keep the virus from adversely affecting your asthma.

What to do about the flu

Antiviral medications can help you avoid coming down with influenza even when you've had a flu shot. Flu vaccines consist of the World Health Organization's (WHO) best guess of the viruses from the preceding year that may cause the flu during next year's winter season. However, the WHO's predictions aren't always accurate. As a result, a flu shot may not fully protect you against the viral strains that cause the current year's flu epidemic, thus making antiviral medications extremely beneficial.

Consider the following measures when dealing with viral infections:

✔ If your have persistent asthma, ask your doctor about receiving an annual flu vaccine to reduce the risk of suffering from an influenza respiratory infection that could aggravate your asthma symptoms.

✔ New antiviral medications, such as zanamivir by inhalation (Relenza) and oseltamivir phosphate by oral tablet (Tamiflu), can stop the flu dead in its tracks and get you back on your feet sooner if you take these drugs within the first two days of developing flu symptoms. Common flu symptoms include high fever, muscle aches, fatigue, and increased respiratory symptoms. Using these antiviral products can reduce the respiratory complications that accompany viral infections, making these medications especially beneficial if you have asthma.

✔ If your young child or infant experiences repeated viral infections that cause coughing and wheezing episodes, and your family medical history includes *atopy* (the genetic susceptibility for the immune system to produce antibodies to common allergens, which leads to allergy symptoms), make sure your doctor evaluates your child for the possibility of asthma. (See Chapter 14 for more information about asthma and children.)

Chapter 12

Controlling Asthma with Medications

*T*reatment with medications, which doctors refer to as *pharmacotherapy,* is a crucial component of your asthma management plan (see Chapter 10). As with the other aspects of your asthma management plan — self-monitoring (most commonly by using a peak flow meter, as I explain in Chapter 13); keeping track of your symptoms (usually with a symptom diary; see Chapter 10); avoiding possible asthma triggers (Chapter 11); and educating yourself about your disease (Chapter 13) — adhering to your doctor's instructions for taking prescribed medications is vital in effectively treating your condition.

Physicians who care for people with asthma and allergies are very aware that patients prefer not to take medications on a regular basis. However, asthma is more than the coughing, wheezing, or other symptoms that you may experience off and on. If you have persistent asthma — like the majority of asthmatics in the United States — some degree of airway inflammation and hyperreactivity (increased sensitivity) is always present, even when you feel fine. Controlling that inflammation is the key to keeping your condition from getting out of hand and developing severe asthma episodes.

Asthma is a chronic condition requiring chronic treatment. Therefore, you should treat your asthma the way people with high blood pressure or heart disease or diabetes treat their conditions: by taking medications preventively, on a regular basis. Most asthmatics get into trouble with their disease from too little rather than too much treatment. As I explain in Chapter 10, patients who take their medications as directed can prevent the majority of emergency room visits and hospitalizations that asthma causes.

BERGER BIT

Understanding the medicine that you take

An informed patient is a healthier person. Remember: Making sure that you understand all aspects of your treatment is your responsibility as a patient. Don't hesitate to inquire about medications your doctor prescribes for your asthma (or any ailment, for that matter). I advise knowing the following information about your prescription before you leave your doctor's office and begin using a medication:

✔ The name of the medication, the prescribed dose, how often you should take it, and over what period of time you must use it. Your doctor may provide an instruction card with this information. This card can greatly assist you in communicating with other doctors about the medications you're taking, and it may prove vital in an emergency situation. Likewise, ensuring that the product's name is clearly written is important, because the drug and brand names of many medications sound alike.

✔ The way the drug works, any potential adverse side effects that may result, and what you should do if any of these side effects occur.

✔ What you should do if you accidentally miss a dose or take an extra dose of the medication.

✔ Any cautions about potential interactions between your prescription and other medications you already take or may take, including over-the-counter (OTC) antihistamines, decongestants, pain relievers, vitamins, or nutritional supplements.

✔ Any effects your prescription may have on various aspects of your life, such as your job, school, exercise or sports, other activities, sleeping patterns, and diet.

✔ If the medication is for your child, make sure that you know how your child's dosage may differ from an adult's.

✔ If you're pregnant or nursing a child, make sure that you inform your doctor about these situations.

✔ Be sure your doctor knows about any adverse reactions you've had to any drugs in the past, including both prescription and OTC preparations. (See Chapter 20 for more information on adverse drug reactions.)

Use only those products that are clearly identified to treat the symptoms you experience. You should also always carefully read the product instructions and only take the medication as those instructions say or according to your doctor's directions.

Occasionally, doctors need to prescribe medications "off label" (beyond the manufacturer's official recommendations) in order to achieve maximal improvement in a particular patient's condition. Our patient's health and well-being is our primary commitment, and sometimes treatments need to be individualized, such as using high-dose inhaled topical corticosteroids in cases of severe persistent asthma (see Table 12-1) or using an H-2 antihistamine (such as Tagamet or Zantac) together with H-1 antihistamines (such as Claritin, Allergra, or Zyrtec) to treat urticaria (hives), as I explain in Chapter 18.

In addition to the printed information that doctors may provide concerning the drugs they prescribe, you can also request materials from the National Council on Patient Information and Education, 666 11th St. NW, Suite 810, Washington, DC, 20001-4542; phone 202-347-6711.

Your physician's goal is to determine the most appropriate medications to help you achieve the best possible control of your symptoms and your best possible lung function without adverse side effects. Therefore, you should routinely take the drugs that your doctor prescribes, because they're essential to managing your condition and because they can help significantly improve your quality of life. Without using the medications that your doctor prescribes, you're likely to have a much more difficult time controlling your asthma.

Effective asthma pharmacotherapy should help you achieve the following goals in managing your condition:

✔ Prevent and control your asthma symptoms

✔ Reduce the frequency and severity of your asthma episodes

✔ Reverse your airway obstruction and maintain improved lung function

In this chapter, I explain and discuss the types of medications that doctors prescribe to treat asthma, the brand names of those drugs, and how they work. I also provide tips on taking these medications and explain the different delivery systems used to administer many of these products.

The Long and Short of Asthma Medications

Asthma pharmacotherapy involves two basic classes of medications. These medications are

✔ **Long-term control medications:** Doctors prescribe these products as part of a regular regimen (most often with daily doses) to achieve and maintain control of the underlying airway inflammation that characterizes asthma.

✔ **Quick-relief medications:** At times, you may need these products — often called *rescue drugs* — to provide prompt relief of severe and sudden airway constriction and airflow obstruction that can occur when your asthma symptoms unexpectedly worsen.

Your doctor may prescribe products from both classes of medications as part of your long-term asthma management program (see Chapter 13). The specific combination of products that your doctor prescribes depends on the severity of your asthma and other factors, such as

✔ **Your age.** As I explain later in this chapter, doses and products for infants, toddlers, children under 12, and the elderly often vary from those that doctors prescribe for adults and children over 12.

> ✔ **Your medical history and physical condition.** For example, your doctor may adjust dosages and/or products if you're pregnant or nursing a child.
>
> ✔ **Any other ailments that may affect you, as well as other medications you may take to treat those conditions.**
>
> ✔ **Any sensitivities you may have to particular drugs or to certain ingredients in the formulations of particular medications.**

Taking long-term control medications

If used in an appropriate, consistent manner, long-term control medications can reduce existing airway inflammation and may also help prevent further inflammation from occurring.

Long-term control medications include the following categories of drugs:

> ✔ Anti-inflammatory drugs such as inhaled topical corticosteroids, oral corticosteroids, and inhaled mast cell stabilizers (cromolyn and nedocromil) that act as anti-inflammatories
>
> ✔ Long-acting bronchodilators, such as inhaled salmeterol, formoterol, and oral forms of albuterol
>
> ✔ Sustained release methylxanthine bronchodilators, such as oral theophylline
>
> ✔ Leukotriene modifiers, such as oral montelukast, zafirlukast, and zileuton

The following sections explain how each of these drugs works, the circumstances under which doctors prescribe them, and the medicines' generic and brand names.

Corticosteroids

Corticosteroids provide the most potent and consistently effective long-term control for asthma. With their anti-inflammatory action, these drugs can

> ✔ Decrease swelling in your airways
>
> ✔ Reduce mucus production in your airways
>
> ✔ Make your airways less hyperresponsive ("twitchy") to asthma triggers

Corticosteroids may also prevent irreversible damage (known as *remodeling* — replacing healthy tissue with scar tissue) to the airway (see Chapter 10).

Toning your lungs, not your muscles

The attempts by some athletes to build up muscle mass by abusing anabolic steroids (related to *testosterone*) cause many people to harbor a negative perception about all steroids. However, not all steroids cause such health risks. In fact, the corticosteroids in inhaled topical and oral corticosteroid products are a completely different type of drug than anabolic steroids, which are actually male hormones. The confusion is largely due to the common use of the term *steroid,* which really is a general term for any of the hormones with related chemical structures produced by specific glands in the body. These hormones include testosterone from the *testes,* estrogen from the *ovaries,* and corticosteroids (related to *cortisone*) from the *cortex* (outer layer) of the *adrenal gland* (glands above the kidneys).

The most accurate description used by the majority of medical professionals is actually the proper term *corticosteroid* for the types of inhaled topical and oral products that I describe in this section of the chapter.

Inhaled topical corticosteroids

Doctors generally consider inhaled topical corticosteroids the *primary controller* or *maintenance therapy* for patients with moderate and severe persistent asthma, because of the drugs' anti-inflammatory properties. Likewise, doctors use these drugs as a primary controller because the inhaled forms of medications usually offer the best means of delivering drugs directly to the airways with minimal side effects. Consistent and appropriate (as determined by your doctor) use of inhaled topical corticosteroids can also reduce the need for oral (or *systemic*) corticosteroids, which may cause serious adverse side effects when used long-term.

Inhaled topical corticosteroids usually start reducing airway inflammation after a week of regular administration, reaching their full effect within four weeks. However, although these drugs can work well as preventives, if you develop severe symptoms — from a sudden high exposure to potent asthma triggers, for example — you need to use a quick-relief medication (usually a bronchodilator that your doctor prescribes) as part of your asthma management plan.

Doctors can prescribe inhaled topical corticosteroids as a metered-dose inhaler (MDI), a dry powder inhaler (DPI), or compressor-driven nebulizer (CDN) formulation. Because the pressurized canisters of different concentrations of some of these MDI medications are packaged in plastic sleeves of the same color, it's especially important to know which strength your doctor specifically prescribes for you (see Table 12-1).

Table 12-1   Inhaled Topical Corticosteroid Medications

Active Ingredient	Formulation	Brand Name	Total Usual Daily Child Dose (Under 12)	Total Usual Daily Adult Dose
Beclomethasone	MDI: 42 mcg/puff, or 84 mcg/puff (Vanceril DS) HFA P&B (MDI): 40 mcg (QVAR)	Beclovent, Vanceril, Vanceril DS, QVAR-HFA	42 mcg: Low dose: 2-8 puffs Med. dose: 8-16 puffs High dose: More than 16 puffs 84 mcg: Low dose: 1-4 puffs Med. dose: 4-8 puffs High dose: More than 8 puffs HFA: (not established for children under 12)	42 mcg: Low dose: 4-12 puffs Med. dose: 12-20 puffs High dose: More than 20 puffs 84 mcg: Low dose: 2-6 puffs Med. dose: 6-10 puffs High dose: More than 10 puffs HFA: 40 mcg: Low dose: 1-3 puffs Med. dose: 3-5 puffs High dose: More than 5 puffs
Budesonide	Turbuhaler (DPI): 200 mcg/dose Respules (CDN): 0.25 mg, 0.5 mg per 2 mL unit dose	Pulmicort Turbuhaler, Pulmicort Respules	DPI: Low dose: 1 inhalation Med. dose: 1-2 inhalations High dose: More than 2 inhalations CDN (12 months-8 years): Initial dose: 0.5 mg, starting as single dose or 0.25 twice per day, not to exceed 1 mg High dose (for patients on oral corticosteroids who need to convert to inhaled corticosteroids): Total of 2 mg per day.	DPI: Low dose: 1-2 inhalations Med. dose: 2-3 inhalations High dose: More than 3 inhalations CDN: Low dose: 0.5 mg twice per day Med. dose: 1 mg twice per day High dose: 2 mg twice per day
Flunisolide	MDI: 250 mcg/puff	Aerobid, Aerobid-M	Low dose: 2-3 puffs Med. dose: 4-5 puffs High dose: More than 5 puffs	Low dose: 2-4 puffs Med. dose: 4-8 puffs High dose: More than 8 puffs

Active Ingredient	Formulation	Brand Name	Total Usual Daily Child Dose (Under 12)	Total Usual Daily Adult Dose
Fluticasone	MDI: 44, 110, 220 mcg/puff Flovent Diskus (DPI): 50, 100, 250 mcg/dose Flovent Rotadisk (DPI): 50, 100, 250 mcg/dose	Flovent	MDI: Low dose: 2-4 puffs of 44 mcg Med. dose: 4-10 puffs of 44 mcg or 2-4 puffs of 110 mcg High dose: More than 4 puffs of 110 mcg or more than 2 puffs of 220 mcg DPI: Low dose: 2-4 inhalations of 50 mcg Med. dose: 2-4 inhalations of 100 mcg High dose: More than 4 inhalations of 100 mcg or more than 2 inhalations of 250 mcg	MDI Low dose: 2-6 puffsof 44 mcg or 2 puffs of 110 mcg Med. dose: 2-6 puffs of 110 mcg High dose: More than 6 puffs of 110 mcg or more than 3 puffs of 220 mcg DPI Low dose: 2-6 inhalations of 50 mcg Med. dose: 3-6 inhalations of 100 mcg High dose: More than 6 inhalations of 100 mcg or more than 2 inhalations of 250 mcg
Fluticasone with salmeterol	Diskus (DPI) in 3 formulations: 100, 250, or 500 mcg of fluticasone with 50 mcg of salmeterol	Advair	Not yet approved for children under 12	1 inhalation twice per day
Mometasone	Twisthaler (DPI): 200 mcg/dose	Asmanex*	Recommended dose is 1 inhalation per day	Recommended dose is 1-2 inhalations per day
Triamcinolone	MDI: 100 mcg/puff	Azmacort	Low dose: 4-8 puffs Med. dose: 8-12 puffs High dose: More than 12 puffs	Low dose: 4-10 puffs Med. dose: 10-20 puffs High dose: More than 20 puffs

*Awaiting approval in the U.S.

Doctors usually divide the daily dosage into the daily dosage into two doses. In some cases, you may take your daily dosage in one dose, depending on your doctor's advice.

Note: mg = milligram; CDN: compressor-driven nebulizer; DPI: dry powder inhaler; HFA (hydrofluoroalkane): see the "Necessity is the mother of HFA" sidebar later in this chapter; P & B: press and breathe.

Although all available evidence indicates that inhaled topical corticosteroids are highly effective and safe for use by children, some concern exists about the possible temporary effects on the rate of growth in children who use these products. If your child uses one of these products, make sure your child's physician is aware of this fact so that your child's growth can be accurately monitored.

In order to avoid the rare occurrence of an oral yeast infection or hoarseness (due to yeast infection in the throat) as a result of using inhaled topical corticosteroids, make sure that you thoroughly rinse your mouth with water after using any of these products. It's also essential to use a holding chamber (see "Delivering Your Dose: Inhalers and Nebulizers," later in this chapter) with an MDI formulation of inhaled corticosteroids to improve delivery of the medication to the airways of the lungs to further reduce the risk of developing an oral yeast infection or hoarseness of the throat.

Table 12-1 lists inhaled topical corticosteroid medications that are currently approved for use in the U.S. The Second Expert Panel on the Management of Asthma, as contained in the National Institutes of Health (NIH) Guidelines for the Diagnosis and Management of Asthma, recommends the dosages that I list throughout this chapter.

Oral corticosteroids

In severe asthma cases, early use of oral corticosteroids can prevent relapses and reduce the need for hospitalization, and they are also essential for treating patients who don't respond quickly to bronchodilators. Doctors may also use oral corticosteroids to gain prompt control of asthma when starting long-term therapy (see Chapter 13).

If overused, these drugs can cause systemic adverse side effects, including fluid retention, altered blood sugar levels, weight gain, peptic ulcers, mood alteration, high blood pressure, reduced bone density, and impaired immune functioning. For this reason, oral corticosteroids are often the last medications that doctors add to your pharmacotherapy and the first ones they remove — after they determine that your symptoms are under control. If you suffer from severe, persistent asthma, your doctor may choose to prescribe a course of alternate-day, single morning oral corticosteroid therapy to control symptoms while reducing the risk of adverse side effects.

Table 12-2 lists the oral corticosteroids that doctors in the U.S. commonly prescribe for asthma treatment.

Table 12-2		Oral Corticosteroid Medications		
Active Ingredient	*Formulation*	*Brand Name*	*Total Usual Daily Child Dose (Under 12)*	*Total Usual Daily Adult Dose*
Methylprednisolone	2, 4, 8, 16, 32 mg tablets	Medrol	0.25-2 mg per kg of the child's weight in a single daily dose or single dose every other day as needed for control of symptoms. Doctors may also prescribe a short course "burst" of 1-2 mg per kg of the child's weight per day, for a maximum of 60 mg per day, for 3-10 days	7.5-60 mg in a single daily dose or single dose every other day as needed for control of symptoms. Doctors may also prescribe a short course "burst" of 40-60 mg per day as a single dose or 2 divided doses for 3-10 days
Prednisolone	5 mg tablets	Prednisolone		
Prednisolone	5 mg/5 mL solution 15 mg/5 mL solution	Prelone		
Prednisolone	1 mg/mL solution	Pediapred		
Prednisone	1, 2.5, 5, 10, 20, 25 mg tablets; 5 mg/5 mL solution	Deltasone, Prednisone		

Note: 1 kg (kilogram) = 2.2 pounds; mg = milligram; mL = milliliter.

Mast cell stabilizers

As I explain more extensively in Chapter 1, mast cells are important players in the inflammatory process. These cells exist in large numbers in your lungs and nose. When triggered (usually by allergens), mast cells release several substances, including histamine and leukotrienes, which cause inflammation and also lead to airway constriction and increased mucus production.

Mast cell stabilizers used in long-term treatment of asthma, such as inhaled cromolyn and nedocromil, inhibit the release of mast cell mediators, thus preventing or reducing inflammation. (See Chapter 10 for an explanation of airway inflammation.) However, to properly prevent asthma symptoms, both cromolyn and nedocromil need to reach deep into your lungs.

If your airways are already inflamed or constricted, you may need a one-week course of oral corticosteroids (or 30 days of inhaled topical corticosteroids) to sufficiently reduce the existing airway inflammation to ensure that the inhaled cromolyn or nedocromil work effectively as preventive medications. Your doctor may also prescribe a bronchodilator for you to use prior to inhaling cromolyn or nedocromil for the first month that you take these drugs.

Although appropriate long-term, routine use of cromolyn and nedocromil can reduce the intensity of your asthma symptoms, neither drug is helpful in managing an asthma episode if one occurs. If you suffer an asthma attack, you may need to use a short-term rescue bronchodilator, as your asthma management plan specifies. However, even during an asthma episode, your doctor may advise you to continue using cromolyn or nedocromil to maintain the drug's preventive effect, in addition to any other prescribed treatment.

Cromolyn

Cromolyn can be effective in certain patients, either alone or in conjunction with a bronchodilator, in preventing the symptoms of persistent mild-to-moderate asthma. Doctors sometimes prescribe cromolyn in a nasal formulation (Nasalcrom) to prevent allergic rhinitis symptoms (see Chapter 7).

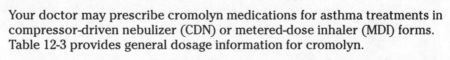

Your doctor may prescribe cromolyn medications for asthma treatments in compressor-driven nebulizer (CDN) or metered-dose inhaler (MDI) forms. Table 12-3 provides general dosage information for cromolyn.

Because cromolyn has an excellent safety profile and produces no significant side effects, doctors use it to treat young children (in CDN form) and pregnant women (in MDI form). Cromolyn especially helps suppress symptoms triggered by unavoidable exposures to asthma triggers, such as animal dander, pollen, and viral respiratory infections. Your doctor may prescribe this drug during pollen season, winter months, or if you experience routine exposures to pets.

Table 12-3		Mast Cell Stabilizer Medications		
Active Ingredient	*Formulation*	*Brand Name*	*Total Usual Daily Child Dose (under 12)*	*Total Usual Daily Adult Dose*
Cromolyn	MDI: 1 mg per puff CDN: 20 mg per ampule	Intal	MDI: 1-2 puffs four times per day or as needed prior to exercise or allergen exposure (ages 5-11) CDN: 1 ampule four times per day or as needed prior to exercise or allergen exposure (ages 2-11)	MDI: 2-4 puffs four times per day or as needed CDN: 1 ampule four times per day or as needed prior to exercise or allergen exposure
Nedocromil	MDI: 1.75 mg per puff	Tilade	MDI: 1-2 puffs four times per day or as needed prior to exercise or allergen exposure (ages 6-11)	2-4 puffs four times per day or as needed prior to exercise or allergen exposure

Note: mg = milligram; CDN: compressor-driven nebulizer; MDI: metered dose inhaler.

Cromolyn is usually more effective for treatment of infants and young children when the medication is delivered to the lungs by a compressor-driven nebulizer (CDN) rather than a metered-dose inhaler (MDI).

To prevent pollen-induced symptoms, start taking inhaled cromolyn one week before the beginning of pollen season. Taking inhaled cromolyn 30 minutes before exposure to animal dander — during (preferably) brief visits with people who have pets, for example — can often reduce the risk of developing asthma symptoms.

Cromolyn can prevent or reduce exercise-induced asthma (EIA) symptoms if you take it 15 to 30 minutes before exercising.

Nedocromil

Although chemically distinct from cromolyn (see the preceding section), nedocromil can also provide similar long-term anti-inflammatory benefits. As with cromolyn, nedocromil maintains an excellent safety profile. The main differences between the two drugs include the following:

✔ At regular dosage levels, nedocromil proves more effective than cromolyn, because it can start preventing airway inflammation in three days. In contrast, cromolyn may take from one to six weeks to produce its anti-inflammatory effect. (Refer to Table 12-3 for dosage information.)

✔ At recommended doses, doctors find nedocromil a more effective tool than cromolyn for preventing symptoms of EIA.

✔ Only patients over age 6 who suffer mild persistent asthma should use nedocromil.

✔ Nedocromil is only available as an MDI formulation.

Some patients find the taste of nedocromil unpleasant. To reduce the aftertaste, your doctor may recommend using a holding chamber (see "Delivering Your Dose: Inhalers and Nebulizers," later in this chapter) or sipping water before or after inhaling nedocromil.

Long-acting beta$_2$-adrenergic (beta$_2$-agonist) bronchodilators

Doctors prescribe long-acting beta$_2$-adrenergic bronchodilators for long-term prevention of asthma symptoms, usually in addition to anti-inflammatory medications such as inhaled topical corticosteroids and/or occasionally mast cell stabilizers (cromolyn or nedocromil). In addition to relaxing your airway smooth muscles, thus providing a bronchodilator effect, long-acting beta$_2$-adrenergic bronchodilators can also increase the anti-inflammatory effect of other medications, if you use them on a consistent, long-term basis.

Because long-acting bronchodilators can dilate the airways for up to 12 hours per dose, doctors often prescribe these products to control nighttime asthma symptoms. Doctors can prescribe these drugs in metered-dose inhaler (MDI), dry powder inhaler (DPI), and tablet forms (see Table 12-4).

Serevent, a long-acting bronchodilator in DPI (Serevent Diskus) and MDI formulations (see Table 12-4), works well to prevent episodes of nighttime asthma and exercise-induced asthma (EIA), if taken 30 minutes before exercising, and also enhances the effect of inhaled topical corticosteroids when used together. Serevent Diskus is approved for use in patients as young as 4 years of age. Both the MDI and the Diskus device contain the same medication. However, one inhalation of the Diskus is equal to two puffs of the MDI.

Never consider long-acting beta$_2$-adrenergic bronchodilators as a substitute for an anti-inflammatory medication. Long-acting bronchodilators should only be used as an addition to anti-inflammatory treatment. Using long-acting bronchodilators with inhaled topical corticosteroids enables you to reduce your inhaled topical corticosteroid dose, while maintaining equal or better control of your asthma. Studies provide strong evidence that adding a long-acting bronchodilator to your pharmacotherapy enhances the effectiveness of your existing inhaled topical corticosteroid medication.

The introduction of Advair (refer to Table 12-1), a combination of an inhaled topical corticosteroid (fluticasone) with a long-acting beta$_2$-adrenergic bronchodilator (salmeterol), represents a *complementary* (an enhanced anti-inflammatory effect compared to either therapy alone) combination of medications. According to recent studies of patients with persistent asthma who had previously been treated with inhaled topical corticosteroids, Advair (initially available in a Diskus DPI device) improved lung functions by 25 percent on average as compared to 15 percent with fluticasone (Flovent) alone and 5 percent with salmeterol (Serevent) alone. Because it has been found that the beneficial effect of Advair (in a single inhalation device) is comparable to taking fluticasone and salmeterol at the same time (in separate individual products), Advair represents a significantly more convenient and effective form of combination asthma therapy.

Effectively using these long-acting products may also reduce your need for quick-relief bronchodilators. However, long-acting bronchodilators such as salmeterol (Serevent) take longer to kick in (ranging from 10 to 30 minutes and reaching peak effectiveness in four to six hours) and don't work well as rescue medications if asthma episodes develop. Formoterol (Foradil), not yet approved in the U.S., is a long-acting bronchodilator with a more rapid onset of action; it starts working in most patients within one to three minutes.

Table 12-4	Long-Acting Beta$_2$-Adrenergic Bronchodilators			
Active Ingredient	*Formulation*	*Brand Name*	*Total Usual Daily Child Dose (under 12)*	*Total Usual Daily Adult Dose (12 yrs and older)*
Salmeterol	Diskus (DPI): 50 mcg/ inhalation MDI: 21 mcg/puff	Serevent	DPI: 1 inhalation twice per day (ages 4-11) MDI: Not yet approved for children under 12*	DPI: 1 inhalation twice per day MDI: 2 puffs twice per day
Albuterol (sustained release)	4 or 8 mg extended-release tablets	Volmax, Proventil Repetab	0.3-0.6 mg per kg of child's weight, not to exceed 8 mg total per day (ages 6-11)	1 tablet (4 or 8 mg) twice per day, not to exceed 32 mg total per day
Formoterol	Aerolizer (DPI)	Foradil*	One 12 mcg capsule by inhalation twice per day (ages 6-11)	One 12 mcg capsule by inhalation twice per day

*Awaiting approval in the U.S.

Note: 1 kg (kilogram) = 2.2 pounds; mcg = microgram; CDN: compressor-driven nebulizer; DPI: dry-powder inhaler; MDI: metered dose inhaler.

If you experience an asthma attack, continue using the quick-relief medication your doctor prescribes, as your asthma management plan directs. If you have a heart condition, make sure your doctor knows this before prescribing long-acting beta₂-adrenergic bronchodilators for you. In some cases, use of these products can cause elevated heartbeat.

Methylxanthines

The principal methylxanthine drug that doctors prescribe for asthma treatment is *oral theophylline,* which is related to the caffeine family. Since the development of more effective products, such as inhaled corticosteroids and safer inhaled bronchodilators (which achieve more consistent results and produce fewer adverse side effects), doctors don't prescribe theophylline as much as in the past. Table 12-5 provides general dosage information for methylxanthine medications.

Doctors most often use theophylline in conjunction with inhaled topical corticosteroids. Your doctor may add theophylline to your pharmacotherapy in order to reduce the frequency and severity of your persistent asthma symptoms and possibly to decrease the amount of inhaled topical corticosteroids you may need to take.

Because of the drug's long-acting effects, which can last from 8 to 24 hours, doctors often use theophylline to control nighttime asthma symptoms, particularly for patients with mild to moderate persistent asthma.

Although doctors consider theophylline safe, the drug can cause a variety of undesirable side effects, such as nausea, vomiting, stomach cramps, diarrhea, and tremors. These undesirable side effects have occasionally been implicated in poor school performance by children who were taking theophylline for their asthma. If you're taking a theophylline medication (usually in the form of tablets or capsules) and experience any of these types of side effects, you should immediately report those symptoms to your doctor.

Various factors, such as viral infections, alcohol, heart failure, and taking other medications, can impede your liver's ability to eliminate theophylline from your system. This impediment can result in higher than desirable levels of the drug in your body, leading to the side effects that I mention in the preceding paragraph, or more serious adverse side effects, such as increased irritability, insomnia, or behavioral problems — symptoms similar to the effects you experience after drinking too much coffee. In rare cases, excessive theophylline levels in your blood can create toxic central nervous system effects, potentially causing a coma, convulsions, or even death.

Conversely, factors such as smoking, an overactive thyroid, a high protein diet (featuring red meat) and certain medications, including phenobarbitol, rifampicin (Rifampin), and phenytoin (Dilantin), can increase your liver's rate of metabolizing and processing theophylline, thus often requiring an increase in dosage of the drug.

Make your doctor aware of any other medications that you take for asthma, as well as any other ailments, if he or she considers theophylline for your pharmacotherapy. Your physician may use a standard blood test to determine whether the level of theophylline in your body is optimal.

If you suffer an asthma attack, don't take theophylline as a rescue medication. Instead, use an appropriate quick-relief bronchodilator to relieve your acute symptoms.

Table 12-5		Methylxanthine Medications		
Active Ingredient	**Formulation**	**Brand Name**	**Total Usual Daily Child Dose (under 12)***	**Total Usual Daily Adult Dose ***
Theophylline	400, 600 mg tablets	Uni-Dur Uniphyl	Starting dose of 10 mg per kg of child's weight per day.	Starting dose of 10 mg per kg of patient's weight per day;
Theophylline	100, 200, 300, 450 mg tablets	Theo-Dur	Under 1 year: Maximum 5 mg per kg of child's weight per day.	Usual max: 800 mg per day.
Theophylline	100, 200, 300, 400 mg capsules	Theo-24	Over 1 year: Maximum 16 mg per kg of child's weight per day.	
Theophylline	50, 75, 100, 125, 200, 300 mg capsules	Slo-bid Gyrocaps		

*Dosages apply to all methylxanthine products
Note: 1 kg (kilogram) – 2.2 pounds; mg – milligram

Leukotriene modifiers

Leukotrienes are potent biochemical substances that play a significant role in asthma attacks. When a precipitating factor triggers the release of these chemicals, leukotrienes cause airway constriction, increase mucus secretions, and attract and activate inflammatory cells in your airway. *Leukotriene modifiers* are a class of drugs that inhibit or stabilize leukotriene activity, thus decreasing airflow obstruction, airway constriction, and mucus production. Ultimately, inhibiting or stabilizing leukotriene activity reduces asthma symptoms. (If you're loco for more leukotriene information, see Chapter 2.)

The long-term, routine use of leukotriene modifiers can possibly reduce the amount of inhaled topical corticosteroids or other inhaled medications that you may need to control your asthma symptoms.

Leukotriene modifiers generally begin to work within a few hours. However, these drugs often require a few days to a week to reach their full effect.

Leukotriene modifiers can sometimes reduce respiratory reactions in patients with sensitivities to aspirin and non-steroidal anti-inflammatory drugs (NSAIDs). If you suffer from these types of sensitivities, however, continue avoiding aspirin, non-steroidal anti-inflammatory drugs (NSAIDs), and newer prescription NSAIDs, known as COX-2 inhibitors, while taking leukotriene modifiers, because reactions still might occur. As with other allergies, avoidance is still the best approach when dealing with any type of drug sensitivity.

Leukotriene modifiers available in the U.S. include montelukast (Singulair), zafirlukast (Accolate), and zileuton (Zyflo). Table 12-6 provides dosage information on these products.

Table 12-6			Leukotriene Modifiers	
Active Ingredient	**Formulation**	**Brand Name**	**Total Usual Daily Child Dose (See Formulation Details)**	**Total Usual Daily Adult Dose**
Montelukast	10 mg tablet (ages 15 and older) 5 mg chewable tablet (ages 6-14) 4 mg chewable tablet (ages 2-5)	Singulair	One 5 mg chewable tablet (ages 6-14) per day (in the evening) One 4 mg chewable tablet* (ages 2-5) per day (in the evening)	One 10 mg tablet per day (in the evening)
Zafirlukast	20 mg tablet (12 and older) 10 mg tablet (ages 6-11)	Accolate	One 10 mg tablet twice per day (ages 7-11)	One 20 mg tablet twice per day
Zileuton	300 mg, 600 mg tablet	Zyflo	Not approved for children under 12	2,400 mg daily: Two 300 mg tablets or one 600 mg tablet four times per day

*Soon to be approved in the U.S.

Note: 1 kg (kilogram) = 2.2 pounds; mg = miiligram

Doctors can prescribe leukotriene modifiers in tablet form, which for some patients means they're easier to take. As a result, you may find taking these medications on a regular basis more convenient than other medications.

Because certain leukotriene modifiers can inhibit particular liver activities, make sure your doctor is aware of any other medications that you take. For example, in some cases, your liver may have trouble processing certain antibiotics and anti-seizure medications if you take leukotriene modifiers. If you take zileuton, make sure your doctor monitors your liver. In some people, zileuton impairs liver function. Likewise, avoid taking zileuton if you have an existing liver condition or experience difficulty controlling your alcohol intake. Because of its potential effects on your liver, zileuton may also interfere with theophylline, warfarin (Coumadin), an anti-blood clotting medication used to reduce the risk of strokes, or beta-blockers (used for treating high blood pressure or migraine headaches), such as propranolol (Inderal).

Phenobarbital or rifampin can increase your liver metabolism, thus breaking down certain other medications such as montelukast more rapidly if you take them concurrently. For this reason, your doctor should closely monitor your respiratory symptoms if you're taking montelukast with these medications because your asthma may potentially not be as well controlled.

Co-administration of zafirlukast with other medications can affect the blood levels of zafirlukast. When used in combination with theophylline, zafirlukast blood levels may decrease by as much as one-third, while with aspirin, zafirlukast blood levels can increase by close to 50 percent. Lower blood levels of zafirlukast may result in less than optimal control of your respiratory symptoms; elevated levels can produce side effects such as headache, or in some cases, nausea. Therefore, as I mention throughout this book, you should always make sure that your doctor knows about all medications you're taking, even OTC preparations, for any and all ailments.

Leukotriene modifiers aren't rescue medications. If you suffer an asthma attack, use a quick-relief bronchodilator as your asthma management plan specifies. However, continue taking your prescribed leukotriene modifiers during your asthma episode, because the drug often enhances the effectiveness of quick-relief medications.

Using quick-relief medications

The primary function of quick-relief drugs, also known as *rescue medications,* is to promptly reverse acute airflow obstruction and relieve constricted airways during an asthma episode. Your doctor may also prescribe a quick-relief product, such as an inhaled beta$_2$-adrenergic bronchodilator, prior to exercise to prevent symptoms of exercise-induced asthma (see Chapter 11).

Quick-relief medications include

- Short-acting beta$_2$-adrenergic bronchodilators
- Anticholinergics (see "Anticholinergics," later in this chapter), which may provide added relief when combined with inhaled short-acting beta$_2$-adrenergic bronchodilators
- Oral corticosteroids that doctors prescribe for use in asthma attacks (see "Oral corticosteroids," later in this chapter)

Short-acting beta$_2$-adrenergic (beta$_2$-agonist) bronchodilators

Adrenaline-like drugs, short-acting beta$_2$-adrenergic bronchodilators rapidly relax the smooth muscles in your airways, causing your airways to dilate (open), usually within five minutes of inhaling the medication. Inhaled or aerosol forms of these drugs provide the most effective, prompt relief of acute bronchospasms, and many doctors consider beta$_2$-adrenergic bronchodilators the medication of choice for treating asthma symptoms that suddenly worsen and for preventing exercise-induced asthma (EIA).

Although relatively mild, especially when used in inhalation forms (in contrast with oral or injectable formulations), the principal side effects of short-acting beta$_2$-adrenergic therapy can be tremors, increased heart rate, and palpitations. These side effects occur as a result of the drug's direct stimulation of the heart and skeletal muscles, and they often go hand in hand with the drug's bronchodilator action, especially at high and/or frequent dosages.

Recently, with improved chemical technology, a new version (isomer) of albuterol known as *levalbuterol* (Xopenex) has been developed. This medication provides the same level of bronchodilation at one-fourth the dose of albuterol. Therefore, the dose-dependent side effects are reduced, making this medication particularly useful in especially sensitive groups, such as children (*off-label;* see the "Understanding the medicine that you take" sidebar earlier in this chapter) and the elderly, when given by compressor-driven nebulizer (CDN).

Table 12-7 gives you general dosage information for short-acting beta$_2$-adrenergic bronchodilators.

Holding chambers (spacers) and nebulizers work especially well, ensuring that your lungs receive short-acting bronchodilator medications. (See "Delivering Your Dose: Inhalers and Nebulizers," later in this chapter, for more information).

Table 12-7 Short-acting $Beta_2$-Adrenergic Bronchodilators

Active Ingredient	*Formulation*	*Brand Name*	*Total Usual Daily Child Dose (Under 12)*	*Total Usual Daily Adult Dose*
Albuterol	MDI: 90 mcg/puff, 200puffs/canister Rotohaler (DPI; Ventolin): 200 mcg/capsule CDN solution with calibrated dropper: 5 mg/mL (0.5%) CDN unit dose bottle (nebule) 2.5 mg/3mL (0.083%) Tablets: 2, 4 mg Syrup: 2 mg per 5 mL	Ventolin, Proventil (both available in MDI, CDN, tablet, and syrup), Proventil HFA	MDI: Two puffs 4 times per day or as needed prior toexercise DPI: One capsule every 4-6 hours or as needed prior to exercise CDN solution: 0.05 mg per kg of child's weight in 2-3 cc of saline solution every 4-6 hours CDN unit dose (2-11 years, over 15 kg weight): 2.5 mg (one unit dose/nebule) 3-4 times per day Tablets: (ages 6-11) Starting dose: One 2 mg tablet 3-4 times per day, maximum of 24 mg per day Syrup: 1 teaspoon every 6 hours	MDI: Two puffs 4 times per day or as needed prior to exercise DPI: One capsule every 4-6 hours or as needed prior to exercise CDN: 1.25-5 mg in 2-3 cc of saline solution every 4-8 hours CDN unit dose: 2.5 mg (one unit dose/nebule) 3-4 times per day Tablets: Starting Dose: One 2 mg or 4 mg tablet 3-4 times per day, maximum of 32 mg per day Syrup: 1-2 teaspoons every 6 hours
Bitolterol	MDI: 370 mcg/puff 300 puffs/canister CDN: 2 mg/mL (0.2%) solution Usual dose 1.25 mL = 2.5 mg Increased dose 1.75 mL = 3.5 mg Decreased dose 0.75 mL= 1.5 mg (each mL contains 2 mg of bitolterol)	Tornalate	MDI: Not approved for children under 12 CDN: Not approved for children under 12	MDI: Two puffs every 8 hours, not to exceed 2 puffs every 4 hours or as needed prior to exercise CDN: 0.5-3.5 mg (0.25-1 mL) in 2-3 mL of saline solution every 4-8 hours
Levalbuterol	CDN: 0.63 mg/3 mL nebule 1.25 mg/3 mL nebule	Xopenex	Not approved for children under 12	Low dose: 0.63 mg per nebule every 6-8 hours High dose: 1.25 mg per nebule every 6-8 hours if symptoms are acute or unresponsive to low dose

(continued)

Table 12-7 (continued)

Active Ingredient	Formulation	Brand Name	Total Usual Daily Child Dose (Under 12)	Total Usual Daily Adult Dose
Metaproterenol	MDI: 0.65 mL/puff, 200 puffs/canister CDN: 0.4%, 0.6% vials Tablet: 10 mg, 20 mg Syrup: 10 mg per Tsp	Alupent	MDI: Not approved for children under 12 CDN: Not approved for children under 12 Tablet: (ages 6-9) 10 mg every 6 hours; (ages 9 and above) 20 mg every 6 hours Syrup: (ages 6-9) 1 teaspoon every 6 hours; (ages 9 and above) 2 teaspoons every 6 hours	MDI: 1-2 puffs every 2-4 hours or as needed, 1-2 puffs 5 minutes before exercise CDN: Low dose: 0.4% vial every 4 hours as needed High dose: 0.6% vial every 4 hours as needed Tablet: 20 mg every 6 hours Syrup: 2 teaspoons every 6 hours
Pirbuterol	MDI: 200 mcg/puff 400 puffs/canister Autohaler (breath-activated MDI): 200 mcg/puff 400 puffs/canister	Maxair	Not approved for children under 12	2 puffs 4 times per day or as needed, or as needed prior to exercise. Should not exceed 12 puffs per day
Terbutaline	MDI: 90 mcg/puff 300 puffs/canister Tablets: 2.5, 5 mg	Brethaire, Brethine, Bricanyl	MDI: Two puffs 4 times per day or as needed prior to exercise Tablets: (ages 12-15) One 2.5 mg tablet 3 times per day, maximum of 7.5 mg	MDI: Two puffs 4 times per day or as needed prior to exercise Tablets: One 5 mg tablet 3 times per day, maximum of 15 mg

Note: 1 kg (kilogram) = 2.2 pounds; mcg = microgram; mg = milligram; mL = milliliter; CDN: compressor-driven nebulizer; DPI: dry powder inhaler; HFA (hydrofluoroalkane): see the "Necessity is the mother of HFA" sidebar later in this chapter; MDI: metered dose inhaler; P&B: press and breathe.

If your short-acting bronchodilator isn't providing rapid relief of symptoms, the following factors may be causing a problem:

- **You're not using the product properly.** Make sure that your doctor shows you the proper technique for using your inhaler and reviews your technique during office visits.

- **Your canister may be empty.** To check whether you need a new canister, remove the container from the actuator sleeve and put it in water (a sink works well for this test). If the canister starts floating to the top, it's likely close to empty.

- **The mouthpiece (where you inhale) may be dirty or blocked.** Keep your inhaler clean. (See "Delivering Your Dose: Inhalers and Nebulizers," later in this chapter, for more information.)

To prevent EIA, your doctor may recommend that you inhale a dose of your prescribed short-acting beta$_2$-adrenergic bronchodilator 15 to 30 minutes before you begin to exert yourself.

If you take more than eight puffs per day or use more than one canister (usually 200 puffs) of a short-acting bronchodilator per month, your asthma isn't adequately controlled, and you should see your doctor to adjust your asthma management plan. You may need to take long-term anti-inflammatory medication, such as inhaled topical corticosteroids, on a regular basis to control your asthma. Overusing your short-acting beta$_2$-adrenergic bronchodilator (more frequently than once every one to two hours) is a sign that your asthma symptoms are worsening. If you must use your short-acting bronchodilator more often than once every one or two hours, contact your doctor immediately.

In my 20 years of practice, I've never seen the overuse of inhaled short-acting beta$_2$-adrenergic bronchodilators correct worsening asthma symptoms. In fact, overusing your short-acting bronchodilator almost always makes your condition worse, because frequently using this medication doesn't address the real source of the problem — the underlying airway inflammation. (See the sidebar "Quick fix versus long-term asthma management" for more information on overusing your short-acting bronchodilator.)

Using short-acting bronchodilators while also taking beta-blockers, such as Inderal, Lopressor, and Corgard (frequently prescribed for migraine headaches, high blood pressure, glaucoma, angina, or hyperthyroidism), may cancel out the benefits of both medications. If you need both medications, your doctor may recommend alternatives to beta-blockers or may prescribe ipratropium bromide as an alternative quick-relief medication for your asthma symptoms (see "Anticholinergics," later in this chapter). This potentially adverse interaction between medications is a particularly good example of why it's vital to make sure that all your physicians know the medications that you're taking for all your medical conditions.

I strongly advise against using over-the-counter (OTC) inhaled bronchodila-tors such as AsthmaHaler, Bronkaid Mist, Primatene Mist, or similar products. In many cases, these OTC products provide much shorter relief than prescription inhaled short-acting beta$_2$-adrenergic bronchodilators, and they often contain epinephrine (adrenaline) or similar drugs. Although epinephrine is used in emergency treatment and in self-injection kits, such as EpiPen or AnaKit, for cases of severe asthma attacks and anaphylaxis (a potentially life-threatening reaction that affects many organs simultaneously), routine use of the drug can cause serious adverse side effects, including shakiness, an increase in blood pressure, or a rapid or irregular heartbeat. Because of this danger, you should especially avoid using OTC bronchodilators if you have a heart condition.

Quick fix versus long-term asthma management

Controlling asthma means treating the underlying airway inflammation. Don't substitute the quick fix of an inhaled short-acting beta$_2$-adrenergic bronchodilator for consistent, routine use of the appropriate long-term asthma medications that your doctor prescribes for controlling your asthma.

Think of your asthma as a smoldering campfire in your lungs. If you only pay attention to the embers *after* they flare up, containing the flames becomes a serious problem. The goal of your asthma management plan should instead be to get your asthma under control to the extent that you only rarely use bronchodilators on an as-needed basis — usually to reduce the risk of symptoms when exposed to unavoidable asthma triggers or precipitating factors, especially exercise.

Also, beware of relying on inhaled short-acting bronchodilators, because the quick relief these products provide can also give you the false impression that your asthma is just a set of symptoms, rather than a serious, underlying medical problem. Imagine having a high fever and only taking a pain reliever to reduce your discomfort. You may temporarily feel better, but if the underlying cause of your high temperature is a severe inflammation, such as appendicitis, treating only the symptoms can lead to a very serious situation — in this case a ruptured appendix — because you may not realize the gravity of your condition, thus delaying necessary treatment.

Likewise, if zapping your wheezing with an inhaled short-acting beta$_2$-adrenergic bronchodilator is the only way you deal with your persistent asthma, you may feel fine for a short while. However, if you use your peak flow meter (see Chapter 13) to check your peak expiratory flow rate (PEFR), or if your doctor performs a spirometry procedure (see Chapter 10), you quickly realize that your airflow is significantly decreased and your lung functions are below normal. When based solely on how they're feeling, the majority of asthma patients tend to underestimate the magnitude of their airway obstruction. Often, it isn't until they can objectively measure their airflow, typically by using a peak flow meter, that they really become aware of their deteriorating condition.

Anticholinergics

Anticholinergic drugs block *acetylcholine* (neurotransmitter that stimulates mucus production) and therefore help reduce mucus in your airways. These drugs also relax the smooth muscle around the large and medium airways of the lungs. Inhaled anticholinergics often work especially well when doctors combine their use with short-acting beta$_2$-adrenergic bronchodilators to dilate your airways.

On their own, anticholinergics don't prevent exercise-induced asthma (EIA) symptoms, and they have little effect on asthma symptoms that allergens trigger.

Anticholinergic medications are usually most effective for patients who have partially reversible airflow obstruction or produce greater amounts of mucus. Doctors frequently use these products on patients with chronic bronchitis and emphysema, collectively referred to as *chronic obstructive pulmonary disease* (COPD). Ipratropium bromide, a quick-relief drug that doctors often prescribe in conjunction with a short-acting beta$_2$-adrenergic bronchodilator for dilating the airways, has an excellent safety profile and few potential adverse side effects. These can include drying of the mouth and airway secretions and, in rare cases, wheezing. It's important not to spray this product in your eyes, as doing so can temporarily blur your vision. This drug can provide greater bronchodilation when combined with a bronchodilator such as albuterol into a single inhaled product (Combivent). Table 12-8 provides general dosage information for anticholinergic medications.

Table 12-8	Anticholinergic Medications			
Active Ingredient	**Formulation**	**Brand Name**	**Total Usual Daily Child Dose (under 12)**	**Total Usual Daily Adult Dose**
Ipratropium	MDI: 18 mcg/ puff 200 puffs/ canister Nebulizer (CDN): 0.5 mg 2.5 mL (0.02% vial)	Atrovent	Not approved for children under 12	MDI: 2-3 puffs every 6 hours, not to exceed 12 puffs per day CDN: 1 vial every 6-8 hours
Ipratropium + albuterol	MDI: 370 mcg/puff 300 puffs/ canister	Combivent	Not approved for children under 12	Two puffs 4 times per day

Note: mcg = microgram; mL = milliliter; CDN: compressor-driven nebulizer; MDI: metered dose inhaler.

Oral corticosteroids

In addition to their use as long-acting medications, oral corticosteroids can also play a quick-relief role in your asthma management. During moderate-to-severe asthma episodes, your doctor may use oral corticosteroids to rapidly gain control over worsening symptoms. In such cases, oral corticosteroids can help your other quick-relief medications work more effectively, resulting in a more rapid reversal or reduction of airway inflammation, speeding recovery, and reducing the rate of relapse.

A short course of oral corticosteroids generally lasts three to ten days, depending on the severity of your symptoms and your response to treatment. If you use oral corticosteroids longer than two weeks, doctors frequently taper off the dosage to minimize side effects, instead of stopping the drug abruptly. This slow tapering of oral corticosteroid dosage allows most patients to regain their ability to produce their own natural corticosteroids from the cortex (outer layer) of their adrenal gland. I strongly advise that you don't suddenly stop taking oral corticosteroids without checking with your physician first.

Delivering Your Dose: Inhalers and Nebulizers

Learning how to use inhalers and nebulizers is a vital aspect of effectively treating your asthma. If your medication doesn't go where it's supposed to go, you don't benefit from it. One of the unique aspects of treating a respiratory condition is that the proper use of an inhaler is just as important as the medication itself in the inhaler: The objective is to get the medication to the area of your lungs where it can work most effectively.

The major advantages of delivering drugs directly into your lungs with inhaled delivery systems include the following:

✔ You can more effectively administer higher concentrations of medication into your airways.

✔ You can reduce the risk of systemic side effects that may occur when you use oral forms of these medications.

✔ The onset of relief from inhaled drugs is usually more rapid than with oral products.

Using a metered-dose inhaler

A metered-dose inhaler (MDI) consists of a canister of pressurized medication that fits into a plastic actuator sleeve and connects to a mouthpiece. An MDI propels medication at over 60 miles per hour (a lot faster than my first car!), and that medication needs to make a sharp turn to effectively get into the airways of your lungs. Therefore, most of the medication sprayed from the MDI never even reaches your lungs. For example, the spray can coat your mouth, the end of your tongue, or the back of your throat. In the best-case scenario, your small airways receive only 10 to 20 percent of the inhaled drug. Inhalers help millions of people with asthma breathe easier, but properly using inhalers is crucial to their success. Many people around the world experience difficulty controlling their asthma because they use their inhalers incorrectly.

Necessity is the mother of HFA

You're probably familiar with the issue of replacing ozone-depleting chlorofluorocarbons (CFCs) with less damaging propellants in refrigerators, air conditioning systems, and aerosol sprays, particularly in hair, deodorant, and fragrance products. This issue especially affects people with asthma because many MDI formulations use CFCs as propellants. A temporary medical exemption allows pharmaceutical companies to continue using CFCs. This exemption is presently scheduled for phase-out by 2005, but it may be extended.

As a result, pharmaceutical companies continue to develop more environmentally-friendly propellants for MDI products. Hydrofluoroalkane (HFA), a new nonchlorinated propellant, recently won FDA approval for use in inhaled medications. Proventil HFA is the first ozone-friendly product on the market with this propellant, which delivers medication to the lungs more effectively than the CFC propellants developed in the 1950s.

The HFA MDI delivers medication in a plume, with less velocity than the standard CFC-propelled MDI, which may explain why the HFA propellant proves more effective. Imagine — but please don't attempt — trying to steer a car around a tight curve on a narrow road at 60 miles per hour. Unless you slow down, you may wind up in someone's front lawn (or worse).

This driving scenario is similar to what happens with medication that you inhale from a CFC-propelled MDI: At best, 10 to 20 percent of the spray actually makes its way around the various curves of your respiratory tract and into your airways where it can help you (and this estimate assumes you're using the proper inhaler technique!). In most cases, because of a lower velocity propellant spray, a non-CFC propelled product allows more of the medication to get into the smaller, more peripheral airways of your lungs.

Metered-dose inhaler instructions

When prescribing your inhaled medication, your physician should instruct you on how to properly use an MDI. Likewise, he or she should review your inhaler technique at subsequent office visits. The following, however, are some important instructions that apply to using most MDI products:

1. **Remove the cap and hold the inhaler upright.**

2. **Shake the inhaler.**

3. **Tilt your head back slightly and breathe out slowly.**

4. **Depending on your physician's specific instructions, open your mouth with your head 1 to 2 inches away from the inhaler or position the inhaler in your mouth.**

5. **Press down on the inhaler to release medication as you start inhaling or within the first second of inhaling; continue inhaling as you press down on your inhaler.**

   Breathe in slowly through your mouth, not your nose, for three to five seconds. Press your inhaler only once while you're inhaling (one breath for each puff). Make sure you breathe evenly and deeply.

6. **Hold your breath for 10 seconds to allow the medicine to reach deep into your lungs.**

7. **Repeat puffs as your prescription dictates.**

   Waiting one minute between puffs may permit the second puff to reach into the airways of your lungs better.

Getting the right dose from your MDI

Two important factors that can affect the dosage of medication you receive from your MDI include the following:

✔ **Loss of prime:** People who use inhalers often keep several around the house or office so that backup medication is always handy. Keeping too many back-up inhalers around can lead to infrequent inhaler activation and *loss of prime*. Loss of prime occurs when the inhaler's propellant evaporates or escapes from the metering chamber after days or weeks of nonuse. If you haven't used an inhaler recently, you should waste a puff of medication into the air before inhaling your first dose to ensure that your medicine contains its full potency.

✔ **Tail-off:** In a misguided attempt to economize, many inhaler users try to squeeze every last drop of medication from their metered-dose inhalers. However, research indicates that this practice may actually contribute to the documented rise in asthma deaths and poor quality of life for some people with asthma because of a phenomenon known as *tail-off*. As an MDI reaches its empty stage, dose reliability becomes increasingly unpredictable. Therefore, I strongly urge you not to use your MDI beyond the labeled number of doses, even if you think that some medication remains.

Using holding chambers

Doctors recommend holding chambers (also known as *spacers*) for younger children, as well as people who can't use an MDI correctly. A *holding chamber* is a hollow device that extends the space between the opening of the inhaler and your mouth. The holding chamber traps and suspends particles of medication as the inhaler releases them, allowing you to inhale your dose over a span of one to six breaths, depending on the particular device you use.

I recommend using a holding chamber when taking inhaled topical corticosteroids with an MDI to minimize the possibility of developing an oral yeast infection and to improve delivery of the medication to your lungs.

Holding chambers come in various shapes and sizes. Several of these devices (such as AeroChamber and E-Z Spacer) have both a mouthpiece for adults, as shown in Figure 12-1, and a mask for infants and small children, as shown in Figure 12-2.

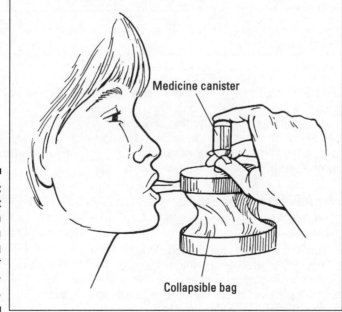

Figure 12-1:
An adult using an MDI with a holding chamber and mouthpiece.

Medicine canister

Collapsible bag

Using a dry-powder inhaler

Dry-powder inhalers (DPIs), as their name implies, dispense medication in a dry-powder formulation. DPIs come in different shapes and sizes and can deliver bronchodilators as well as anti-inflammatory medications.

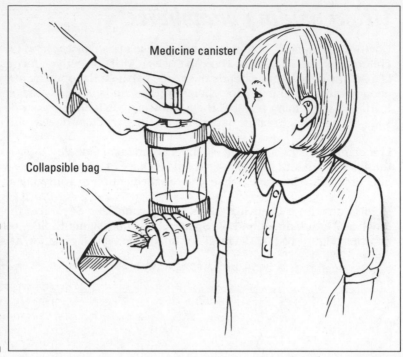

Medicine canister

Collapsible bag

Figure 12-2:
A child
using an
MDI with a
holding
chamber
and mask.

DPIs are easy to use and very effective, if you operate them properly. The medication particles in the dry powder are so small that they can easily reach the tiniest airways. Keep in mind that, unlike most metered-dose inhalers (MDIs), with a few types of DPIs, you may not taste or feel the medication when using the device. If you've administered the medication properly, however, you will receive its benefit.

Dry-powder inhaler instructions

Although DPIs don't require using a holding chamber, you'll need to use your DPI in a specific way. Because every DPI works a little differently, you should make sure you know how to use the one your doctor prescribes for you. As with an MDI (see "Metered-dose inhaler instructions"), your physician should instruct you on how to properly use your DPI and should review your inhaler technique at subsequent office visits. The following are important, general instructions on the proper use of most DPIs:

1. **Follow the manufacturer's instructions to prime your DPI and then load a prescribed dose of the dry-powder medication.**

2. **Breathe out slowly and completely (usually for three to five seconds).**

3. **Put your mouth on the mouthpiece and inhale deeply and forcefully.**

4. **Hold your breath for 10 seconds and then exhale slowly.**

5. **Repeat the procedure as outlined by your physician until you've taken the correct number of doses.**

Getting the right dose from your DPI

In addition to the steps in the previous section, you should keep the following points in mind in order to obtain the most benefit from your DPI:

✔ Your DPI is breath activated. That means you can control the rate at which you inhale the dry powder medication. However, you do need to inhale with sufficient force (minimal flow rate) in order to assure delivery of the medication to the smallest airways of your lungs. In order to be truly effective, using a DPI requires closing your mouth tightly around the mouthpiece of the inhaler and inhaling steadily, deeply, and forcefully.

✔ Make sure the dry powder in your DPI stays dry, to avoid caking or clumping, which can affect the reliability of the dose that is delivered. For DPIs with caps, make sure you always replace the cap after using the product. It's also important never to wash a DPI that still contains medication.

✔ In contrast with the operation of an MDI, you don't need to shake your DPI just before using it in order to assure delivery of the proper dose of medication to the airways of your lungs. In fact, shaking some DPIs can result in losing dry powder from those types of devices.

Some of the benefits of using a DPI include the following:

✔ Children as young as 4 years of age can use these devices.

✔ For many people who have poor MDI technique or who have difficulty coordinating the steps required for properly inhaling medication from an MDI, a DPI is often an excellent alternative, especially for children.

✔ One inhalation from a DPI often provides the same dosage of a comparable medication as with two puffs from an MDI.

✔ Because some DPIs have dose counters, it's easier to tell when your inhaler is almost empty.

✔ Cold temperatures don't reduce the effectiveness of DPIs.

✔ DPIs don't use CFCs, so they don't damage the planet's ozone layer.

Using nebulizers

A nebulizer is an air compressor connected to a generator. Nebulizers deliver medication as a mist that is easy to inhale, and it often brings rapid symptom relief. Nebulizers are especially useful when a child is too young or too sick to use other devices. In addition to standard, home plug-in models, you can purchase portable nebulizers with battery packs or cigarette lighter adapters to use in a vehicle while traveling.

Doctors may prescribe nebulizer therapy for adults to reduce or eliminate hospital or emergency room visits, especially for severe persistent asthma sufferers. Many nebulizer users find that the device allows them more effective relief than metered-dose inhalers. Therefore, if you are experiencing sudden-onset, severe asthma attacks on a frequent basis, you may benefit greatly from having a nebulizer prescribed for home use.

Here are some general guidelines for using a nebulizer with a mouthpiece:

- Place your mouth over the mouthpiece and breathe in and out.

- Make sure that you breathe through your mouth and not your nose.

- You or your child can use a face mask that covers your mouth and nose with your nebulizer.

- When using a nebulizer on your child, don't "blow by" or mist the medication in your child's face. A nebulizer requires a closed system to provide effective treatment (see Chapter 14).

- Use all the medication in your nebulizer. (Doing so normally takes 7 to 15 minutes, depending on the type of nebulizer you are using.)

Cleaning your medication delivery system

Rinse daily and wash weekly your inhaler, chamber, and nebulizer with a mild detergent to keep them clean and free of medication build-up. (Don't forget about inhalers that have been sitting in a drawer or handbag for a long time.) Remember to always keep the cap on your inhaler when you're not using it. If the cap accidentally becomes dislodged, make sure you that you properly clean your inhaler before using it again. Don't use harsh chemicals in washing your delivery devices, and make sure to follow manufacturer's instructions for maintenance and care.

Special Issues in Using Asthma Medications

When prescribing medications for asthma (or any other medical condition) in older adults, young children, surgical patients, and pregnant women, physicians often need to make special adjustments in dosages and products, as I explain in the following sections.

For details on how doctors adjust pharmacotherapy for young children with asthma, see Chapter 14. For important information on taking asthma and allergy medications while pregnant, turn to Chapter 15.

Asthma medications and older adults

Because asthma often coexists with chronic bronchitis in elderly patients, your doctor may need to prescribe a two- to three-week trial therapy with oral corticosteroids to determine the extent of reversible airflow obstruction (improvement), as measured by spirometry (see Chapter 10), before prescribing appropriate and effective long-term asthma medications.

Elderly patients can be at an increased risk for potential adverse side effects from asthma medications for many reasons. The following bullets are examples of more common side effects and issues for older people with asthma:

✔ As you age, your response to the use of bronchodilators may change. For this reason, elderly asthma patients may experience increased sensitivities to adverse side effects of beta$_2$-adrenergic medications, including tremors and an increased heart rate. If you have heart disease, your doctor may consider prescribing a combination inhaler containing a beta$_2$-adrenergic medication (short-acting bronchodilator) with an anticholinergic (for example, Combivent; see Table 12-8) to reduce the need for additional doses of beta$_2$-adrenergics.

✔ High-dose inhaled topical corticosteroid use can potentially reduce the bone mineral content in some asthma patients (particularly the elderly) who may have pre-existing osteoporosis and/or a sedentary lifestyle. If this sounds like you, your doctor may recommend taking calcium supplements, vitamin D, and (for women) estrogen replacement therapy.

✔ Make sure your doctor is aware of any type of past or current prostate condition before taking any anticholinergic medications, because these drugs may aggravate a pre-existing prostate problem.

✔ Because they are more likely to use beta-blockers and/or aspirin, elderly patients are potentially at risk for worsening of asthma due to adverse drug interactions resulting from using these types of medications. For more information on drug sensitivities and adverse drug reactions that can affect your asthma, see Chapter 11.

✔ Some older patients who may have impaired liver functions may require a reduced dose of theophylline in order to prevent accumulation of this drug in the bloodstream, which can lead to potential side effects. In addition, drug interactions that can cause problems with asthma medications in this age group include some commonly prescribed antibiotics (erythromycin) and cimetidine (Tagamet). Always make sure your doctor is aware of any possible liver conditions that may be affecting you, especially if you take theophylline.

Surgery and asthma medications

Because using anesthesia during surgery may depress lung functions, you should make your surgeon aware of your asthma and the medications you take to control it. (Your surgeon should evaluate both your lung functions and medication use prior to surgery.)

Your doctor may prescribe a short course of oral corticosteroids to improve your lung function starting just prior to surgery. If you have been taking oral corticosteroids in the six months prior to surgery, your doctor may also prescribe intravenous hydrocortisone on a set schedule during surgery, with a rapid taper of the dose within 24 hours after your procedure.

Treating asthma in the future

Based on the extensive experience I've gained during the last two decades while conducting clinical trials of new asthma drugs, I believe that more effective and innovative products are on the horizon. In fact, the pharmaceutical industry, with significant governmental guidance and support, continues to develop new approaches to treating asthma, such as:

✔ Improving existing medications and delivery devices.

✔ Developing innovative therapies in order to prevent airway inflammation from initially occurring.

✔ Treating asthma patients with anti-interleukin drugs (see Chapter 2). Research clinics have identified several interleukins (proteins that affect the way your immune system functions) as possible players in the inflammatory process. In fact, many studies are looking at inhibiting this aspect of interleukin activity as a way of preventing airway inflammation.

✔ Administering anti-IgE therapy to reduce levels of IgE antibodies in the body.

(IgE antibodies are involved in the reaction that results in the release of chemicals, such as histamine and leukotrienes, from the mast cells that line your respiratory tracts to induce the symptoms of an allergic reaction.)

✔ Finding ways of genetically modifying the disease-producing processes in our bodies that contribute to developing conditions such as allergies and asthma.

I expect the newer products to address the underlying airway inflammation that characterizes asthma even more successfully than has been possible until now. As a result, you can expect medications that more effectively treat the root cause of asthma, thus reducing the frequency and severity of symptoms that you experience. That would bring us a step closer to the goal of having patients achieve normal lung functions and complete control of symptoms with less need for taking medications on a regular basis. When that happens, maybe this chapter won't need to take up as many pages in future editions of this book.

Chapter 13

Managing Asthma Long-Term

The key to controlling your asthma, rather than letting your asthma control you, is to treat your condition on a consistent and preventive basis. Doing so means managing your asthma for the long-term, rather than only dealing with symptoms and episodes temporarily.

Asthma isn't something that you usually outgrow. Extensive studies over the past 15 years have shown that asthma is an on-going physical condition that doesn't just disappear forever when you feel better. Keep in mind that your asthma can vary in its symptoms and severity over the course of your lifetime. However, just like the color of your eyes or your own individual fingerprint pattern, once you have asthma, it remains as another of your distinctive, although unseen, physical characteristics.

The airways of your lungs get bigger as you grow, so mild airway obstruction may not affect you as much as you get older. Also, as you mature, your sensitivities may not be sufficient to cause clinical symptoms that you might notice. However, it's not uncommon for people who feel that they "outgrew" their asthma as children or teenagers to experience symptoms of the disease later in life, particularly in response to certain triggers (see Chapter 11).

Developing and sticking to a long-term asthma management strategy is a priceless investment in your overall health and quality of life, especially if you have persistent asthma. The fundamental point of this approach is to address the root cause of your symptoms — the underlying airway inflammation that characterizes asthma — thus enabling you to achieve the goals of long-term asthma management that I list in Chapter 10.

In most cases, I find that after patients realize how much better they can feel by effectively managing their asthma on a long-term basis, they won't put up with going back to the ineffective, short-term, crisis-management ways of dealing with their disease.

Looking at What a Long-Term Management Plan Includes

A comprehensive long-term management plan for persistent asthma should include the following elements:

- Objective testing and monitoring of your lung functions to initially diagnose your condition and to continuously assess the effectiveness of your treatment (see Chapter 10).

- Avoiding and controlling exposures to asthma triggers and precipitating factors (see Chapter 11).

- Developing a safe and effective pharmacotherapy program that results in minimal or no adverse side effects. The program includes taking appropriate long-term preventive medications on a routine basis to control your asthma and using appropriate short-term, quick-relief rescue medications if your symptoms suddenly get worse (see Chapter 12).

- Initiating pharmacotherapy with a *stepwise* (step-up or step-down) approach (see the next section).

- Consulting with an asthma specialist, such as an allergist or pulmonologist (lung doctor) when advisable (see Chapter 10).

- Tailoring your asthma management plan to your specific circumstances and condition and continuing education for you and your family about asthma and your specific condition (see "Understanding Self-Management," later in this chapter).

Understanding Asthma Severity and the Stepwise Approach

Experts from different fields of medicine have classified the severity of asthma — whether allergic or nonallergic — into four levels. These asthma severity levels provide the basis for the stepwise management of the disease.

Bear in mind, however, that these levels of severity aren't permanent or static. Asthma is a condition that can change throughout your life. The primary goal of the stepwise approach that I describe in this chapter is to get your asthma to the lowest classification possible. Therefore, effectively treating your condition is crucial: Otherwise, your asthma severity may move up the classification scale to the point where you could potentially suffer from severe, relentless symptoms that adversely affect your quality of life.

As described in the National Institutes of Health (NIH) Guidelines for the Diagnosis and Management of Asthma, the four levels of asthma severity are:

✔ **Mild intermittent:** Symptoms occur no more than twice a week during the day and no more than twice a month at night. Lung-function testing (see Chapter 10) shows 80 percent or greater of the predicted normal value, compared to reference values based on your age, height, sex, and race, as established by the American Thoracic Society. In addition, your peak expiratory flow rate (PEFR) shouldn't vary by more than 20 percent during episodes and from the morning to the evening. Between episodes, you may be *asymptomatic* (not have noticeable symptoms), and your PEFR should be normal. If your asthma is at this level, a worsening of symptoms is usually brief, lasting a few hours to a few days, with variations of intensity.

✔ **Mild persistent:** Symptoms occur more than twice a week during the day, but less than once a day, and more than twice a month at night. Lung-function testing shows 80 percent or greater of the predicted normal value. Your PEFR may vary between 20 and 30 percent. If your asthma is at this level of severity, then worsening of symptoms can begin to affect your activities.

✔ **Moderate persistent:** Symptoms occur daily and more than once a week at night, requiring daily use of a short-acting bronchodilator. Lung-function testing shows a 60 to 80 percent range of the normal predicted value. Your PEFR can vary more than 30 percent. Symptoms can get worse at least twice a week, with episodes lasting for days and affecting your activities.

✔ **Severe persistent:** Symptoms occur continuously during the day and frequently at night, limiting physical activity. Lung-function testing is 60 percent or less of the normal predicted value. Your PEFR may vary more than 30 percent, and frequent aggravations of your condition can develop.

When diagnosing your condition, your doctor should identify your asthma's level of severity. I advise you to see which of the severity levels your condition most resembles, based on the definitions that I list in this section. Your own symptoms and lung functions may not always fit neatly into one of these particular severity levels. Your doctor, therefore, should evaluate your individual condition and develop a treatment plan for you based on the specific characteristics of your asthma. Keep in mind, however, that based on symptom criteria and the results of lung-function testing, the vast majority of asthma patients have some form of persistent asthma — mild, moderate, or severe — requiring long-term control therapy.

If the symptoms you're experiencing seem to indicate that you have persistent asthma, I strongly advise having your lung functions evaluated by spirometry if you haven't already done so (see "Assessing Your Lungs," later in this chapter, as well as in Chapter 10). For a spirometry evaluation, you may need to ask your doctor for a referral to an asthma specialist, such as an allergist or pulmonologist (lung doctor), because in many cases, primary care physicians don't have easy access to office spirometers.

Using the Stepwise Approach

Asthma severity levels are steps in the staircase to controlling asthma, as shown in Figure 13-1. The basic concept of stepwise management is to initially prescribe long-term and quick relief medications, based on the severity level that's one step higher than the severity level you're experiencing (see Table 13-1). By using this approach, your doctor can usually help you gain rapid control over your symptoms. After your condition has been under control for a month (in most cases), your physician will probably reduce the level of your medications by one level *(step down)*.

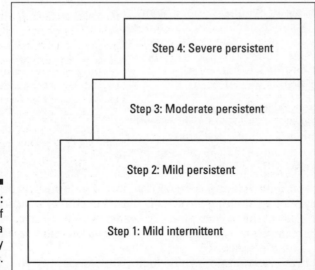

Figure 13-1:
The steps of asthma severity levels.

Using the stepwise approach to asthma management means that you *step up* your medication therapy to gain control, and then *step down* your medical treatment to maintain control. Like waltzing, after you and your doctor master the steps, you should be able to move around the dance floor of life with the ease and grace of Fred Astaire or Ginger Rogers. Regular monitoring of your peak expiratory flow rate (PEFR) and follow-up visits with your doctor, however, are vital to ensuring that you stay in step, as I explain in the next section.

The information contained in Table 13-1 is based on the National Institutes of Health (NIH) Guidelines for the Diagnosis and Management of Asthma. Please remember that these are guidelines. Your doctor should always evaluate your own specific condition and prescribe individualized treatment accordingly.

Table 13-1	Stepwise Approach for Managing Asthma in Adults and Children Older Than 5 Years of Age	
Step	**Long-Term Control**	**Quick Relief**
Step 1: Mild intermittent	**No daily medication needed**	**Short-acting bronchodilator:** Inhaled beta$_2$-adrenergics as needed for symptoms. Intensity of treatment may vary depending on the severity of your symptoms. (If you're using a short-acting inhaled beta$_2$-adrenergic more than twice a week, you may need to initiate long-term control therapy. You should consult your doctor in this case.)
Step 2: Mild persistent	**One daily medication:** Anti-inflammatory medication, either inhaled topical corticosteroid (low doses) or mast cell stabilizers, such as cromolyn or nedocromil. (Children often begin with a trial of a mast cell stabilizer.) Your doctor may also consider anti-leukotriene modifiers such as zafirlukast and montelukast. Your physician may also consider a methylxanthine product such as sustained-release theophylline as an alternative treatment, but not as preferred therapy.	**Short-acting bronchodilator:** Inhaled beta$_2$-adrenergics as needed for symptoms. Intensity of treatment may vary depending on the severity of your symptoms. (If you're using a short-acting inhaled beta$_2$-adrenergic more than twice a week, you may need additional long-term control therapy. You should consult your doctor in this case.)

(continued)

Table 13-1	*(continued)*	
Step	*Long-Term Control*	*Quick Relief*
Step 3*: **Moderate persistent**	**Daily medication:** Anti-inflammatory medication, inhaled corticosteroid (medium dose), or inhaled corticosteroid (low to medium dose), adding a long-acting bronchodilator, especially for nighttime symptoms — either long-acting inhaled beta$_2$-adrenergics, sustained release theophylline, or long-acting beta$_2$-adrenergic tablets. **If needed:** Anti-inflammatory medication, inhaled cortico-steroid (medium-high dose) and long-acting bronchodilator, especially for nighttime symptoms — either long-acting inhaled beta$_2$-adrenergics, sustained release theophylline, or long-acting beta$_2$-adrenergic tablets.	**Short-acting bronchodilator:** Inhaled beta$_2$-adrenergic as needed for symptoms. Intensity of treatment may vary depending on the severity of your symptoms. (If you're using a short-acting inhaled beta$_2$-adrenergic more than twice a week, you may need additional long-term control therapy. You should consult your doctor in this case.)
Step 4*: **Severe persistent**	**Daily medication:** Anti-inflammatory medication, inhaled corticosteroid (high dose), and long-acting bronchodilator — either long-acting inhaled beta$_2$-adrenergics, sustained release theophylline, or long-acting beta$_2$-adrenergic tablets; and, if required, long-term use of corticosteroid tablets or syrup.	**Short-acting bronchodilator:** Inhaled beta$_2$-adrenergics as needed for symptoms. Intensity of treatment may vary depending on the severity of your symptoms. (If you're using a short-acting inhaled beta$_2$-adrenergic more than twice a week, you may need additional long-term control therapy. You should consult your doctor in this case.)

*If your asthma severity is at Step 3 or Step 4, I recommend consulting an asthma specialist, such as an allergist or pulmonologist (lung doctor), to achieve better control of your condition.

Stepping down

If you're on long-term maintenance control at any level, your doctor should review your treatment every one to six months. A gradual stepwise reduction in treatment may be possible after your symptoms are under good control, meaning that you feel good, have maintained improved lung function, and experience no asthma symptoms.

The goal of the stepwise approach is to use early and aggressive treatment to gain rapid control over your asthma symptoms so that your doctor can reduce your medication to the lowest level required to maintain good control of your condition.

Stepping up

If you find yourself frequently resorting to your quick-relief medications, your symptoms are *not* under good control, and your doctor should consider increasing your treatment by one step. In assessing whether to step up your therapy, your doctor will probably evaluate the following aspects of your current treatment step:

- ✔ Your inhaler technique. (See "Evaluating your inhaler technique," later in this chapter.)

- ✔ Your level of adherence in taking the medications that your doctor prescribes. Remember: Taking your prescriptions as your doctor instructs is vital. If you're having trouble with a product (because of potential side effects) or you don't understand your doctor's instructions, make sure that you tell your physician so that he or she can take appropriate measures to insure that your treatment is as safe and effective as possible.

- ✔ Your exposure level to asthma triggers, such as allergens and irritants and precipitating factors, such as viral infections and other medical conditions. You should control your exposure to asthma triggers and precipitating factors as much as possible, no matter what step of treatment you're receiving. (See Chapter 11 for information on controlling asthma triggers.)

Make sure that your asthma management plan clearly explains at what point you should contact your physician if your symptoms worsen.

Treating severe episodes in stepwise management

Your doctor may consider prescribing a rescue course of oral corticosteroids at any step if you suddenly experience a severe asthma episode and your condition abruptly deteriorates. (Chapter 12 provides more information on oral corticosteroids.)

In some cases, severe episodes can occur even if your asthma is classified as intermittent. In many instances, patients with intermittent asthma may experience severe and potentially life-threatening episodes, often because of upper respiratory viral infections (such as the flu or colds), even though these patients may otherwise have long periods of normal or near-normal lung functions and few clinically perceptible asthma symptoms.

Assessing Your Lungs

Objective measurements of your lung functions are essential for monitoring the severity of your asthma. Just as you check the oil level in your car on a regular basis (rather than waiting for the flashing red warning light), you and your doctor should also regularly check the functioning of your airways to determine whether you are at the right step of asthma medication. In addition to recording your asthma symptoms in a daily symptom diary (see the next section), you should also obtain objective measurements of lung functions with spirometry and peak flow monitoring.

What your doctor should do: Spirometry

A spirometer is a sophisticated machine that your doctor or asthma specialist, such as an allergist or pulmonologist (lung doctor), uses for measuring airflow from your large and small airways before and 15 minutes after you've inhaled a short-acting bronchodilator. The spirometer helps your asthma specialist diagnose whether you have asthma and also allows your physician to follow your asthma's clinical course.

For adults and children over age 4 or 5, spirometry currently provides the most accurate way of determining whether airway obstruction exists and whether it's reversible. For information on other types of lung function tests your doctor may recommend and to find out more about diagnosing asthma in children under age 4, see Chapter 10.

What you can do: Peak flow monitoring

Just as diabetics check their blood sugar levels with a monitoring device and people with hypertension often take their own blood pressure, you can keep an eye on your lung functions at home with a peak flow meter. The readings from this handy tool (see Figure 13-2) can be vital in diagnosing asthma and its severity and can also help your doctor prescribe medications and monitor the effectiveness of your treatment. Peak flow monitoring can also provide important early warning signs that an asthma episode is approaching.

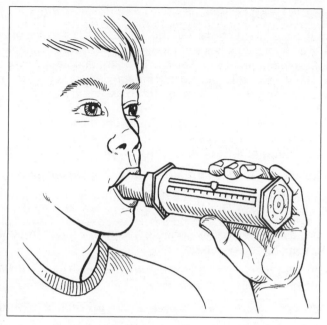

Figure 13-2:
A patient
using a peak
flow meter.

Children over 4 or 5 who have asthma generally can also use this small, hand-held device to measure their own peak expiratory flow rate (PEFR). If your kids constantly question your judgment (as mine do about almost every-thing), using a peak flow meter can help get youngsters to understand when their condition may require them to limit their activities. If your child under-stands that it's the PEFR — not just you or your doctor — telling him or her that it's not advisable to go to soccer practice on that particular day because of worsening asthma symptoms and a resulting PEFR reduction, you may have more success in helping to control your child's asthma.

Explaining and using peak flow meters for children

I often advise parents to explain to their kids that when their peak flow rate is down, it's like having an injury in their lungs. You can reinforce this analogy by telling your child that although the underlying airway inflammation isn't visible — unlike the injury to a sprained ankle, for example — the problem still needs proper treatment, just as a sprain needs to heal before resuming normal activities.

By the same token, when your child's PEFR is between 80 to 100 percent of his or her personal best, you can breathe easier about encouraging sports and other physical activities that are vital aspects of improving their overall health and fitness, including their lung functions. Make sure, however, that you and your child know how to manage potential symptoms of exercise-induced asthma (EIA), as I explain in Chapter 14.

Using a peak flow meter at home

Here are some basic instructions and tips for using most types of peak flow meters (several different makes and models are currently available). Remember, however, to follow the instructions that come with your specific device. You should also ask your doctor for specific advice on the most effective way you can use your peak flow meter to assess your condition.

Generally, you use a peak flow meter by following these steps:

1. **Move the sliding indicator at the base of the peak flow meter to zero.**

2. **Stand up and take a deep breath to fully inflate your lungs.**

3. **Put the mouthpiece of the peak flow monitor into your mouth and close your lips tightly around it.**

4. **Blow as hard and as fast as possible, like you're blowing out the candles on your birthday cake.**

5. **Read the dial where the red indicator stopped. The number opposite the indicator is your peak flow rate.**

6. **Reset the indicator to zero and repeat the process twice more.**

7. **Record the highest number that you reach.**

Finding your personal best peak flow number

Your personal best peak flow number is a measurement that reflects the highest peak flow number that you can expect to achieve over a two to three week period after a course of aggressive treatment has produced good control of your asthma symptoms. Your best number is usually the result of step-up therapy.

To determine your personal best peak flow number, take two peak flow readings a day during an entire week when you're doing well and record the best result. You should take one reading prior to taking medication in the morning and another reading between noon and 2:00 in the afternoon after taking an inhaled short-acting bronchodilator. Compare your personal best peak flow number with the measurement that your physician predicts, which is based on national studies for children or adults of particular heights, sexes, and ages. This number can help you determine how your measurements compare with the norm. When your asthma is well controlled, your PEFR should consistently read between 80 and 100 percent of your personal best.

If your peak flow measurements fall below 80 percent, early and aggressive intervention with medications and strict avoidance of potential asthma triggers may be necessary to prevent worsening symptoms. Ignoring a declining peak flow reading can lead to serious symptoms and may result in the need for emergency treatment.

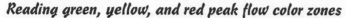

Reading green, yellow, and red peak flow color zones

The peak flow zone system involves green, yellow, and red areas, which are similar to a traffic signal. Using your peak flow meter on a regular basis should enable you and your doctor to treat symptoms before your condition deteriorates further.

You or your doctor may want to place small pieces of colored tape next to the actual numbers on your peak flow meter itself, corresponding with the green, yellow, and red zones that your doctor provides as a graph on your written asthma peak flow diary.

Table 13-2 explains how to read the peak flow color zones.

Table 13-2	The Peak Flow Color Zone System	
Zone	*Meaning*	*Points to Consider*
Green zone	Readings in this area are *safe.*	When your reading falls into the green zone on your meter, you've achieved 80 to 100 percent of your personal best peak flow. No asthma symptoms are present, and your treatment plan is controlling your asthma. If your readings consistently remain in the green zone, you and your doctor may be able to consider reducing daily medications.
Yellow zone	Readings in this area indicate *caution.*	When your readings fall into the yellow zone, you're only achieving 50 to 80 percent of your personal best peak flow. An asthma attack may be present, and your symptoms may be about to get worse. You may need to step-up your medication temporarily.
Red zone	Readings in this area mean *medical alert.*	Readings in the red zone mean that you've fallen below 50 percent of your personal best peak flow. These readings often signal the start of a moderate to severe asthma attack.

If your readings are often in the yellow zone, even after taking the appropriate quick-relief medication that your asthma management plan specifies, you should contact your doctor. If your readings are in the red zone, you should use your quick-relief bronchodilator and anti-inflammatory medications immediately (based on your specific and individualized asthma management plan) and contact your doctor if your PEFR doesn't immediately return to and remain in the yellow or green zones.

Assessing Your Condition

In addition to obtaining an objective measurement of your lung function with measuring devices, another important aspect of controlling your asthma is keeping track of a variety of other indicators. Your most valuable tracking device is usually a daily symptom diary. In fact, you should develop a rating system (in consultation with your doctor) for use in your diary that assesses your symptoms on a scale of 0 to 3, ranging from no symptoms to severe symptoms.

Keeping symptom records

Besides serving as a record of your PEFR readings, your daily symptom diary should monitor and record the following:

- Your signs and symptoms, as well as their severity
- Any coughing that you experience
- Any incidence of wheezing
- Nasal congestion
- Disturbances in your sleep, such as coughing and/or wheezing that awaken you
- Any symptoms that affect your ability to function normally or reduce normal activities
- Any time you've missed school or work because of symptoms
- Frequency of use of your short-acting beta$_2$-adrenergic bronchodilator (rescue medication)

Tracking serious symptoms

Your daily symptom diary is also the place to monitor occurrences of symptoms that are severe enough to make you seek unscheduled office visits, after-hours treatments, emergency room visits, and hospitalizations. Therefore, you also want to note the date and kind of treatment that you seek.

You should record the following types of serious symptoms:

- Breathlessness or panting while at rest
- The need to remain in an upright position in order to breathe
- Difficulty speaking

✔ Agitation or confusion

✔ An increased breathing rate of more than 30 breaths per minute

✔ Loud wheezing while inhaling and/or exhaling

✔ An elevated pulse rate of more than 120 heartbeats per minute

You should also record exposures to triggers and/or precipitating factors that may have caused asthma flare-ups, including

✔ Irritants such as chemicals or cigarette or fireplace smoke

✔ Allergens such as plant pollen, household dust, molds, and animal fur

✔ Air pollution

✔ Exercise (Chapter 11 provides more information on exercise-induced asthma)

✔ Sudden changes in the weather, particularly cold temperatures and chilly winds

✔ Reactions to beta-blockers (such as Inderal or Timoptic), aspirin, and related products, including NSAIDs and food additives — particularly sulfites (see Chapter 11)

✔ Other medical conditions, such as upper respiratory viral infections (colds and flu), gastroesophageal reflux (GER), and sinusitis (see Chapter 11)

Monitoring your medication use

Recording all the side effects that you experience when taking your prescribed medication is also of great value. Various asthma medications include many levels of side effects that a person can potentially experience as a result of taking those medications. However, in most cases, patients who understand their asthma management plan and take their medications according to instructions have few, if any, adverse side effects from using products to control their asthma symptoms. The tables in Chapter 12 provide extensive details on asthma medication products.

Evaluating your inhaler technique

Your doctor should show you the correct way to use your inhaler and have you demonstrate your inhaler technique at each office visit. In the best of cases when using inhalers, only 10 to 20 percent of the topical inhaled drug gets into the areas of your lungs where it can really do some good. (See Chapter 12.)

Because such small amounts of inhaler medications actually reach the airways of your lungs, understanding how to use your inhaler properly is vital to your treatment. Improper inhaler use is often the reason why some patients have difficulty controlling their asthma symptoms. (Chapter 12 provides detailed instructions on using your inhaler.)

Understanding Self-Management

It takes two (at least) to treat asthma. You and your physician (as well as your other health care providers) are partners in controlling your asthma. Other members of your asthma partnership can include nurses, pharmacists, and other health professionals who treat you or assist you in understanding and finding out more about effectively managing your condition.

If you have asthma, your family also — in a sense — has the condition. Asthma isn't contagious; rather, your family also has the condition because all of you may need to deal with the various issues associated with the treatment of your medical condition. In fact, studies show that family support can be a major positive factor in the success of any asthma treatment plan. Particularly important to your asthma treatment is making sure that the people you live with (as well as coworkers, fellow students, or anyone you're around much of the time) help you reduce your exposure to asthma triggers and to precipitating factors. I explain in detail the most common triggers and precipitating factors to avoid in Chapter 11.

If your child has asthma, you should also be a partner with your child's doctor and other medical professionals in the management of your youngster's condition. (Chapter 14 provides details on managing asthma in children.)

Developing your treatment goals

I strongly advise you to participate in developing treatment goals with your doctor. Make sure that you understand how your asthma management plan works and that you can openly communicate with your doctor about the effects and results of your treatment.

Making sure that your plan is tailored to your specific, individualized needs, as well as those of your family, is also very important. Doing so can include taking into account any cultural beliefs and practices that can have an impact on your perception of asthma and of medication therapy. I recommend openly discussing any such issues with your physician, so that together, you can develop an approach to asthma management that empowers you to take control of your condition. In my view, ensuring that your plan is tailored to fit you and your family results in a more motivated patient, which almost always means a healthier individual.

Evaluating for the long-term

Successfully managing your asthma also means constantly assessing your asthma management plan to determine whether it provides you with the means to achieve your asthma management goals.

Always keep in mind that asthma is a variable, complex, multifaceted condition. Just as many other aspects of your life can change and vary over time, your asthma may also manifest in different ways throughout your life. Remember: Your goal is lifetime management of your condition.

Learning about your asthma

The education process concerning asthma and its treatment should begin as soon as you're diagnosed. I believe that your doctor should make sure that you have a thorough understanding of all aspects of your condition. Ignorance is not bliss when it comes to managing your asthma and/or allergies effectively. Your process of education should include factors such as the following:

- Knowing the basic facts about asthma.

- Understanding the level of your asthma severity, how it affects you, and advisable treatment methods.

- Teaching you all the elements of asthma self-management, including basic facts about the disease and your specific condition, proper use of various inhalers and nebulizers, self-monitoring skills, and effective ways of avoiding triggers and allergy-proofing your home.

- Developing a written, individualized daily and emergency self-management plan with your input (see Chapter 10).

- Determining the level of support you receive from family and friends in treating your asthma. It's also important for your doctor to help you identify an asthma partner from among your family members, relatives, or friends. This person should find out how asthma affects you and should understand your asthma management plan so that he or she can provide assistance (if necessary) if your condition suddenly worsens. I advise including your asthma partner in doctor visits when appropriate.

- Asking your doctor and/or other members of your asthma management team for guidance in setting priorities when implementing your asthma management plan. If you need to make environmental changes in your life, such as allergy-proofing your home (which may include relocating a pet, taking up the carpets, installing air filtration devices, and many other steps that I explain in Chapter 11), you may want advice on which steps you need to take soonest and which steps can wait.

Improving Your Quality of Life

Taking asthma medication doesn't mean that you can afford to ignore other aspects of your health. Effectively managing your asthma for the long term also requires being healthy overall. The better you take care of yourself, the more success you'll have in treating your asthma and living a full, normal life.

Here are some important, commonsense guidelines that I think all asthma patients should consider when developing an asthma management plan.

✔ **Eating right**. A healthy, well-balanced diet is especially important for people who have asthma. Fresh fruits, meats, fish, grains, and vegetables should be important parts of your diet.

✔ **Sleeping well**. If you experience asthma symptoms during the night that disturb your sleep, tell your doctor. These types of symptoms should be treated, and they may indicate that you're susceptible to precipitating factors such as gastroesophageal reflux (GER) or asthma triggers such as dust mites in your bedroom (see Chapter 11).

✔ **Staying fit**. When patients are in good physical condition, their asthma is often easier to control. You don't have to sit on life's sidelines just because you have asthma. Your doctor can prescribe medications that you can take preventively to control symptoms of EIA, thus enabling you to enjoy many types of exercise and sports activities in spite of your asthma. (Chapter 12 provides information on appropriate products for controlling EIA.)

✔ **Reducing stress**. By effectively controlling your asthma, you'll feel less anxious about your condition, thus reducing the overall levels of stress in your life and further helping you manage your asthma.

Expecting the best

With effective, appropriate care from your doctor and your own motivated participation as a patient, your asthma management plan should enable you to lead a full and active life. However, if following your asthma management plan properly still doesn't allow you to participate fully in the activities and pursuits that matter to you, openly communicate this to your physician so that he or she can adjust your plan and maximize the effectiveness of your treatment.

If, as sometimes happens, your doctor deals only with your asthma symptoms — instead of initiating the type of long-term approach that I discuss in this chapter — you may want to consider requesting a referral to an asthma specialist. You should expect to be able to effectively control your asthma, and your doctor should certainly help you achieve this goal.

Chapter 14

Asthma and Allergies during Childhood

As parents, we all know that no one is more precious to us than our children. Therefore, we all want to treat any ailment that affects our youngsters as effectively as possible. If your child has asthma, the good news is that with a proper diagnosis, appropriate management, and your understanding of the disease, you can help your child effectively control his or her asthma.

Unfortunately, some parents (and even some doctors) don't understand asthma well enough to recognize or diagnose the disease properly. Too often, this misunderstanding results in the misdiagnosis of children with asthma as instead having chronic bronchitis or recurring colds. In these cases, children may not receive the appropriate treatment for the underlying airway inflammation that characterizes asthma, and their symptoms may worsen, leading to severe asthma episodes that may require emergency measures to treat.

In fact, asthma — the most common chronic childhood disease in the United States — affects at least five million children. Current estimates are that only half of these youngsters receive an accurate diagnosis and effective treatment for their condition.

Although the U.S. boasts the most advanced health care system in the world, the number of children with asthma ages 4 and younger has more than tripled since 1980. Likewise, the number of people in the U.S. who suffer from asthma has almost doubled since 1980.

Here are some other vital statistics about the state of childhood asthma in the U.S.:

- ✔ Acute asthma attacks are the most common reason for emergency treatment of children.

- ✔ In the last three decades, the hospitalization rate for children with asthma has more than tripled.

- ✔ Asthma accounts for 20 percent of missed school days, second only to viral upper respiratory infections such as the common cold.

These alarming asthma statistics don't need to continue. Treating your child's asthma early and aggressively, as well as practicing long-term preventive maintenance, can make the difference between a sickly youngster and a healthy, well-adjusted kid who rarely experiences the problematic symptoms of this disease.

Understanding Your Child's Asthma

Asthma is a chronic inflammatory disease of the airways that can make getting air in and especially out of the lungs difficult. Besides the serious health risks that asthma can pose for your child, properly managing the disease is vital for your youngster's overall growth: Anything that restricts proper breathing can impair his or her physical and mental development.

Asthma often begins in childhood and affects boys more commonly than girls. Most children who develop asthma experience their first symptoms of the disease before they reach their third birthday.

Look for the following signs and symptoms as possible asthma indicators in your child. (Keep in mind, however, that not every child with the disease experiences all of these signs and symptoms.)

- ✔ Persistent coughing, wheezing, and recurring or lingering chest colds.

- ✔ An expanded or over-inflated chest and hunched shoulders.

- ✔ Signs of coughing, wheezing, or extreme shortness of breath during or after exercise. These symptoms may signal the onset of exercise-induced asthma, or EIA (see "Participating in PE — exercise and asthma," later in this chapter).

- ✔ Coughing at night, in the absence of other symptoms such as a cold.

Because you may find recognizing the preceding symptoms more difficult when observing infants and young children, I also suggest watching for the following signs of possible asthma trouble:

- ✔ Lethargic activity and reduced responses, including not recognizing or responding to parents.

- ✔ Difficulty in nursing or eating.

- ✔ Soft, shallow crying.

- ✔ Nasal flaring (rapidly moving nostrils), which can be a sign of severe asthma.

- ✔ Deep and rapid rib muscle movements, also known as *retractions*, which can occur when an infant or young child is having trouble breathing properly.

- ✔ *Cyanosis*, due to severe airway obstruction blocking the normal flow of oxygen into the lungs, causes a very pale or blue skin color. This can occur in a very severe asthma attack and requires emergency treatment.

In addition to these signs, you also need to consider the presence of *atopy* (the genetic susceptibility for the immune system to produce antibodies to common allergens, which leads to allergy symptoms) as a key predisposing factor for your child developing asthma (see Chapters 2 and 10).

Atopic conditions, including food allergies (see Chapter 19), allergic rhinitis (hay fever — see Chapter 4), and atopic dermatitis (eczema — see Chapter 16), can indicate a potential predisposition for asthma, especially in infants and young children. In fact, more than three-quarters of all children who develop asthma also have allergies. In many cases, allergic reactions associated with the response to inhalant and ingested allergens can also cause flare-ups in a child with asthma.

Inheriting asthma

If you think that your child may have asthma, consider your family's medical history. Two-thirds of asthma patients have a close relative with the disease. Likewise, if you or your child's other parent has asthma, your child's chances of developing asthma are 25 percent; if *both* you and your child's other parent have asthma, your child's odds of developing asthma double to 50 percent.

However, asthma in your family doesn't guarantee that your child will develop asthma. Your child inherits the *tendency* to the disease, not the disease itself. If neither you nor your child's other parent has asthma, the odds of your child developing this disease are no greater than 15 percent.

Asthma triggers for children

Although hereditary factors may increase the likelihood of your child developing asthma, environmental triggers and other precipitating factors usually bring on the symptoms of the disease (see Chapter 11 for more detailed information on these triggers and precipitating factors). Most physicians agree that viral respiratory infections are the most common triggers of asthma attacks in most infants and young children.

The most serious air pollutant and irritant in terms of asthma is tobacco smoke. Parents absolutely should not smoke around a child, especially if the youngster has asthma. Even if your child is out (for example, at school), you should still avoid smoking in the home. The lingering odor of tobacco smoke can still trigger your child's asthma symptoms.

According to numerous studies, exposure to maternal smoke is a major risk factor in the early onset of asthma in infancy. In fact, an infant whose mother smokes is almost twice as likely to develop asthma.

All in the asthma family

If your child is asthmatic, your whole family must deal with the condition. No, asthma's not contagious. However, the rest of the family needs to know how to deal with your child's medical condition.

When your small child can't breathe, he or she is in grave danger. Because a toddler or infant can't communicate what's happening to him or her, serious trouble can strike unless the rest of the family watches and understands how asthma symptoms show up. Therefore, as a parent, you must find out all you can about asthma and its symptoms, testing, and treatment. Your child depends on you!

Controlling — not outgrowing — asthma

The idea that children eventually "outgrow" asthma is a dangerous myth, and withholding treatment hoping that somehow your child's asthma will go just away is a misguided approach. As children grow, their lungs and airways become larger. If the amount of airway obstruction stays the same, the blockage may proportionally constitute a smaller part of the total airway diameter, thus resulting in fewer symptoms as an adult. Your child's sensitivities, however, may not entirely disappear, and the possibility exists that a lack of treatment could result in irreversible airway changes. Clear and compelling evidence shows that early diagnosis and treatment results in fewer asthma symptoms.

Your child's asthma symptoms may diminish or may no longer be apparent, but the increased airway sensitivity remains — just as your child's fingerprints stay the same even though his or her body grows and develops. Asthma isn't a disease that you can really cure; it's a condition that you must control.

Treating early to avoid problems later

In my practice, many adult patients are referred to me with severe asthma. In many cases, I believe that their conditions might not have deteriorated to such an extent if their asthma had only been properly treated during childhood. The first two years after asthma has been diagnosed generally are considered to be the time when aggressive medical treatment can dramatically improve the potential for maintaining normal lung functions in your child.

Unfortunately, some parents only focus on immediately treating serious asthma attacks instead of managing the child's condition on a consistent, everyday basis. I feel that this approach is misguided. Don't watch and wait to see how asthma affects your child: If your child has a persistent cough, shortness of breath, lingering colds, or other early signs of asthma (see the symptoms and signs I list in the first part of this section), make sure that a doctor checks your child's lung functions. This testing can help to determine whether asthma is the cause of your child's symptoms. Treating your child's asthma early and aggressively often can be the most effective way of insuring that the disease won't adversely affect your child's health over the long term.

Diagnosing Childhood-Onset Asthma

When dealing with a child, particularly one who is very young, what may seem an obvious and easily identifiable asthma diagnosis is not always the case. Asthma is a complex condition with many possible combinations of symptoms that can vary widely from patient to patient. In fact, your child's symptoms can change over time.

The process of diagnosing your child's condition should include the following steps:

- A complete medical history
- A physical examination
- Lung function tests
- Any other test that your doctor considers necessary to determine the nature of your child's ailment

To diagnose your child's asthma, your doctor should establish the following key points:

- ✔ Your child experiences episodes of airway obstruction.
- ✔ The airway obstruction is at least partially reversible.
- ✔ Your child's symptoms result from asthma, not other potential conditions that I explain in the "Other reasons that kids wheeze" section, later in this chapter.

Taking your child's medical history

A thorough and complete medical history is vital to diagnosing your child's condition. In addition to asking about the symptoms and signs of childhood asthma that I describe in "Understanding Your Child's Asthma," earlier in this chapter, your doctor may also inquire about the following:

- ✔ Any family history of allergies and/or asthma. (As I explain in the "Inheriting asthma," section of this chapter, genetics play a major role in asthma development.)
- ✔ Any exposures your child receives to common asthma triggers such as inhalant allergens and irritants — especially cigarette smoke — or any other substances, as well as the precipitating factors that I describe in "Asthma triggers for children," earlier in this chapter.
- ✔ Any times your child has been hospitalized for respiratory problems. Your doctor should also ask about any medications that your child takes, whether for respiratory symptoms or for other conditions.

Examining your child for signs of asthma

The focus of a physical exam for children with suspected asthma usually involves the following:

- ✔ Examining your child's breathing passageways, from nose to chest. (See Chapter 10 for details of physical exams.)
- ✔ Observing your child's rate and rhythm of breathing. Your doctor will listen with a stethoscope (auscultation) to the chest and back over areas of your child's lungs, to check for the following signs and sounds of airway obstruction: wheezing or other sounds not usually associated with normal breathing, unusually prolonged exhalations, and rapid, shallow respirations (panting), in more severe cases.

 ✔ Looking for evidence of atopic diseases, such as allergic rhinitis (hay fever), food allergies, or atopic dermatitis (eczema), which may indicate a predisposition to asthma.

 ✔ Checking for signs of hunched shoulders, chest deformities, and skin and muscle retractions (or "sucking-in") between (intercostal) or under (subcostal) your child's ribs.

Testing your child's lungs

After taking your child's medical history and performing a physical examination, your doctor may conduct lung-function tests if your child is over 4 or 5 years old. These tests are vital in diagnosing asthma because they can provide objective measurements of the extent to which your child's lung functions may have been limited or affected by airway obstruction.

To diagnose asthma in children over age 4 or 5, doctors often use a procedure known as spirometry. *Spirometry* involves using a spirometer (pulmonary function machine) to measure your child's airflow, before and 15 minutes after he or she inhales a short-acting bronchodilator, to determine reversibility (improvement in lung function). See Chapter 10 for more details on spirometry.

Spirometry tests are difficult, if not impossible, to perform on children under 4 years old. However, by age 6, most children are quite capable of performing accurate and reliable spirometry (if they *feel* like it!). To properly diagnose an infant or young child with asthma, your doctor may need to rely on your child's medical history and physical examination. In some cases, your doctor may prescribe a trial course of nebulized beta$_2$-adrenergic bronchodilator and/or anti-inflammatory medications to evaluate your child's response.

Other reasons that kids wheeze

All that wheezes is not asthma. Although the misdiagnosis of asthma (often as bronchitis) is a frequent problem in treating childhood respiratory conditions, in some cases, other ailments can cause symptoms that resemble asthma. These other ailments include

 ✔ Viral bronchiolitis (RSV), an often serious respiratory infection that can occur in the first two years of life, may resemble an acute asthma attack. This disease characteristically occurs during the winter months in children under 2 years of age. Studies have shown that over half of children who experience infections of viral bronchiolitis and who have a family history of allergy go on to develop asthma.

 ✔ Viral and/or bacterial bronchitis or pneumonia.

- ✔ Congenital heart disease, often leading to congestive heart failure.

- ✔ Abnormal development of blood vessels, known as *vascular rings,* around the trachea (windpipe) and esophagus.

- ✔ Cystic fibrosis.

- ✔ Vocal cord dysfunction (VCD).

Numerous cases also exist in which children suddenly start wheezing because a coin, food particle, or other foreign body has become lodged in their windpipe, respiratory tube, or esophagus. If you suspect that a foreign object is lodged somewhere in your child's respiratory system, seek medical help immediately.

Special Issues Concerning Childhood Asthma

After your child's asthma has been diagnosed, your child's doctor should develop an appropriate asthma management plan, in consultation with you and your child (if he or she is old enough to participate). Your child's plan should consist of specific avoidance, medication, monitoring, and assessment measures, and it should also provide steps that you and/or your child can take in case his or her asthma symptoms suddenly worsen.

The basic components of an appropriate and effective asthma management plan include

- ✔ **Reducing your child's level of exposure to asthma and allergy triggers.** I describe these triggers in "Asthma triggers for children," earlier in this chapter. (For detailed tips and information on avoidance measures, trigger control, and allergy-proofing, see Chapter 11.)

- ✔ **Peak flow monitoring.** Your doctor should show you and your child (if your youngster is over 4 years old) how to use a peak flow meter. (See "Peak flow meters and school-age children" later in this chapter.) Using this simple device at home and school to measure peak expiratory flow rates (PEFR) can help detect early deterioration of asthma, prompting you or your child to make the appropriate change in your child's medications or, if needed, to seek medical attention.

Children and their parents very often do not perceive the early symptoms of worsening asthma without a peak flow meter. This failure to appreciate the severity of their worsening asthma can result in a crucial delay in initiating proper medical treatment. (For detailed instructions on using peak flow meters, see Chapter 13.)

✔ **Monitoring and assessing your child's lung functions during regular office visits.** These tests and assessments, as well as the PEFR numbers that you (or your child) record in an asthma symptom diary (see Chapter 10) are vital to tracking how your child's condition develops and responds to prescribed treatment.

✔ **Long-term preventive medications that control your child's underlying airway inflammation, congestion, constriction, and hyperresponsiveness.** (See Chapter 10 for details of asthma mechanisms.)

✔ **An asthma management plan for your child's school or day care.** (See "Asthma at School and Day Care," later in this chapter.) Prepare an emergency asthma management plan, which specifies short-term, fast-acting rescue medications for use only in the event that your child's condition suddenly deteriorates. This type of action plan should also clearly explain how to adjust your child's medications in response to particular signs, symptoms, and PEFR levels. Likewise, this action plan should tell you (or your child) when to call for medical help.

✔ **An ongoing process of asthma education for you, your child, and your family.** This education can involve information and resources that your doctor, clinic staff, and patient support groups provide or recommend, as well as relevant books, newsletters, videos, and other helpful materials that you and your family gather. (See the appendix at the back of this book for information on these resources.)

Teaming up for your child's asthma treatment

I strongly advise that you integrate any treatment your youngster may receive from an asthma specialist (an allergist or pulmonologist) and your child's asthma management plan with the general care that your pediatrician, family doctor, and/or primary care physician provides.

A team approach by your child's physicians should eliminate the risk of different doctors prescribing treatments for various childhood ailments that may, in combination, produce adverse side effects for your child.

Managing asthma in infants (newborns to 2 years old)

The most difficult part of treating an infant with asthma is that the child isn't old enough to tell you what's wrong. Unfortunately, no devices are currently available for practicing physicians to use in order to measure infants' lung functions. Special techniques do exist at a few major medical centers but at this time are considered for research purposes and are not used in clinical practice. Therefore, determining the extent and type of your baby's respiratory problems can present some unique challenges. In these cases, the diagnosis is based mainly on medical history (including family history), physical examination, and response to medical therapy.

Depending on your child's condition, your doctor may prescribe some of the following medications to control your baby's asthma:

✔ If your infant's asthma symptoms are mild or intermittent, his or her doctor may prescribe an inhaled, short-acting beta$_2$-adrenergic in a nebulizer or an oral beta$_2$-adrenergic syrup to reduce airway obstruction.

✔ If your child suffers from more severe symptoms, your doctor may prescribe a daily, long-term preventive medication, such as cromolyn (Intal) via nebulizer or inhaler; nedocromil (Tilade) via inhaler; an inhaled corticosteroid (Flovent, Vanceril) via inhaler; or nebulizer form (Pulmicort Respules). Because of your child's young age, administering any of these medications with an inhaler requires using a holding chamber (spacer) and a mask. Occasionally, your child's doctor may also recommend theophylline in a syrup, tablet (crushed), or capsule (sprinkled) form (see Chapter 12 for information on asthma medications and delivery devices).

Physicians prescribe theophylline syrup or suggest emptying beaded contents of a theophylline capsule on food such as applesauce so that your baby can easily ingest the medication.

✔ In the event that your child suffers a severe asthma episode, your child's doctor may prescribe a short course of oral corticosteroids, available in syrup form (Prelone, Pediapred) or as a tablet (prednisone).

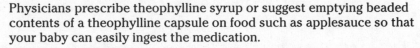

Listening to your children

Because children under 2 years old aren't able to use a peak flow meter, you may consider using a stethoscope to listen to your child's lungs. Some parents find that using a stethoscope can help them detect an asthma attack in their infant or young child at an earlier stage and might enable them to more accurately report their youngster's asthma symptoms to their child's physician.

Consult your child's physician to see whether using a stethoscope can help you. Likewise, you should also receive instructions on using the device properly. Keep in mind that a stethoscope detects breathing problems only if your child's lung function drops by about 25 percent.

Using a nebulizer with your infant or toddler

If your doctor prescribes nebulizer therapy for your infant or toddler, make sure that you, as well as any other person who may be taking care of your child (such as a nanny, babysitter, and/or daycare provider), understand how to use a nebulizer appropriately and effectively. Using this device may challenge an older child, but for an infant or toddler who may be struggling to breathe, using a nebulizer can prove especially difficult. Chapter 13 provides more detailed instructions and tips on using nebulizers properly and effectively.

When using a nebulizer with a very young child (your doctor should give you specific advice based on your child's condition), make stress reduction — for both you and your child — your first consideration. Try making the use of the nebulizer a more pleasant experience and maybe even a special daily occasion. Hold and cuddle your child first, and then slowly but firmly move the mask closer to your youngster's face.

If your child isn't experiencing sudden-onset severe respiratory symptoms, you may be able to introduce the mask initially, before running the air compressor component of the machine. The air compressor can be noisy, and it may frighten your child at first. If your child suffers more severe symptoms, hold the mask fairly close to his or her face and then slowly move it closer until the mask is properly in place.

Delivering nebulizer doses properly

Keep in mind that a "blow by" (holding the nebulizer several inches from your child's face and merely misting the medication) doesn't help your child because the medication doesn't effectively enter his or her airways, which is where your child needs the medicine. In order to properly deliver your child's medications, the nebulizer must work as a closed system, with the mask fitting snugly on your child's face, covering both the nose and mouth.

As with many other situations that involve very young children, you can use music, appropriate toys, a special cartoon video, or other types of entertainment as a helpful distraction for your little one.

If all else fails, remain firm and steady, and make sure that your child receives the necessary medicine. Even the smallest infants ultimately learn that nebulizer treatments make them feel better. Eventually, that realization makes the time you spend administering nebulizer therapy more effective, comfortable, and rewarding for both you and your child.

Treating toddlers (ages 2 to 5 years): Medication challenges

Few medications are available in the U.S. for children ages 2 to 5 years. The FDA has recently approved the use of montelukast (Singulair), a leukotriene modifier (see Chapter 12), in a 4 milligram chewable tablet, for use in this age group. However, inhaled topical corticosteroids and long-acting inhaled beta$_2$-adrenergic (beta$_2$-agonist) bronchodilators (or non-sedating antihistamines for allergic rhinitis) are not specifically formulated for children under 4 years. Therefore, nebulizer use can be extremely important during the toddler and early school-age years (see Figure 14-1).

The lack of specific medications for children under age 4 is a serious concern for doctors and parents. This age group has experienced the highest increases in asthma rates in recent years yet is the last group to receive attention in the development of new asthma medications.

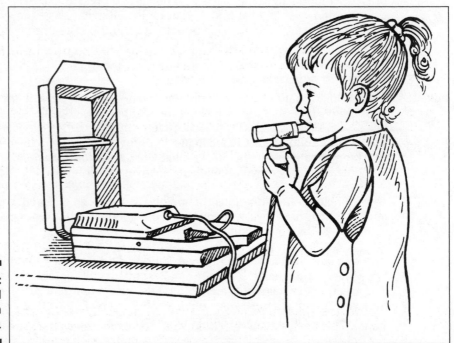

Figure 14-1:
Young child
using a
nebulizer.

Kids are people, too!

Conducting clinical trials with young children — especially those under 4 years — is very costly and time-consuming compared to clinical trials involving children over 12 years and adults. Because of the great need for pediatric patient participation, I believe that more parents of asthmatic infants and toddlers need to volunteer with their children for clinical trials. Doing so can help develop new and better medications that benefit all children. In addition, you and your child will probably learn a great deal about asthma and its management, and I'm sure you'll love all the attention you'll receive while participating in these studies. Pharmaceutical companies also need to make a commitment to conduct trials for younger children; these trials may cost more and prove difficult, but the lives and health of young children depend on such studies.

Fortunately, the U.S. Congress has recently established a program of incentives to encourage pharmaceutical manufacturers to conduct clinical trials of medications, including those for asthma, in the pediatric age group. In fact, recent FDA regulations require pharmaceutical companies to submit detailed plans for studying formulations specifically for children (for example, syrups and chewable tablets) when seeking approval for development of new drugs. Hopefully, this program will lead to improved medical treatments for young children with asthma and other allergic diseases.

Because very few effective asthma medications have gone through the drug development process for FDA approval for use with children under 4 years of age, many doctors prescribe drugs that haven't been studied extensively for use in that age group. Therefore, determining the appropriate dosages of asthma medications for toddlers can prove challenging. Children react differently to medications than do adults, and determining the correct dosage for children isn't as simple as assuming that the toddler receives half of an adult dose.

Peak flow meters and school-age children (ages 5 to 12)

By the time children reach age 5, they can generally use a peak flow meter at home. This device allows you and your doctor to assess the state of your school-age child's lungs. Using a peak flow meter each morning and night can help you and your child manage his or her asthma in the following ways:

- ✔ Provide an objective way of tracking your child's response to his or her asthma medications.

- ✔ Enable you to discuss your child's condition in terms of specific criteria, thus enhancing communication between you and your child's doctor.

✔ Teach both you and your child about what works in terms of treatment and which triggers may cause problems.

✔ Warn you and your child that an asthma episode looms near. Establishing your child's personal best peak flow rate enables you and your child to tell when problems occur, because you can note when the rate goes down according to the green, yellow, and red zones of the peak flow zone system.

For more information on using peak flow meters, turn to Chapter 13.

Teens and asthma: Using inhalers

Many teens with asthma feel different and insecure because of their disease. Unfortunately, adolescent anxieties about fitting in and being cool can result in teen asthmatics ignoring or not properly managing their disease. In some cases, adolescents may even allow their symptoms to worsen rather than simply taking a whiff or two from their inhalers.

To avoid these types of potentially dangerous asthmatic situations, allow your teenager a voice in the management of his asthma. Depending on the severity of your adolescent's asthma, your doctor and teenager can work together to develop a plan for adjusting medication therapy in order to control symptoms, thus avoiding serious episodes that may seem especially embarrassing for a teen. Some asthma medications last 12 hours (see Chapter 12) and therefore your adolescent can use them at home in the morning and the evening, minimizing the need for your teen to be seen using medication while at school.

Your child may also benefit from participating in a support group with other teenage asthmatics. Above all, I believe that encouraging open and honest discussions with children about their conditions, to ensure that they feel better informed and more respected, is vital to their asthma treatment and maintenance. Participation in setting goals for therapy, developing a treatment plan, and reviewing its effectiveness can also help teenagers build a positive self-image, increase personal responsibility, and gain problem-solving skills, thus making them more likely to make better decisions about managing their condition.

Asthma at School and Day Care

If your child has asthma, inform the teachers, administrators, and school nurse about your child's condition. Some schools and day care centers institute asthma management programs that provide the following:

✔ Policies and procedures for administering students' medications.

✔ Specific actions for staff members to perform within the program. These may include establishing clear policies on taking medications during school hours, designating one person on the school staff to maintain each student's asthma plan, and generally working with parents, teachers, and the school nurse (if one is available) to provide the most support possible for students with asthma, especially so they can have access to medications they may need while at school.

✔ An action plan for treating students' asthma episodes.

Whether or not the school or day care center administers such a program, I advise taking the following steps to insure that your child's school days are as healthy, safe, and fulfilling as possible:

• Meet with school staff to inform them about any medications your child may need to take while on campus, as well as any physical activity restrictions that your doctor may advise. (Properly managing their condition allows most children with asthma to participate in sports and physical education classes.)

• File treatment authorization forms with the school office and discuss what school personnel must do if your child suffers an asthma emergency. Also, provide instructions on how to reach you and your child's physician in the event of an emergency.

• Inform school personnel of allergens and irritants that can trigger your child's asthma symptoms and request that the school remove the sources of those triggers, if possible.

Make sure your child understands that everyone's asthma is different and that asthma medications shouldn't be shared. Exchanging asthma medications among kids can cause dangerous problems because individual prescriptions vary according to the severity of each child's asthma and other factors.

Don't let children use each other's inhalers, because doing so can also spread potential infections, such as colds and flu. Chapter 12 contains specific information about asthma medications.

Indoor air quality (IAQ) at school and day care

From about the age of 2, most children spend the majority of their waking hours at school or day care. Therefore, ensuring that these environments are as free of potential asthma triggers as possible is essential to your child's health.

According to the Environmental Protection Agency (EPA), recent studies indicate that indoor pollutant levels can often be two to five times higher than outdoor levels, occasionally as much as 100 times higher. Irritants and allergens that can affect your child at school often include the following:

- ✔ Outdoor smoke, soot, chemicals, pollens, and mold spores

- ✔ Indoor mold from ventilation ducts as well as indoor irritants such as tobacco smoke, scents from printers and copiers, and fumes from heating, ventilation, and air conditioning (HVAC) systems

Asthmatic symptoms related to poor *indoor air quality* (IAQ) may resemble those that you typically associate with colds, allergic rhinitis (hay fever), fatigue, or flu. For this reason, you may not as easily realize that your child's asthma suffers as a consequence of poor IAQ at school and day care. However, the following tips may provide clues that can help you decide whether IAQ is a factor:

- ✔ Many students, teachers, administrators, and other personnel experience similar symptoms.

- ✔ Your child's symptoms (and those of other affected people) improve or disappear after school or day care.

- ✔ Symptoms begin to appear rapidly following physical changes, such as construction work, painting, or pesticide use, at the school or day care.

- ✔ Your child and other people with allergies or asthma only experience symptoms inside the building.

If you think that your child may experience symptoms related to poor IAQ at school or day care, contact an appropriate staff member about the issue. Your child's school (or school system) may staff an IAQ coordinator or health and safety coordinator who should respond to your concerns.

Participating in PE — exercise and asthma

Living with asthma doesn't mean that your child needs to sit on the sidelines. I believe that participating in physical education (PE) and other opportunities for exercise are vital for a child's development, regardless of whether or not the youngster has asthma. Nonetheless, you need to make sure that the school's PE instructors are aware of your child's condition and that they know what to do in case an asthma episode develops.

PE instructors and coaches should encourage your asthmatic child to partici-pate actively in sports, but they must also realize and respect your child's limitations. In addition, extended running and any exercise that takes place in cold, dry air appears to trigger asthma flare-ups, known as exercise-induced bronchospasms (EIB) or exercise-induced asthma (EIA). Exercise is one of the most common precipitants of asthma symptoms that most doctors see in clinical practice. Over 90 percent of patients identify physical exertion as a major cause of their asthma symptoms. Although EIA can develop at any age and occurs equally among adults and children, it is a much greater problem in kids because of their characteristically greater degree of physical activity. (See Chapter 11 for more information on EIA.)

Your child's doctor may prescribe medications to control and prevent EIA (see Chapter 12), as well as advise appropriate warm-up and cool-down activ-ities that can also reduce the risk of EIA. Also, make sure that your child's PE instructors know what actions to take if your child experiences an asthma attack during exercise. Having an action plan in place prior to an emergency can insure that your child receives the proper treatment when he or she needs it most. Part of that plan should include providing immediate access to your child's rescue drug in case it's needed to treat the onset of any acute respiratory symptoms.

As long as your child sticks to his or her asthma management plan, the dis-ease shouldn't preclude your child from enjoying or even excelling at a wide range of physical activities. Consider the example of Olympic Gold medalist Jackie Joyner-Kersee and many other top athletes with asthma, whom many allergists (including myself) have had the privilege of treating.

Goals of Asthma Treatment for Children

With proper medical management and your love, support, and under-standing, your child can control his or her asthma — instead of the disease controlling your child.

The following key points (which I explain in greater detail throughout this chapter) are vital to ensuring that your child leads a normal life in which asthma plays only a small role:

- ✔ A correct diagnosis is vital to your child's asthma management.
- ✔ Make sure that your child receives appropriate and effective medication for his or her asthma.
- ✔ Do your best to limit your child's exposure to allergens, irritants, and other precipitating factors that may trigger his or her asthma.

✔ Develop (with the help of your child's physician) an individualized, specific asthma management plan that you and your child can follow.

✔ Both parents should find out about and participate in managing their child's asthma. Helping to monitor the disease and providing support — especially in the event of severe episodes — helps to ensure the success of your child's asthma management.

✔ Make sure that you, your child, and your child's doctor assess your child's lung functions on a regular basis.

✔ Ensure that your child's school and day care are aware of the particulars of your child's asthma condition.

Chapter 15

Asthma and Allergies during Pregnancy

*I*f you have asthma and you are pregnant or considering pregnancy, here's some good news for you: With appropriate care, the vast majority of women with asthma have uncomplicated pregnancies.

Although treatment issues related to asthma affect approximately 4 percent of all pregnancies in the United States, very few of these cases involve situations that imperil either the mother or the child she carries. However, the potential for serious asthma-related complications does exist if you don't control your asthma during pregnancy.

Uncontrolled asthma can produce adverse effects, both for you and your baby, because the underlying airway inflammation that characterizes the disease affects your breathing. As I explain in "Breathing for Two" later in this chapter, anything that impairs your ability to take in sufficient oxygen is potentially hazardous, both for you and your unborn child.

Therefore, it's vital that you continue treatment for your disease — under your doctor's supervision — with an appropriate and effective asthma management plan that aims for the following goals of therapy:

✔ Maintaining as close to normal lung functions as possible.

✔ Preventing chronic and troublesome symptoms of asthma, such as coughing, shortness of breath, wheezing — especially upon awakening in the morning, and episodes that disturb your sleep at night.

✔ Maintaining near-to-normal levels of exercise and other physical activities.

- ✔ Preventing sudden aggravations of your asthma symptoms, thus minimizing the need for emergency care and hospitalizations.

- ✔ Providing the most effective medication therapy that results in minimal or no adverse side effects.

- ✔ Giving birth to a healthy, beautiful baby. In spite of what some people may think, most asthmatics go through labor well. Although I'm sure it has happened somewhere, in my 20 years practicing as an allergist, I've never seen labor or delivery set off a severe asthma attack.

Special Issues with Asthma during Pregnancy

Although one-third of pregnant women may experience no change in asthma severity levels during pregnancy, another third of expectant mothers suffer from more severe asthma. For the remaining third of pregnant women, their condition may actually improve. In most cases, asthma severity returns to pre-pregnancy levels by the third month after delivery. The severity of your asthma can vary from one pregnancy to another, and there's no way to predict beforehand how pregnancy may affect your condition.

Your hormones and your asthma

For some women, pregnancy seems to trigger asthma symptoms. In fact, you may not realize that you have asthma until the disease shows up during your pregnancy, because the significant hormonal changes your body experiences during pregnancy may cause increased airway congestion.

Your body's hormonal changes can also induce or aggravate allergic and non-allergic rhinitis and sinusitis during pregnancy. These conditions can, in turn, increase the severity of your asthma.

Therefore, you also need to address allergies and related conditions when you're expecting a child. If you have allergic rhinitis (hay fever) or allergic conjunctivitis (both of which affect many people with allergic asthma), you should try to keep those symptoms under control while you're pregnant.

The basics of managing asthma while pregnant

The first step in avoiding asthma-related complications during your pregnancy is to make sure that your doctor properly diagnoses your respiratory symptoms. (See Chapter 10 for more information.)

If the diagnosis reveals that you have asthma, your doctor should help you develop an effective asthma management plan to help control the symptoms of your disease. This plan should consist of specific avoidance strategies, medications, monitoring, and assessment measures. Your management plan should also provide you with steps to take in case your asthma symptoms suddenly worsen.

I strongly advise you to make sure that you (and your doctors) integrate your asthma management plan and any treatment that you may receive from an asthma specialist (such as an allergist or pulmonologist) with obstetric care from your obstetrician, family doctor, and/or primary care physician. A team approach by your physicians helps eliminate the risk of different doctors prescribing different treatments that can, in combination, produce adverse side effects for you and your baby. Integrated treatment can also ensure more effective control of any other condition or complications — besides asthma and related disorders — that you may experience during pregnancy.

Breathing for Two

During your pregnancy, you're not only eating for two but also breathing for two — yourself and your baby. Contrary to what some people believe, the greatest danger to your unborn child is not the preventive (or *controller*) medication your doctor prescribes to help manage your asthma, but rather the adverse effects that oxygen deprivation can have on your baby if you suffer severe or repeated asthma episodes during pregnancy.

In order to avoid adverse effects during your pregnancy, your asthma management plan needs to address the following areas:

✔ Avoiding or at least minimizing exposure to allergens or irritants that may cause asthma flare-ups. In many cases, effective avoidance measures can reduce the possibility of asthma episodes that require you to take additional medications, especially the frequent need for rescue (or *quick-relief*) drugs.

✔ Assessing your condition with appropriate pulmonary function tests to establish benchmark results against which your doctor can compare later tests to determine the severity of your condition.

✔ Treating your condition with appropriate preventive medications to ensure that you adequately maintain your lung functions and that your baby receives a sufficient supply of oxygen. Preventive medications can also minimize the possibility of asthma episodes that may require emergency treatment or drugs.

Mother Nature's milk

If possible, breastfeeding should be offered to all infants for the nutritional, immunologic, and psychological benefits for newborn children. Breast milk, in contrast to cow's milk in infant formulas, may decrease the potential for allergic sensitization by reducing your baby's exposure to ingested food allergens. In addition, breast milk may reduce the incidence of bronchiolitis (see Chapter 14) and infection-induced asthma during infancy, because the baby receives antibodies against viral infections through the mother's breast milk.

Avoiding asthma triggers, allergens, and irritants during pregnancy

During your pregnancy, you should be especially careful to avoid precipitating factors that may trigger asthma episodes. See Chapter 11 for extensive details on asthma triggers and precipitating factors.

If you suffer from allergic asthma, I strongly recommend that you implement (under your doctor's supervision) an avoidance and allergy-proofing plan that limits your exposure to inhalant allergens as well as airborne irritants — especially tobacco smoke.

A comprehensive avoidance strategy should help to alleviate symptoms of allergic rhinitis and/or allergic conjunctivitis that can also intensify your asthma symptoms. Effective allergy-proofing focuses on your home in general and your bedroom in particular. I provide extensive information and tips on allergy-proofing in Chapter 6.

Allergy testing and immunotherapy during pregnancy

If you're already receiving immunotherapy (allergy shots) when you become pregnant, your doctor may advise you to continue with the treatment because, in many cases, it can help prevent allergy attacks that may make your asthma worse. Stopping immunotherapy altogether could result in your symptoms becoming worse, thus requiring additional medication therapy during your pregnancy, in order to keep your allergy and asthma symptoms under control. Frequently, your doctor may advise reduced doses of immunotherapy to minimize potential risks of allergy-shot reactions.

If you are already pregnant and are considering having allergy testing to determine which allergens trigger your symptoms, or if you're thinking about starting immunotherapy, your doctor will probably advise you to wait until after your baby is born before performing allergy testing or initiating allergy shots.

Managing nasal conditions associated with pregnancy

Expectant women often experience worsening of their pre-exisiting rhinitis or develop certain nasal and upper respiratory symptoms for the first time. As with the changes in asthma severity levels that I explain in "Your hormones and your asthma" earlier in this chapter, in many cases these increased or newly acquired nasal symptoms result from hormonal changes that occur only during pregnancy.

Poorly managing these nasal conditions can complicate your asthma and, in severe cases, interfere with sleeping, eating, your emotional well-being, and your overall quality of life. Contending with the unpleasantness of impaired sleep, sneezing, runny nose, itchy eyes, inflamed sinuses, ear infections, and sinus headaches while pregnant is a challenge that you (and your family) want to avoid.

The following sections provide information and tips for managing the most common nasal conditions associated with pregnancy.

Allergic rhinitis

If avoidance and allergy-proofing don't provide sufficient control of your hay fever symptoms, your doctor may advise using nasal cromolyn spray. However, avoid using oral decongestants during the first trimester of your pregnancy. After the first trimester, your doctor may consider prescribing antihistamines such as chlorpheniramine (Chlor-Trimeton) and tripelennamine, as well as decongestants such as pseudoephedrine (Sudafed), depending on your condition and the severity of your allergy symptoms.

Many people treat hay fever symptoms with over-the-counter (OTC) decongestants and antihistamines. But during your pregnancy, you always need to check with your doctor before taking any medications, including OTC products. In many cases, particularly with antihistamines, second-generation prescription products such as Claritin and Zyrtec are actually safer and cause less drowsiness than many of the first-generation OTC drugs.

Vasomotor rhinitis of pregnancy

Vasomotor rhinitis of pregnancy is a nonallergic upper-respiratory syndrome that usually only develops during pregnancy, mostly from the second month to term. The associated symptoms of nasal congestion, nasal dryness, and nose bleeds usually disappear after delivery.

Buffered saline nose sprays can provide effective relief for vasomotor rhinitis of pregnancy . Exercise can sometimes help relieve this condition. If nasal congestion persists, however, your doctor may advise using pseudoephedrine (Sudafed) as a decongestant.

Sinusitis

The incidence of sinusitis in pregnant women is six times higher than in the rest of the population. These often-painful sinus infections can develop as complications of rhinitis and viral upper respiratory infections, such as the common cold.

Sinusitis can trigger asthma symptoms and, in some cases, may complicate your asthma to the point that it doesn't respond to treatment. Poorly managed sinusitis can also worsen to the point where sinus surgery becomes necessary.

To reduce the risk of sinus infections, your doctor may advise using a nasal douche cup, nasal bulb syringe, or other type of nasal wash device at home to irrigate your nostrils with warm saline solution, thus relieving pressure and congestion in your nasal passages. Ask your doctor for specific instructions on using these devices.

If your doctor prescribes medication to clear a sinus infection, amoxicillin is probably his or her first choice, unless you're allergic to penicillin. If you are allergic to penicillin, your doctor may prescribe some type of erythromycin-based medication.

Exercise and asthma during pregnancy

Most asthmatics experience some degree of exercise-induced asthma (EIA), particularly as a result of activities that involve breathing cold, dry air (such as running outdoors). Consult with your doctor to evaluate what level and type of exercise benefits you most during your pregnancy.

Activities that allow you to breathe warmer, humidified air (such as swimming in a heated pool) may be less likely to trigger symptoms of EIA. In order to lessen the occurrence of EIA episodes, ask your doctor about medications that can help control airway inflammation when you exercise and prevent symptoms of this condition. (See Chapter 12 for information on these products.)

With proper treatment and management, asthma doesn't have to keep you from your regular physical activities during pregnancy.

Assessing your asthma during pregnancy

In addition to closely monitoring your lung functions through office spirometry (see Chapter 10 for an explanation of this process), your doctor may also advise measuring your airflow at home using a portable peak flow meter to assess your peak expiratory flow rate (PEFR).

Although PEFR measurements generally don't provide complete information by themselves to fully evaluate the severity of your asthma, they certainly can provide a valuable insight into the daily course of your asthma. (I provide detailed instructions on using peak flow meters in Chapter 13.)

Monitoring your baby's condition

During the beginning of your second trimester, your doctor may use an ultrasound to establish a benchmark for assessing your baby's growth. If your asthma is moderate or severe, your doctor may advise further ultrasound scans during your third trimester.

During the third trimester, weekly assessment of your baby is often recommended. However, if your doctor suspects problems, he or she may need to check the baby's well-being more often. Your doctor should encourage you to record the baby's activity, or kick counts, on a daily basis.

During labor, your doctor needs to closely monitor the baby. In most cases, doctors follow the baby's progress through close electronic monitoring. Also, make sure that the staff measures your PEFR when you're first admitted to the hospital for labor and again every 12 hours thereafter until you deliver.

In rare cases, mothers who enter labor with severe or uncontrolled asthma may require more intensive monitoring, either by continuous, electronic monitoring of the baby's heart rate or relatively frequent *auscultation* (listening through a stethoscope to the baby's heart rate).

Taking asthma medications while pregnant

In general, you need to continue your course of asthma medications through your pregnancy, labor, and delivery. The specific medication plan that your doctor prescribes depends on the severity of your asthma.

The primary goal of pharmacological asthma management during pregnancy is to use the minimum level of medication necessary — with minimal risk of adverse side effects — to control the underlying airway inflammation.

The preferred medications for treatment of asthma while pregnant are:

✔ Inhaled products that deliver the drug directly to your airway in higher, and thus more effective, concentrations than oral medications. Inhaled drugs also reduce the risk of systemic side effects. To find out more about asthma medications, their use, and their side effects, turn to Chapter 12.

✔ Drugs that have a long history of safe use in pregnant women and have been studied extensively in published clinical trials.

The drugs your doctor prescribes in order to safely control your asthma during pregnancy could include the following:

✔ In all asthma cases, your doctor should prescribe an inhaled $beta_2$-adrenergic ($beta_2$-agonist) bronchodilator to use in case your asthma symptoms suddenly worsen, or preventively as needed prior to exercise.

✔ For mild asthma, occasionally using inhaled $beta_2$-adrenergics usually suffices for asthma control. In some cases, your doctor may also recommend regularly using inhaled cromolyn sodium (Intal).

✔ If your asthma symptoms primarily show up at night, your doctor may advise that you use sustained-release theophylline or a long-acting oral or inhaled $beta_2$-adrenergic to control your condition.

✔ Mild to moderate persistent asthma usually requires a regimen of constant preventive doses of inhaled topical corticosteroids, sometimes in combination with a long-acting bronchodilator. In milder cases, your doctor may prescribe theophylline, as well as cromolyn sodium, as alternate choices. However, in more severe cases, you may require short bursts of oral prednisone if a combination of bronchodilators, inhaled topical corticosteroids, and cromolyn sodium fails to keep your asthma symptoms under control.

✔ Managing severe persistent asthma may require higher doses of inhaled topical corticosteroids, often in combination with long-acting bronchodilators. Maintaining this aggressive regimen usually allows your doctor to minimize your use of oral corticosteroids.

✔ In rare cases of uncontrolled asthma during pregnancy, you may require an alternate-day or single-daily morning dose of oral corticosteroids to reestablish control of your symptoms. Make sure that an asthma specialist, in consultation with an obstetrician who specializes in high-risk pregnancies, monitors this course of medication. As soon as your symptoms are under control, your doctors should taper off the dosage of oral corticosteroids and gradually replace them with the regular use of inhaled topical corticosteroids to reduce the risk of adverse side effects to you or your baby.

Handling asthma emergencies while pregnant

Your doctor should instruct you how to recognize the signs of worsening asthma and how to treat these episodes early with appropriate medications. Also, make sure that you can tell when a deteriorating situation may require emergency medical attention, and know what you need to do if that happens. (Chapter 10 provides details on the emergency management of asthma.)

The most important points to keep in mind when dealing with an asthma emergency during pregnancy are:

- ✔ If you're exposed to any allergens or irritants (especially tobacco smoke), get away from those allergy triggers as quickly as possible. Otherwise, your condition may deteriorate.

- ✔ Even if you have days when you're feeling better, don't stop taking your preventive medications during your pregnancy, unless your doctor instructs otherwise.

- ✔ If your symptoms worsen, don't resort to frequently overusing your $beta_2$-adrenergic ($beta_2$-agonist) inhaler. Doing so probably won't improve your condition and may even make matters worse.

- ✔ If your condition doesn't improve rapidly after one or two doses of your $beta_2$-adrenergic inhaler or if your condition continues to deteriorate, seek appropriate medical care, as detailed in your asthma management plan.

Part IV

Allergic Skin Conditions: Beauty Is Only Skin Deep

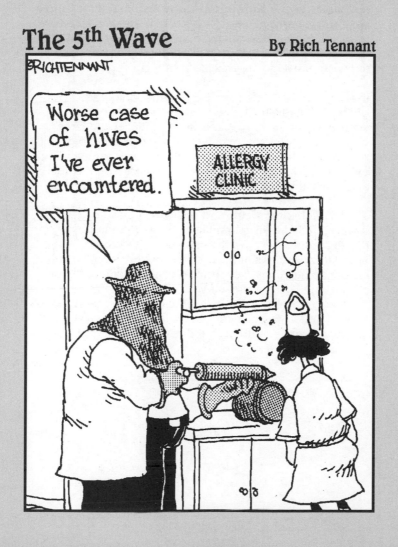

In this part . . .

Whether or not beauty is only skin deep may be a topic for another ...*For Dummies* book. However, the important information that I provide in this part of the book includes advice on dealing with allergic conditions that affect your body's largest organ — your skin.

In Chapter 16 you find out why many people refer to atopic dermatitis (allergic eczema) as the "itch that scratches or the scratch that itches," what may trigger your condition, how to relieve your symptoms, and steps you may be able to take to prevent your eczema from recurring.

In addition to vital tips on dealing with poison ivy, Chapter 17 explains the very extensive range of substances in your everyday life (such as nickel and latex) that can trigger your contact skin (topical) reactions. I also discuss important preventive measures for avoiding exposures, as well as advisable treatments for relieving symptoms if they do occur.

The third chapter of this part deals with urticaria (hives) and angioedema (deep swellings), two of the more perplexing problems known to allergists — especially because most cases of these skin eruptions aren't a result of allergic reactions. Nevertheless, as I explain in Chapter 18, it's important to consult your doctor to determine whether your hives or angioedema may indicate a more serious underlying ailment and to find effective ways of managing your condition so it doesn't adversely affect your quality of life.

Chapter 16

Atopic Dermatitis

• •

In This Chapter

▶ Understanding atopic dermatitis

▶ Diagnosing skin conditions

▶ Preventing outbreaks

▶ Managing your skin condition

• •

*A*topic dermatitis is more than just dry, itchy skin. It can severely affect your quality of life — especially in the case of children who suffer from this condition — and can lead to complications such as bacterial and viral skin infections.

Atopic dermatitis (in Greek, *derma* is skin, and *itis* means inflammation), also known as *atopic eczema* (in Greek, *eczema* means to erupt or boil out) or *allergic eczema* (*atopy* refers to the genetic predisposition to develop allergies; see Chapter 1) frequently occurs in conjunction with allergic respiratory diseases, such as allergic rhinitis (commonly referred to as *hay fever,* as I explain in Chapter 4) and can also precede other allergic symptoms. Therefore, finding out that you have atopic dermatitis can provide the first clue that you're at a higher risk of developing other allergies and asthma.

Key points to keep in mind about atopic dermatitis include the following:

✔ An estimated 15 million people in the United States suffer from atopic dermatitis, and more than half of these individuals already have or will develop asthma or allergic rhinitis.

✔ More than 90 percent of patients with chronic atopic dermatitis are infected with the bacteria *Staphylococcus aureus* (a staph infection), which affects only 5 percent of people who don't have atopic dermatitis.

✔ Approximately 10 percent of infants and children in the U.S. suffer from this skin problem, which can begin as early as two months of age. Atopic dermatitis symptoms often become less severe as you mature, with reduced itching and scratching and lesions that aren't as severe.

> ✔ In children who have undergone double-blind, placebo-controlled oral food challenges (see Chapter 19), milk, egg, peanut, soy, wheat, and fish accounted for close to 90 percent of the food allergens found to worsen their symptoms of atopic dermatitis. In many of these cases, if parents make sure that their children's food allergies are identified — and the children avoid the implicated food — symptoms of atopic dermatitis and other allergies can be greatly reduced and in some instances may potentially stop altogether.

The Body Allergic

Many people think that allergies only affect the respiratory tract (the nose, throat, and lungs), producing the familiar symptoms of asthma and allergic rhinitis. However, the immune system's tendency to trigger allergic reactions when exposed to allergens can show up in other organs of the body.

As I explain in Chapter 1, anything that causes an allergic reaction that triggers the release of histamine and other potent mediators of inflammation is a problem, because these chemicals are at the root of most allergy symptoms. Doctors view atopic dermatitis as a serious medical problem because the allergic reaction targets your body's largest organ — your skin. (Keep that anatomy fact in mind for your next game of Trivial Pursuit.)

The Itch That Scratches or the Scratch That Itches?

Although the heading of this section may seem like a "chicken or egg" question, the hallmark of atopic dermatitis is what doctors call the *itch-scratch cycle*. A related characteristic is a lowered itch threshold, which means that an individual is much more prone to feeling itchy.

These key aspects of the disease can initiate a vicious cycle of incessant itching: The inflammation caused by atopic dermatitis dries out the skin, producing an itchy feeling. This itchiness leads a person to scratch the itch, resulting in more irritation and inflammation, which further dries out the skin, making it even itchier, resulting in more scratching and increasingly damaged skin. Eventually, the skin is weakened to the point where fissures and cracks develop, allowing irritants, allergens, bacteria, and viruses to enter, triggering allergic reactions or causing infections.

Other defining characteristics of atopic dermatitis include

✔ Chronic or chronically relapsing *lesions* (irritated reddening) of the skin. On adults, these lesions commonly result in scarred, thickened skin with creased, accented lines, particularly in areas such as the palms and inside the elbows. These areas can develop a leathery texture.

With infants and children, these lesions may also affect the face, extremities, the creases of knees and elbows, and the trunk and neck areas, but not the diaper area (see Figure 16-1).

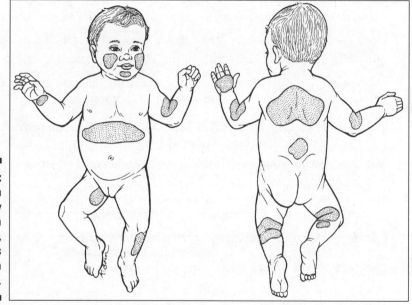

Figure 16-1:
Eczema can affect many areas of a child's skin, as this illustration shows.

✔ Chronic hand eczema may be the most common symptom of atopic dermatitis in many adult cases, but eczema can also affect the neck, feet, and creases of the knees and elbows.

✔ A personal or family history of asthma, allergic rhinitis, allergic conjunctivitis, food allergies, and atopic dermatitis often is associated with atopic dermatitis. However, in cases involving infants or young children, evidence of other allergies may not be as obvious. When diagnosing atopic dermatitis in younger children, doctors may also look for minor signs, such as

• *Xerosis* (dry skin)

• *Ichthyosis* (white, dry, and scaly skin)

• Severely lined palms

- Susceptibility to skin infections, especially herpes simplex (a virus that often causes fever blisters) and *Staphylococcus aureus* (a bacterial "staph" infection that causes *impetigo,* a contagious bacterial skin infection)

- Dry skin around nipples

If your doctor suspects that you suffer from atopic dermatitis, your physical examination also includes an evaluation of the following potential signs and symptoms:

✔ Red and scaly skin, abrasions, and pimples

✔ The extent, location (on your body), and severity of skin lesions

✔ Any crusting or oozing pustules that may indicate infection, scaling, or scarring of the skin around the lesions

Also, your doctor may look for evidence of atopy (allergic conditions) by determining the presence of the following additional signs and symptoms:

✔ Allergic shiners: Dark circles under your eyes that can provide evidence of allergic rhinitis (see Chapter 4).

✔ Dennie-Morgan infraorbital fold: A small skin fold under the eyes.

✔ Recurrent conjunctivitis: Redness over the eyeballs and on the underside of your eyelids, as well as swollen, itchy, and watery eyes (see Chapter 4 for more information on this allergy).

✔ Side effects, such as furrowed or thin, shiny skin, a result of chronic overuse of topical corticosteroid medications. (I explain the appropriate uses of these medications later in this chapter.)

Naming your disorder

Most patients (and even some doctors) often use the terms *eczema* and *atopic dermatitis* interchangeably. However, in medical terms, *eczema* refers more generally to a severe, inflammatory itchy skin condition (sometimes also described as the "itch that rashes") that is one of the most common symptoms of atopic dermatitis as well as other conditions, including:

✔ Skin inflammations, such as seborrheic dermatitis, irritant dermatitis, and contact dermatitis (see Chapter 17). In particular, doctors often need to evaluate patients over 16 with eczema symptoms for contact dermatitis.

✔ Scabies, herpes simplex infections, recurrent *Staphylococcus aureus* ("staph" infection), and HIV.

✔ Psoriasis and other nonallergic, noninfectious chronic inflammatory skin conditions.

If you have eczema, your doctor may advise you to undergo certain medical tests to determine whether the underlying cause of your skin inflammation has an allergic basis or is instead the result of an infectious organism. Your physician may also supplement these tests by taking small samples of a lesion for culture and identification of suspected bacterial, viral, or fungal agents.

Most people with eczema have unusually high levels of total IgE antibodies and eosinophils (see Chapter 2). Therefore, your doctor may further recommend allergy skin testing and/or specific IgE RAST blood testing (see Chapter 8) to identify any particular allergens that may be triggering your skin symptoms

Infant issues

Atopic dermatitis rarely occurs in infants under 6 weeks of age. If a baby has an eczema rash in the first month of life, your doctor needs to evaluate the infant for the possibility of an immunodeficiency disorder. In the vast majority of cases, your doctor isn't evaluating your baby for AIDS (just one out of a whole multitude of immune deficiency diseases) but is instead attempting to rule out other types of diseases, as I explain in Chapter 2.

Other special considerations for infants with skin conditions include

- ✔ **Diaper dermatitis:** This type of skin rash isn't a typical allergic reaction. A skin infection or contact dermatitis is a more probable cause of diaper rash.

- ✔ **Seborrheic dermatitis:** With babies, distinguishing seborrheic dermatitis from atopic dermatitis may prove difficult. If your infant's armpit, diaper area, and top of head (cradle cap) show signs of eczema, *seborrheic dermatitis* is the more likely cause.

Atopic dermatitis and children

The earlier the onset of atopic dermatitis, the more severe the problem. Because 60 percent of patients with atopic dermatitis develop signs of this disease before their first birthday, this condition is especially problematic for parents caring for affected infants and young children. Youngsters with atopic dermatitis often infect their skin by scratching themselves with fingernails that are full of all sorts of bacteria. As any parent knows, kids can get really dirty very fast. Keeping infants and young children from scratching their itchy skin is one of the main challenges in treating and managing atopic dermatitis — they just don't understand why they shouldn't scratch. Later in the chapter, I provide tips on how to break or at least control the itch-scratch cycle — the key to managing atopic dermatitis.

True story

As a child, I suffered from atopic dermatitis, so I can truly relate to children with this type of allergy. Atopic dermatitis is a miserable condition and is an especially serious and traumatic problem for children. I remember scratching incessantly at night. Wearing shorts and short-sleeve shirts was embarrassing because I didn't want people to see the bleeding behind my knees and inside my elbows. Fortunately, my condition improved with age. However, I still have occasional flare-ups of my atopic dermatitis, mostly on my hands and fingers, because my profession as a physician requires me to repeatedly wash my hands, which has a constant drying effect on my skin.

Infants and children who show signs of atopic dermatitis (such as eczema) are often at a greater risk of subsequently developing other allergies. If your child has eczema and other signs of atopic dermatitis, watch out for other types of symptoms, such as coughing, a scratchy throat, or runny nose. Instead of indicating a cold, these symptoms may serve as early warning signs of allergic rhinitis and/or asthma.

Treating Atopic Dermatitis

Successful management of atopic dermatitis requires a systematic, multi-pronged approach based on these key steps:

- ✔ Moisturizing and softening your skin to keep it from drying out.

- ✔ Identifying and eliminating (as much as possible) irritants, allergens, sources of infection, and causes of emotional stress.

- ✔ Using topical corticosteroid preparations, such as hydrocortisone (Hytone), triamcinolone (Kenalog), mometasone (Elocon), and fluticasone (Cutivate) to control the inflammatory symptoms of allergic reactions. Your doctor may also prescribe other medications, depending on your condition.

The only way to manage atopic dermatitis is to control the itching. To illustrate this point, I often ask parents of children with atopic dermatitis to compare the appearance of their children's arms and legs with their backs. Although your children's limbs may appear extremely scratched and inflamed, their backs usually look far better. (Kids have a hard time reaching around to scratch their backs — if they can't scratch it, they won't damage it.) Therefore, keeping your children's fingernails short, instituting effective topical measures (such as using emollient soaps and moisturizers), and administering prescribed topical and/or oral medications are all essential to help control itching and keep the scratching damage to a minimum.

Moisturizing your skin

The first line of defense against atopic dermatitis is maintaining moist skin. In many cases, making sure that your skin doesn't dry out provides dramatic relief of your symptoms. I suggest developing a regular routine of skin care that includes taking baths with products that help your skin absorb moisture and applying creams and ointments immediately after bathing to lubricate and moisturize your skin. An effective skin moisturizing routine may also reduce your need for topical corticosteroid medications.

One of the simplest and most effective ways to relieve symptoms of atopic dermatitis is to take lukewarm soaking baths for 20 to 30 minutes. Avoid hot baths or showers because the heat increases itching and skin dryness.

Keep these other points in mind when bathing:

- ✔ Adding oatmeal (Aveeno) or baking soda to your bath water may provide a soothing effect, but doing so won't help moisturize your skin.

- ✔ Use mild bar soap (Dove, Basis) or a non-soap cleanser with neutral pH (Cetaphil). Avoid using bubble bath or bath oils because they can form a barrier that prevents the bath water from moisturizing your skin. If you find oil especially soothing, add it to your bath after you get in the water to seal in the moisture.

- ✔ Dry yourself gently by patting your skin with a soft towel; avoid rubbing briskly.

- ✔ Apply emollient cream (Eucerin, Aquiphor) or lotion (Keri) to retain your skin's moisture within three minutes after drying off. Even Crisco shortening has been used effectively as an inexpensive moisturizer.

I strongly advise against using lotions with high water or alcohol content because these products usually evaporate quickly, leaving your skin dry. Likewise, avoid lotions and creams that contain preservatives, solubilizers, fragrances, and astringents because these ingredients can dry and irritate your skin. Check the label to see whether the product contains these ingredients.

Avoiding triggers of atopic dermatitis

As with other allergic conditions, avoidance is a vital aspect of effectively managing atopic dermatitis. Although you may not be able to eliminate or avoid all allergy triggers and irritants in your environment, taking reasonable steps to identify, eliminate, and avoid factors that worsen or aggravate your atopic dermatitis can often provide enough relief to substantially improve your quality of life.

Irritants

In addition to the common irritants of asthma, allergic rhinitis, and sinusitis, which I list in Chapter 7, you also need to avoid materials, substances, and conditions that can trigger the scratch-itch cycle. Materials and situations to avoid include

- **Abrasive clothing:** I usually advise patients to wear open-weave, loose-fitting cotton or cotton-blend clothes. I also suggest laundering new clothes before wearing them to get as many of the chemicals, especially formaldehyde, out of the fabric as possible.

- **Detergent:** Avoid residual detergent in laundered clothes. Try using liquid detergent and adding a second rinse cycle to remove more detergent during washing.

- **Temperature extremes:** In winter, an area humidifier can help keep your skin from drying out and cracking, especially if your home has central heating. In the summer, use air conditioning to maintain a comfortable climate indoors and to remove excess humidity.

- **Sports:** Avoid conditions or activities that involve heavy perspiration, intense physical contact, or heavy clothing. However, children with atopic dermatitis need to remain as normally active as possible. Swimming may serve as an acceptable activity, although children should learn to rinse the chlorine off as soon as they get out of the pool and to apply moisturizer to their skin immediately after drying.

Sunlight can benefit people with atopic dermatitis as long as you don't get a sunburn, overheat, or perspire excessively. However, make sure that you use sunscreen when you expose yourself to the sun. Because sunscreens can irritate your skin, find one that doesn't trigger your atopic dermatitis symptoms.

Allergens

Inhalant allergens such as pollens, molds, dust, and animal dander, which are common triggers of allergic rhinitis, can sometimes trigger symptoms of atopic dermatitis. (I provide an extensive survey of these allergens in Chapter 5.) Key points to keep in mind about inhalant allergens and atopic dermatitis include the following:

- Some patients experience atopic dermatitis symptoms that worsen with seasonal changes, which inhalant allergens, such as ragweed pollen, may cause.

✔ Exposure to dander (especially from household pets), dust mites, and molds may cause perennial atopic dermatitis symptoms. If your symptoms worsen (especially around your face and head) during the night while you sleep, dust mites (see Chapter 5) may be the problem. Consider taking steps to allergy-proof your home, or at least your bedroom, against these microscopic creatures. (See Chapter 6 for avoidance and allergy-proofing steps, as well as more dust mite details.)

Infections

Skin infections and complications can recur regularly with atopic dermatitis. Common infectious agents include herpes simplex (viral), *Staphylococcus aureus* (bacterial), scabies (mite infestation), and *dermatophyte* (fungal) infections. The keys to avoiding these infections are breaking the itch-scratch cycle and maintaining well moisturized skin.

Stress

We all have times when we let upsetting events and pressures get to us. However, if you have atopic dermatitis, feelings of frustration, embarrassment, anger, and hostility may lead you to scratch more, thus worsening your skin's condition.

Professional counseling can help you if your state of mind adversely affects your ability to manage atopic dermatitis.

Taking medications

If your symptoms don't improve as a result of the self-care and avoidance measures that I describe earlier in this chapter, or if your eczema is severe, your doctor may prescribe specific medications to treat your condition.

Topical corticosteroids

Topical corticosteriod medications, applied directly to the affected skin area, are a mainstay of eczema treatment because of their anti-inflammatory action. Doctors currently use seven classes of topical corticosteroids (ranked according to strength, as I explain in Table 16-1) to treat symptoms of atopic dermatitis. These products are available in cream, ointment, and lotion forms. You should keep the following in mind when using topical corticosteroids to treat atopic dermatitis:

✔ Your doctor should instruct you on the proper and safe application of topical corticosteroids. In general, avoid using high-potency preparations on your face, eyelids, armpits, or genital areas. For those areas, use low-potency topical corticosteroids.

✔ Your doctor should prescribe high-potency topical corticosteroids only for a short time and only for use on scarred and thickened skin areas. A two- to three-week course of a low-potency medication generally follows your high-potency prescription.

✔ Use topical corticosteroids with emollients to help keep your skin moisturized.

✔ The lowest potency topical corticosteroid at the lowest dosage that will control your atopic dermatitis symptoms is the preparation that you should use, based on your doctor's recommendation.

Table 16-1   Topical Corticosteroid Classes Ranked from Highest Potency (Group 1) to Lowest Potency (Group 7)

Potency	Active Ingredient	Formulation	Brand Name
Group 1	Clobetasol	0.05% ointment/cream	Temovate
	Betamethasone	0.05% ointment/cream	Diprolene
Group 2	Mometasone	0.1% ointment	Elocon
	Halcinonide	0.1% cream	Halog
	Fluocinonide	0.05% ointment/cream	Lidex
	Desoximetasone	0.25% ointment/cream	Topicort
Group 3	Fluticasone	0.005% ointment	Cutivate
	Halcinonide	0.1% ointment	Halog
	Betamethasone	0.1% ointment	Valisone
Group 4	Mometasone	0.1% cream	Elocon
	Triamcinolone	0.1% ointment/cream	Kenalog
	Fluocinolone	0.025% ointment	Synalar
Group 5	Fluocinolone	0.025% cream	Synalar
	Hydrocortisone	0.2% ointment	Westcort
Group 6	Desonide	0.05% ointment/cream/lotion	DesOwen
	Alclometasone	0.05% ointment/cream	Aclovate
Group 7	Hydrocortisone	2.5% and 1% ointment/cream	Hytone

Before using topical corticosteriods with children, make sure that your doctor explains the potential adverse side effects. In some cases, highly potent topical corticosteroids may be absorbed through the skin into the blood circulation. This can potentially suppress the function of adrenal glands, particularly in children (due to their thinner skin), resulting in rare cases in a reduced rate of growth. Local side effects, at the site of application, can include skin *atrophy* (thinning), stretch marks, and infections. The base used in some types of topical corticosteroid creams and ointments can also cause skin irritations. Notify your doctor immediately if any of these side effects occur.

Antibiotics

In cases where bacterial skin infections occur, your doctor may prescribe a short course of an anti-staphylococcal antibiotic such as a cephalosporin or erythromycin. You may apply some of the antibiotics, such as mupirocin (Bactroban), used to treat local bacterial skin infections, directly to the affected area as topical preparations, but oral antibiotics are generally more effective and have less potential for causing skin irritiation than topical antibiotic preparations.

If your skin infections don't respond to antibiotics, herpes or some other type of viral infection may be the underlying cause. In such cases, your physician may refer you to a dermatologist to diagnose your condition.

Antihistamines

When chemical mediators such as histamine are released into the skin, they act directly on nerve endings and initiate a series of events that result in the sensation that the brain translates into itching. Because antihistamines competitively inhibit or block the action of histamine on receptor sites in the skin, these medications can be useful in controlling symptoms of itchiness by reducing the underlying skin inflammation.

Although some relief of itching is associated with first-generation antihistamines (such as Benadryl), I usually prefer to prescribe non-sedating second-generation antihistamines — instead of over-the-counter (OTC) sedating antihistamines — so that patients don't have to deal with drowsiness on top of their atopic dermatitis symptoms. Many patients handle the non-sedating products well and have no problems sleeping at night.

However, if my patient can't sleep because of the severity of his or her atopic dermatitis symptoms (for example, intense itching), I may take advantage of the drowsy side effects of OTC antihistamines by prescribing an a.m./p.m. dosing regimen: at night, a sedating antihistamine; during the day, a non-sedating one (see Chapter 8 for more information on allergy medications). Taking an OTC antihistamine such as Benadryl in the evening may help my patient relax and sleep (the active ingredient in Benadryl is the same ingredient as in many sleep preparations), thus breaking the itch-scratch cycle (at least at night). During the day, I prescribe a non-sedating antihistamine, such as Allegra or Claritin, or a less sedating one, such as Zyrtec, to keep allergic reactions under control while still enabling my patient to remain active and alert. However, I always caution my patients in these cases that the sedative side effects of the first-generation OTC antihistamine may still persist during the day.

Coal tar

Back in the old days (even before my time), coal tar preparations made from crude coal tar extracts were a mainstay of atopic dermatitis treatment. Although doctors don't use these older preparations much anymore (especially since the development of topical corticosteroids), you can find newer, less-odorous coal tar products that effectively control itching and skin inflammation. In fact, some patients prefer to use coal tar medications as compounds in ointments or creams, such as 5 percent LCD (Liquor Carbonis Detergens), often reducing the need for more potent topical corticosteroid preparations. For example, in cases of scalp eczema, some doctors recommend tar shampoos (T/Gel, Ionil-T) as an effective treatment.

Don't apply tar preparations on newly inflamed skin, your face, or other areas exposed to sunlight. Doing so can cause further inflammation and occasional photosensitivity reaction (see Chapter 17). Although the new coal tar preparations don't stain as much as the older products, be careful when using them near clothing, especially white or light-colored garments. Some doctors recommend that you use the preparation at bedtime and then wash it off in the morning so you don't have to worry about odor or staining during the day.

Dealing with special cases

Your atopic dermatitis condition may require other, more specialized forms of treatment than the ones I describe in the chapter. Your doctor may prescribe some of the following treatments for difficult-to-manage atopic dermatitis:

- **Wet dressings:** These dressings can help prevent you from scratching and may also help absorb the topical corticosteroids through the outer layer of your skin. However, overusing wet dressings may result in dry and cracked skin unless you apply a moisturizer. Occasionally, your doctor may advise using an occlusive (barrier) dressing such as Saran wrap, for short periods of time, to prevent evaporation of the preparation. Only apply these medications with dressings under your physician's supervision, and only use this type of treatment if you suffer from severe and chronic types of atopic dermatitis.

- **Oral corticosteroids:** If you suffer from severe atopic dermatitis, you may require a short course of oral corticosteroids. However, you need to taper off the dosage of oral corticosteroids rather than stopping it abruptly in order to avoid a syndrome called *rebound flaring,* in which your atopic dermatitis symptoms may suddenly reappear.

- ✔ **Phototherapy:** This treatment, which uses ultraviolet (UV) light, can effectively treat some cases of chronic atopic dermatitis. However, only consider phototherapy if it is administered under the supervision of a dermatologist.

- ✔ **Photochemotherapy:** A recently developed treatment that combines UV light and the drug methoxysporalen is known as *photochemotherapy*. Due to potentially serious adverse side effects, this treatment is only indicated for patients with severe, widespread, atopic dermatitis that hasn't responded to other aggressive therapy.

- ✔ **Hospitalization:** If your case of atopic dermatitis is extremely severe, your doctor may need to remove you from environmental allergens, irritants, and emotional stress to effectively treat your unrelenting symptoms.

- ✔ **Phosphodiesterase (PDE) inhibitors:** These drugs work by inhibiting the production of IgE antibodies and decreasing the release of histamine (see Chapter 2). Ongoing research of this new form of atopic dermatitis treatment shows potential benefit in clinical trials. However, at the present time, most doctors (and insurance companies) don't consider PDE inhibitors standard therapy.

- ✔ **Tacrolimus ointment:** Tacrolimus is currently used in oral and intravenous forms to prevent organ rejection in kidney or liver transplant patients. Researchers have recently developed an ointment containing this drug that has been found effective in reducing or eliminating skin rashes in the majority of patients with atopic dermatitis who were tested. In contrast to topical corticosteroid preparations, tacrolimus thus far appears to have no potential to cause skin atrophy (thinning) and is a highly effective therapy for atopic dermatitis. This topical medication, recently approved for treatment of atopic dermatitis, may potentially be of particular benefit in children, among whom an alternative to the chronic use of topical or oral corticosteroids would be extremely preferable. Therefore, it appears that topical tacrolimus ointment (Protopic) may play an important role in the future treatment of atopic dermatitis and other inflammatory skin conditions, such as psoriasis and contact dermatitis (see Chapter 17).

Chapter 17

Contact Dermatitis

● ●

In This Chapter

▶ Understanding the difference between atopic and contact dermatitis

▶ Knowing whether your contact dermatitis is irritant or allergic

▶ Identifying contact dermatitis causes

▶ Managing skin reactions

▶ Avoiding and treating poison ivy

● ●

*I*f you just realized that the lush riverbank where you caught some rays yesterday was full of poison ivy, poison oak, or poison sumac, then this is definitely the chapter for you. In this chapter, I include important information and tips on diagnosing, treating, and avoiding the many manifestations of contact dermatitis that can occur in everyday life.

Contact dermatitis is a condition that occurs when the skin physically contacts an irritant or allergen that triggers a reaction, usually at the site of exposure. The reaction often produces inflammation, resulting in symptoms such as a skin rash, blistering, itching and burning sensations, and cracked or crusting areas of the skin. According to recent studies, contact dermatitis — in various forms — affects more than 10 percent of the U.S. population; and in the workplace, contact dermatitis accounts for almost one quarter of occupational disease cases.

Classifying Contact Dermatitis

Because allergens and irritants both can cause contact dermatitis, the diseases are classified either as *allergic contact dermatitis* or *irritant contact dermatitis*. Each name refers to the types of triggers that cause your reactions, as I explain in this section. Based on historical, clinical, and patch-test findings (see "Diagnosing Contact Dermatitis," later in this chapter), approximately 80 percent of all contact dermatitis cases are due to irritants, while only 20 percent are directly triggered by allergens.

The key to managing any form of contact dermatitis is identifying the irritants or allergens that affect you and avoiding or limiting contact with those substances, if possible.

Treatment for most cases of contact dermatitis involves using cold compresses and topical corticosteroid preparations for symptomatic relief. I provide more details on contact dermatitis relief later in this chapter.

Irritant contact dermatitis

This condition, the result of direct physical injury to the skin, represents the vast majority of cases of contact dermatitis. Irritating or toxic man-made substances such as solvents, acids, or harsh soaps usually cause irritant contact dermatitis. In addition, direct skin contact with plants that possess chemically irritating sap, thorns, spines, nettles, and sharp-edged leaves — such as creeping spurge, poinsettias, castor bean, buttercup, and certain cacti — can also evoke symptoms of irritant contact dermatitis.

Unlike allergic contact dermatitis, the skin reaction that results from irritant contact dermatitis is nonallergic (*non-immunolgic*) and usually begins shortly after (often within minutes) your initial contact with the offending substance.

In some instances, symptoms occur because of repeated contact and long exposure to an irritating substance, such as detergent (in the case of *dishpan hands*). In fact, irritants are capable of causing contact dermatitis in anyone (whether you're allergic or nonallergic) if the irritants are applied against the skin in sufficient concentration for a long enough period of time.

Allergic contact dermatitis

In contrast with irritant contact dermatitis, allergic contact dermatitis only occurs in that smaller percentage of susceptible individuals who are sensitized to particular contact allergens and who in many cases have experienced prior sensitization.

While irritant reactions tend to occur within a few minutes of exposure to an offending substance, frequently cause burning and pain, and are directly dependent on the dose of irritant to which a person is exposed, allergic contact dermatitis — which is due to an immunologic reaction (see the next section) — typically appears 36 to 48 hours following exposure to the allergen, causes itching more often as a primary symptom, and is much less dose-dependent. That means that if you're highly allergic to a contact allergen, you can have a significant reaction even with exposure to only a small dose of the specific contact allergen. Many substances, such as the resin of *Toxicodendron* plants (poison ivy, poison oak, and poison sumac) as well as latex, formaldehyde, and nickel in the items that you use, wear, or come into contact with on a frequent basis, can trigger allergic reactions in sensitized individuals.

Many people label allergic contact dermatitis as eczema. However, unlike atopic dermatitis and other atopic conditions — such as allergic rhinitis (hay fever), food allergies, and asthma, which can appear in various organs — symptoms of allergic contact dermatitis are local, or *topical,* which means that these symptoms occur only where the allergen touches your skin. Indirect reactions can also occur if your hand or finger initially contacts an allergen and then spreads it to other parts of your body. (See the "Signs and Symptoms" section later in this chapter.)

Understanding Allergic Contact Dermatitis Triggers

In contrast with atopic dermatitis, a family history of allergies doesn't play a role in determining whether you have a predisposition to developing allergic contact dermatitis. In fact, nonallergic people are just as likely to develop allergic contact dermatitis as those people who have other allergies. That's because the human immune system has two general ways of responding when it detects the presence of foreign organisms or substances, including allergens:

- ✔ **Humoral immunity:** Also known as the *antibody response,* this process, which involves the production of IgE antibodies (which I explain in Chapter 1), is associated with allergic diseases such as atopic dermatitis, allergic rhinitis (hay fever), food allergies, and certain drug allergies. The allergic reaction usually begins immediately or very soon after allergen exposure, may target different organs of your body, and can range — depending on the type of exposure and your sensitivity level — from barely bothersome to life-threatening.

- ✔ **Cell-mediated immunity (CMI):** This is the way the immune system responds in allergic contact dermatitis. Doctors also use the term *delayed hypersensitivity* (see Chapter 2) to describe this process, in which allergen contact results in an allergic reaction hours or even days after initial contact. (For example, you may not realize you've contacted poison ivy until your drive home from the weekend camping trip.) Although a delayed reaction is rarely life-threatening, it may take longer to subside or disappear than atopic-condition reactions in some cases. Because CMI allergic reactions don't involve the production of specific antibodies by the immune system, prick-puncture skin tests and allergy shots aren't effective diagnostic or treatment procedures when dealing with allergic contact dermatitis. (See Chapter 6 for more information on allergy tests and immunotherapy.)

A rash of allergens

Allergic contact dermatitis triggers abound throughout the modern world. At least 3,000 chemicals in use today can potentially trigger allergic contact dermatitis symptoms. For this reason, manufacturers are constantly testing new products prior to marketing — especially cosmetics, fragrances, and hair dyes — in an attempt to avoid introducing new items that may cause adverse allergic reactions.

Many of the organic and artificial substances and materials that people use in a wide variety of products and industries (agriculture, health care, manufacturing, and so on) can act as allergens if people become sensitized to them. For example, bank tellers and cashiers who constantly handle large amounts of cash can develop contact allergies to some of the chemicals and ink in bank notes and nickel in the coins that they handle. (Keep in mind, however, that bank tellers handle very large numbers of bills and coins all day long. The possibility that your teenagers may suddenly develop an allergy to the cash that you give them is less likely.)

If I listed all the substances, compounds, and products that potentially cause allergic contact dermatitis, I'd have to call this book *Heavy Book Lifting For Dummies;* that's how extensive the list would be. In the following sections, I provide you with a more concise and practical list of the most common chemicals and substances that can affect you.

Toxicodendron

The *Toxicodendron* family of plants, which includes poison ivy, poison oak, and poison sumac, is perhaps the most infamous source of allergic contact dermatitis cases and frequently causes streaky *lesions* (irritated reddening) developing on skin areas brushed by the plant. (Some physicians refer to this type of allergic contact dermatitis as *Rhus dermatitis*.) In fact, almost 85 percent of the U.S. population reacts to the resin from these plants. At the end of this chapter, I give you more specific information on dealing with these plants.

Latex and other rubber compounds

Although poison ivy may make the headlines, you can find many more allergic contact dermatitis triggers without leaving your home, office, or school. For example, look around you — many items in your environment probably contain latex, which is the sap of the Brazilian rubber tree. Both the proteins in the natural tree sap and the chemicals that are added in the manufacturing process to the tree sap can trigger allergic contact dermatitis. Many synthetic rubber compounds can also act as allergic contact dermatitis triggers.

As many as 14 million Americans experience sensitivity to latex and other rubber compounds, and that number may rise because of the increasing use of latex gloves in the health care and food service industries. Other common latex and synthetic rubber-containing items include

- ✔ Office and school products, such as rubber bands and erasers
- ✔ Athletic shoes and other sports equipment items (rubber handgrips on bicycles and tennis racquets, for example)

✔ Baby and children's items, such as rubber toys, balloons, pacifiers, infant bottle nipples, and disposable diaper fasteners

✔ Household items, including carpet backing, pillows, and cushions

✔ Clothes — especially waterproof apparel, such as raincoats, galoshes and boots, rubber gloves, and the elastic in many types of underwear

✔ Medical products (such as surgical gloves, face masks, adhesive bandages, hot water bottles, intravenous tubing, catheters, and syringes)

✔ Contraceptives, such as condoms and diaphragms

For most of the products in the previous list, you can find non-latex alternatives. For example, you can use gloves made of vinyl or Tactylon (a form of plastic) as a common substitute for latex gloves. However, if finding rubber-free products is expensive, impractical, or inconvenient, you may want to consider *patch testing* (see the "Patch testing" section later in this chapter) to confirm that natural rubber is actually triggering your dermatitis. Likewise, you may also want to check whether other rubber chemicals such as those in the thiuram group (commonly used in adhesives and disinfectants) or those in the thiourea group (used in detergents and photocopy paper) may also trigger your skin reaction due to allergic contact dermatitis.

Many fungicides, wood preservatives, anticorrosion agents, surgical dressings, plastics, and adhesives contain non-latex rubber compounds that can also trigger allergic contact dermatitis. These substances often affect workers in health, plastics, chemical, and agriculture industries.

In addition to triggering symptoms of allergic contact dermatitis, *natural rubber latex* (NRL) proteins can attach to the corn starch powder that is used in some latex gloves and can subsequently trigger immediate and serious systemic allergic reactions in susceptible individuals. Doctors refer to this reaction as *Type I IgE-mediated immediate hypersensitivity* (see Chapter 2). This type of systemic reaction occurs from inhaling latex allergen particles in the air, affecting organs other than the skin. Symptoms can include runny nose, sneezing, itchy eyes, scratchy throat, coughing, and in severe cases, wheezing and difficulty breathing, similar to an asthma attack. Widespread hives and angioedema (deep swellings) can also result, possibly progressing to *anaphylaxis* (a potentially life-threatening reaction that affects many organs simultaneously) in some individuals.

If you notice these sorts of nasal or respiratory symptoms when you are exposed to latex, have your doctor check it out. You may be suffering from a more serious type of allergic condition. A history of hand dermatitis from wearing rubber gloves may also be a warning sign of latex sensitivity.

If you have experienced a previous systemic reaction to latex, you should take active measures to avoid future exposure to the substance. Make sure that you notify (in writing) all your health care providers — including your dentist and pharmacist — of your immediate hypersensitivity to latex. I also advise you to remind these professionals of your allergy every time you visit their offices.

If your occupation (in the U.S.) exposes you to latex — for example, by using latex gloves (as a health care worker) or by breathing latex dust as a result of being directly involved in the manufacturing process — you should read recent advisories from the U.S. Occupational Safety and Health Administration (OSHA), which provide you and your employer with guidelines on how to reduce unnecessary exposure to NRL proteins on the job. OSHA bulletins are usually posted in workplaces and can be requested from your local state OSHA office or from the U.S. Department of Labor, Occupational Safety & Health Administration, Office of Public Affairs - Room N3647, 200 Constitution Avenue, Washington, D.C. 20210; (202) 693-1999; www.osha.gov/.

Nickel

Remember what I told you about cashiers who develop allergen sensitivities because of the number of coins that they handle? (See the introductory text in this chapter.) The source of the bank tellers' allergy reactions is nickel, a metallic element that you can find in many of the objects that you touch in your daily life. Allergic reactions to nickel can include an eczema-type rash, itching, and hive-like skin eruptions. The following is more than five cents' worth of important information about nickel:

- At least 10 percent of the U.S. population suffers from a sensitivity to nickel. This sensitivity is ten times more common in women than in men, because women usually wear more costume jewelry than men and generally start wearing it at an earlier age. However, men are more likely to suffer from *occupational* contact dermatitis involving nickel because they are more likely than women to work in fields such as mining, engineering, construction, and as jewelers.

- Ear piercing plays a significant role in the development of an allergic condition from nickel exposure. In many cases, people who suffer from a nickel allergy display scars or eczema around their ear lobes, because many earrings and earring posts contain nickel.

- Other forms of jewelry that contain nickel can also produce allergic skin reactions, such as clasps, fasteners, belt buckles, buttons and rivets on jeans, snaps, and eyeglass frames. Your perspiration leaches nickel out of these objects, allowing the skin to absorb the element and trigger a rash. A common nickel reaction often occurs on the wrist, under your watch.

- Coins, pocket knives, keys, and cigarette lighters and cases that you carry in your pants pockets can produce skin eruptions on your thighs.

- Mascara, eyeshadow, and eye pencils often contain nickel and can therefore cause facial dermatitis in sensitized individuals.

- Other typical sources of nickel contact include door handles, doorknobs, drawer handles, bicycle handlebars, shoe buckles, kitchen utensils and cookware, scissors, knitting needles, umbrellas, and many stationery items such as pens, pencils, and paper clips.

If you're sensitive to nickel, one solution may be to wear only jewelry and accessories with higher gold content. (You can tell people that you're allergic to cheap jewelry.) I also suggest wearing a protective layer between your skin and any items that contain nickel. For example, try carrying items such as coins, keys, pocket knives, and so on in a pouch or other enclosure that prevents nickel from leaching onto your skin.

Paraphenylenediamine (PPD)

Paraphenylenediamine (PPD) is a chemical that manufacturers use in dyes, particularly for darker shades of hair color, fur, and clothing. If you suffer from a sensitivity to this chemical, you may also suffer from a cross-reactivity (see Chapter 1) to related chemicals, such as those in stamp-pad ink, sulfa drugs, color film developer, and epoxy resin. Here are some key points to keep in mind about PPD and allergic contact dermatitis:

✔ Hairdressers can easily develop allergies to PPD. In fact, most hair dye labels advise hairdressers to perform patch tests before using their products.

✔ If you're allergic to PPD, make sure that you inform your health providers — especially your pharmacist — because some people with this allergy may also react to sulfa drugs, such as sulfisoxazole (Gantrisin) and trimethoprim-sulfamethoxazole (Bactrim, Septra).

✔ Because of cross-reactivity, topical and injected anesthetics such as Benzocaine and some other so-called -*caines* (Novocaine, Nesacaine, Pontocaine, Butyn, Butesin) can also trigger allergic contact dermatitis symptoms if you possess PPD sensitivities. Other common -caines, such as Xylocaine, Marcaine, Sensorcaine, Carbocaine, and Nupercaine, aren't as likely to cross-react with PPD.

✔ Sunscreens that contain para-aminobenzoic acid (PABA) can cause allergic contact dermatitis because of a cross-reactivity with PPD or can trigger photoallergic contact dermatitis, a related condition that I explain later in this chapter. In both cases, I advise using sunscreens labeled "PF," which stands for PABA-free. (How's that for technical terminology?)

Ethylenediamine (EDA)

Ethylenediamine (EDA) has been used as a stabilizer in prescription topical anti-infective medications such as Mycolog Cream (often used for treating diaper rash) and similar generic products. EDA is also an ingredient in asthma medications such as aminophyilline and in antihistamines such as hydroxyzine (Ataray), antazoline (Vasocon A), and mepyramine. Also keep the following facts in mind about EDA:

✔ Many people use Mycolog Cream and similar generics to relieve diaper rashes in infants and toddlers. However, the EDA in these types of preparations can act as a sensitizer. Asthma patients who are subsequently given intravenous forms of aminophyilline (theophylline EDA), which doctors occasionally use for treatment of respiratory symptoms, can experience systemic reactions, including systemic contact dermatitis (widespread rashes over the entire body) and even life-threatening systemic allergic reactions. (See Chapter 20 for more information on adverse drug reactions.)

✔ Pharmacists who frequently handle antibiotic compounds can develop sensitivities to EDA that can lead to systemic reactions if they take antibiotics internally.

Formalin

As the liquid form of the gas formaldehyde, formalin can cause allergic contact dermatitis on the hands. A wide variety of products, such as the following, commonly use formalin:

✔ **Clothing**: Drip-dry, permanent press, and water-repellent garments, tanned leather and furs, as well as dry cleaning and spotting fluids, include formalin.

✔ **Cosmetics:** Shampoos, soaps, underarm deodorants, bath preparations, mascara, and so on.

✔ **Antifreeze and anticorrosive agents.**

✔ **Paints, paint removers, varnishes, and polishes.**

✔ **Disinfectants, detergents, and household and industrial cleansers.**

✔ **Paper, ink, and photographic developers.**

✔ **Insecticides, fumigants, and agricultural chemicals.**

Potassium dichromate

Chromates can cause allergic contact dermatitis on the hands and fingers of construction workers, who expose themselves to this metal in cement, mortar, plaster, rust removers, boiler cleaner and even in the leather gloves they might be wearing. In some cases, systemic reactions can also occur if workers inhale dust from work materials. Some sensitized individuals experience rashes on the tops of their feet because of contact with the potassium dichromate that manufacturers use to tan shoes.

Other allergic contact dermatitis conditions

In certain circumstances, the allergic contact dermatitis triggers that I summarize previously in the chapter (yes, that was the short list) can also cause related types of allergic skin conditions in sensitized individuals. In some cases, allergic contact dermatitis results from additional factors such as interaction with sunlight, overuse of topical medications, or even contact with your partner. In addition, urticaria (hives) can result from a contact reaction.

Photoallergic contact dermatitis (PACD)

No, photoallergic contact dermatitis (PACD) isn't the result of looking at a photograph of yourself taken on a bad hair day that makes your skin crawl. PACD is a rash or eczema condition that occurs from an interaction (known as *persistent light reaction*) between ultraviolet (UV) light (sunlight) and topical products that contain substances to which you're sensitized. These products can include

- ✔ **PABA:** You can frequently find this substance in sunscreens. However, using sunscreens with PABA can lead to a rash on the face or other skin areas. Because doctors advise using sunscreens to protect your skin from overexposure to UV rays, I recommend always using PABA-free (PF) sunscreens such as PreSun, Ti-Screen, Shade Sunblock, and many others. Check the labels on sunscreens that you want to use or ask your pharmacist for advice on these products.

- ✔ **Musk ambrette:** This synthetic chemical, used mostly in men's after-shave and cologne, can cause an eczema-type rash in reaction with sunlight. If you are sensitive to this substance, I advise using only fragrance-free products.

- ✔ Topical antibacterials such as sulfa drugs and topical antihistamines such as diphenhydramine cream (Benadryl) can also trigger PACD. If you treat a skin condition with these products and you experience eczema reactions when you're in the sun, ask your doctor to recommend alternative medications. If your doctor gives you a prescription for topical or oral antibiotics, he or she should warn you against sun exposure while taking the medication. (See Chapter 20 for more information on drug interactions.)

Connubial contact dermatitis

Connubial contact dermatitis, also sometimes called *consort contact dermatitis,* applies mostly to couples, as the name suggests. While I'm certainly in favor of sharing as a basis for a healthy relationship, sharing everything isn't wise. Although allergies aren't contagious, sharing personal hygiene products and medications can expose you and your significant other to allergy triggers that may not affect the other person.

Connubial contact dermatitis often results from sharing deodorant, hair products, contact lens solutions, skin products, intimate devices, and other items that come into contact with porous parts of the body (including genital areas). Outbreaks of this type of contact allergy usually result in eczema (and sometimes hives) on the face, neck, hands, or genitals.

Contact urticaria

Urticaria is the medical term for hives. Hives can erupt as a result of allergic and nonallergic reactions to a variety of irritants and allergens. In Chapter 18, I cover hives that erupt because of systemic reactions to foods, insect bites and stings, and drugs, as well as to light, water, temperature extremes, and stress and exercise. That chapter also gives you helpful tips on diagnosing and treating hives and angioedema (a related form of skin swelling).

Doctors classify contact forms of hives as *nonallergic* and *allergic*. The following list focuses on the two most common forms of contact hives:

- ✔ **Nonallergic contact urticaria:** This form of hives can affect people who aren't sensitized to an allergy trigger or irritant. With this disease, hives can erupt soon after your skin contacts substances such as insect and spider hairs, alcohol, sodium benzoate, acetic acid, sorbic acid, balsam of Peru, cobalt chloride, and even over-the-counter topical antibiotics such as neomycin (Neosporin) and bacitracin (Betadine).

- ✔ **Allergic contact urticaria:** With this form of hives, the hives may erupt as a result of skin contact with triggering substances in raw potatoes, fish, and liver (yet another reason not to like liver!), as well as substances in antibiotics, natural rubber, epoxy, and treated wood.

Systemic contact dermatitis

If you overuse topical medications (antibacterial creams, ointments, or topical antihistamines), your skin may absorb some of the allergens that these products can contain. Your immune system may then produce antibodies against those allergens. If you subsequently receive an oral or injected form of the medication to which your body became sensitized as a result of previous allergic dermatitis, severe systemic reactions can potentially occur (as I explain in the "Ethylenediamine" section earlier in this chapter).

Because your body can produce antibodies to allergens in skin care products, I advise against applying creams, lotions, and ointments for every minor skin irritation, rash, or itch that occurs. In many cases, minor skin problems may respond well to simple remedies such as cold compresses and commonsense avoidance practices.

For example, if you develop a rash during hot weather and you've been wearing tight-fitting clothes, slip into something looser and more comfortable. You'll probably perspire less, which means that fewer of the irritants and allergens that may be present in your garments will leach out into your skin. Looser clothing probably also means less direct rubbing or pressure on the area where the rash has developed, which should help the inflammation to subside if it's not the result of a more serious condition.

Apply cold compresses before resorting to topical medications, unless your condition lingers, rapidly worsens, or spreads; or if you're experiencing symptoms of a systemic reaction. In those cases, I would strongly advise seeing a doctor. Depending on the nature, extent, and severity of your condition, you may be referred also to a dermatologist or allergist for further evaluation and treatment.

Diagnosing Contact Dermatitis

Often, the cause of your condition is obvious. However, because most of us constantly come into contact with so many potential irritants and allergens — as ingredients or compounds in a multitude of products at home, work, or school — identifying the true cause of your dermatitis may challenge your doctor at times. In fact, you and your doctor may need to thoroughly examine and investigate many aspects of your life to determine what causes your skin condition.

Diagnosing your skin condition may also require a special form of skin testing known as a *patch test*. Patch testing can help your doctor determine whether your dermatitis is due to allergy and which specific allergens trigger this type of allergic reaction. (Read more about patch testing later in this chapter.)

Symptoms and signs

Characteristic signs of allergic contact dermatitis include a red rash, swollen pimples, blisters, and itchy skin. These symptoms may appear hours to days after your skin contacts an allergen, and they usually develop where the allergen touches your skin. As you may expect, the part of your skin that touches the allergen usually shows the most severe inflammation. Very often, the outline of your rash and the location on your body where it appears can provide your doctor with important clues in diagnosing the specific cause of your allergic contact dermatitis (see Figure 17-1).

Your hands can also transmit allergens to other parts of your body, where the rash and other symptoms develop most noticeably. For example, although allergens or irritants in mascara, eye shadow, eyeliner, and other cosmetics can often cause eyelid eczema, an allergen in fingernail polish may cause the problem in some cases. If you're sensitized to an allergen in fingernail polish and you rub your eyes, the rash may appear on both your upper and lower eyelids.

More ways of skinning your dermatitis

The extent and severity of your allergic contact dermatitis reaction can also depend on other factors that you and your doctor need to consider in the diagnostic process, as I explain in the following points:

- ✔ Skin conditions can coexist. In some cases, allergens in topical products that you use to treat eczema caused by atopic dermatitis can trigger allergic contact dermatitis.

- ✔ If your skin is already inflamed or irritated, it may be more susceptible to contact dermatitis.

- ✔ The sensitivity levels of your skin's different areas can vary greatly. The thinner the skin, the greater the absorption of contact allergens. For this reason, in general, your eyelids, neck, and genital areas are the most sensitive, while palms, soles of feet, and your scalp are more resistant to outbreaks.

- ✔ More than half of all cases of contact dermatitis (whether allergic or nonallergic) affect the hands, due to increased exposure.

- ✔ If enough allergens remain on your skin following an initial reaction, flare-ups can sometimes occur weeks to years after exposure.

Variations on a skin disease

Because eczema is a common symptom of many dermatitis diseases, your physician also needs to consider other possible causes of your symptoms. Other potential causes of eczema could include the following medical conditions:

- ✔ **Seborrheic dermatitis:** This condition usually involves eczema around the scalp and nose. With infants, if the top of the head, armpit, and diaper area show signs of eczema, seborrheic dermatitis is the likely cause.

- ✔ **Atopic dermatitis:** As I explain in Chapter 18, this condition often involves a systemic reaction to allergens that can also trigger other allergies such as allergic rhinitis (hay fever). Doctors also often link atopic dermatitis to food allergies.

- ✔ **Phototoxic dermatitis (PICD):** This nonallergic condition, sometimes called exaggerated sunburn, often results from an interaction between intense sunlight and topical exposure to chemicals in coal tar products, sulfa drugs, and certain dyes. Substances in citrus fruits and celery can also act as precipitants of this condition. Bartenders and other beverage servers who work outside and squeeze limes and lemons into drinks while exposed to intense sunlight can experience forms of PICD (sometimes called *phytodermatitis*), often two to three days after exposure. Symptoms usually include rash, skin swelling, pimples, and blisters.

- ✔ **Irritant contact dermatitis:** As I mention at the beginning of this chapter, this form of contact dermatitis is nonallergic, but symptoms can appear virtually identical to those of allergic contact dermatitis. Irritant contact dermatitis occurs frequently because of the wide variety of substances in our modern world — especially in the workplace — that can irritate the skin.

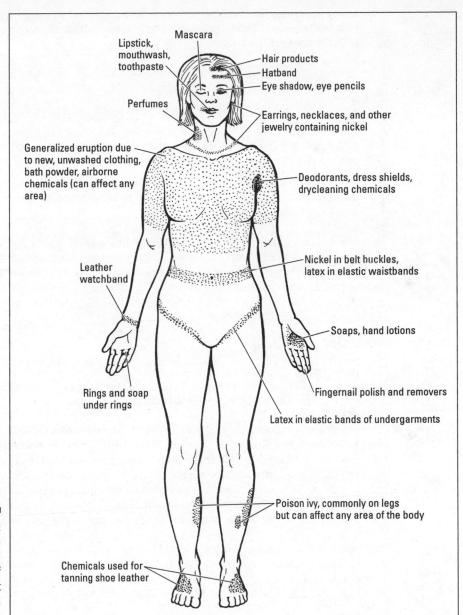

Mascara

Lipstick, mouthwash, toothpaste

Hair products

Hatband

Eye shadow, eye pencils

Perfumes

Earrings, necklaces, and other jewelry containing nickel

Generalized eruption due to new, unwashed clothing, bath powder, airborne chemicals (can affect any area)

Deodorants, dress shields, drycleaning chemicals

Leather watchband

Nickel in belt buckles, latex in elastic waistbands

Soaps, hand lotions

Rings and soap under rings

Fingernail polish and removers

Latex in elastic bands of undergarments

Poison ivy, commonly on legs but can affect any area of the body

Chemicals used for tanning shoe leather

Figure 17-1: Common areas and causes of contact dermatitis.

The skinny on your skin condition

A careful, thorough medical history evaluation is vital to diagnosing the correct cause of your dermatitis condition. Therefore, your doctor may inquire in great detail about many aspects of your life. Your doctor needs this level of information to narrow the range of potential contact allergens

and irritants, from the thousands that you're exposed to every day to the most likely suspects. Try to answer your doctor as thoroughly as possible about subjects such as

- ✔ Your symptoms, your general health, other conditions and illnesses you may have suffered, and your family medical history.
- ✔ Prepare to answer questions about your home, work, or school environments.
- ✔ Your doctor may find other important clues to the nature of your condition in descriptions of your hobbies, recreational activities, and the types of clothing that you wear.
- ✔ Noting the time and place when your symptoms appear can also help your doctor with your diagnosis.

 In some cases, your symptoms may subside before you get to see your physician. In such instances, you may want to take a color photograph — not black and white — of your skin condition (if practical) to show your doctor the extent and severity of your dermatitis.

Patch testing

The most important medical procedure that doctors use in confirming the diagnosis of allergic contact dermatitis is patch testing. This test can also be used to establish the diagnosis of irritant contact dermatitis.

 The patch test involves applying patches that contain small, diluted amounts of suspected allergens directly to the skin. Your doctor uses the results of this test to see whether the applied allergens have caused a small area of allergic contact dermatitis. Think of the patch test process as a miniature reproduction of your skin condition. In most cases, common contact allergens are placed on small aluminum discs and then taped onto the surface of your skin so that several patches with different allergens can all be applied in rows at the same time.

 Your doctor should only perform patch testing after he or she takes a thorough medical examination of your condition and performs a complete physical examination. These procedures enable your doctor to focus on testing the most likely suspects from a list of more than 3,000 substances that trigger allergic contact dermatitis.

 Never agree to a patch test if your dermatitis is severe or widespread. Likewise, your doctor should instruct you to immediately remove any patch that causes severe itching or discomfort.

In some cases, your doctor may ask you to bring materials from your home, work, or school that may contain suspected contact allergy triggers to use in your patch test.

Patch testing is generally done on your upper back in rows, directly onto skin that is free of any signs of dermatitis. In some cases, doctors may alternatively apply patch tests to the upper, outer arm. Each patch contains one suspected allergen, with a corresponding number or letter on the patch that identifies the test substance. The number and types of substances that may be administered in a patch test will depend on what your doctor thinks might be causing your skin problem.

Your doctor will instruct you to keep the patches in place for 48 hours and to avoid wetting them (for example, by taking a shower) during this time period. In addition, while the patches are in place, your doctor will most likely ask you to refrain from strenuous sports or any other types of heavy work or recreational activity that could result in significant perspiration (yes, you can be a couch potato — but only for two days!) Your doctor will also usually ask you to return to the office 48 hours after the patch tests have been applied and will remove the patches and interpret the results of the test at that time.

A positive reaction to the suspected allergen produces small-scale symptoms that mimic your dermatitis condition. Because positive tests can continue producing reactions, these patch test sites are frequently reexamined after 72 hours. Some positive reactions may not occur for 96 hours (four days, in case you're counting) or even one week, as is often the case when testing for neomycin (Neosporin ointment), a common topical antibiotic.

However, because positive reactions can also indicate the presence of other allergic sensitivities — unrelated to your current dermatitis — the patch test results should also correlate with your physical examination and medical history to more conclusively identify the suspected allergen. Experienced physicians know you don't treat the lab results, you treat the patient. Incidental findings that don't correlate with the patient's medical history require further evaluation by a specialist.

The case of the perplexing palm rash

Sometimes a doctor needs to perform some detective work. Here's a case in point: One of my patients noticed a rash on his palms, every week, from Sunday to Tuesday. After determining that the skin inflammation was the result of a form of allergic contact dermatitis, I treated it with a topical corticosteroid cream, and the rash disappeared. However, on the following Sunday, the same type of rash reappeared. After much investigation and questioning, I found that the culprit was the metal rake handle — which contained nickel — that my patient used every Friday and Saturday in his yard. I advised him to use a rake with a wooden handle. Since then, his rash hasn't reappeared (and his yard still looks great!).

Treating Contact Dermatitis

The most effective way of dealing with contact dermatitis in any form — and preventing future episodes — is avoiding whatever causes the problem.

If avoiding the trigger isn't possible or practical, treating the rash and other types of dermatitis outbreaks, as I mention in the next section, with simple home remedies can provide effective relief from mild symptoms.

Doing it yourself

If you experience a limited episode of allergic contact dermatitis, try using cold water compresses. You can make these compresses from any clean, soft, smooth cotton material. Use cool (not hot) tap water or a solution that your doctor recommends, such as Burow's solution, to dampen the compress, and then apply it to your inflamed area. Leave the compress in place for half an hour before removing it. Repeat this procedure two to six times a day, depending on your doctor's specific advice.

If your doctor also prescribes a topical corticosteroid cream, such as hydrocortisone, your compresses facilitates absorption of the cream and can also enhance its anti-inflammatory effect.

In some cases, your doctor may advise you to only use compresses until the skin condition begins to subside. Your doctor may then direct you to discontinue using the compresses and to start applying only the topical corticosteroid cream.

Be nice to your skin. You must keep your skin clean, but avoid using harsh soaps because they can damage your skin's natural protective layer. Likewise, don't overdo bathing (even with gentle soaps), because doing so can dry out your skin, increasing the chance of contacting irritants and allergens that cause inflammation. I recommend frequently (three to four times per day) lubricating your affected area with a lotion or ointment that your doctor recommends. As I explain in Chapter 15, you also need to apply moisturizers immediately after bathing and avoid drying off briskly. Gently using a soft towel to pat yourself dry retains vital moisture.

Turning to medication

The products that physicians usually prescribe to relieve allergic contact dermatitis symptoms include topical corticosteroids and oral antihistamines. In cases of severe symptoms, your doctor may prescribe oral systemic corticosteroids. Likewise, if you suffer from infected skin lesions, your doctor may also prescribe an appropriate course of oral antibiotics.

Topical corticosteroids

Topical corticosteroid products are available in various strengths. Your doctor determines the most appropriate form and dosage for you, however, because different areas of your body may require different potencies, depending on the extent and severity of your dermatitis. Doctors generally make low potency hydrocortisone creams their first choice for the treatment of mild allergic contact dermatitis symptoms. Low potency hydrocortisone creams are also the only products that I recommend using on your face or on the skin of infants and young children. Areas of thicker skin, such as the palms of your hands and the soles of your feet require stronger topical corticosteroid creams. Prolonged use of very high potency topical applications are associated with serious side effects such as systemic absorption and thinning of the affected skin. Therefore, you should use the least potent topical corticosteroid whenever possible. (See Table 16-1 in Chapter 16 for the potency rankings of common topical corticosteroids.)

Usually, your doctor will advise you to apply the product evenly over the affected area. In more severe cases, your doctor may advise using an occlusive (barrier) dressing, such as Saran wrap, to prevent evaporation of the topical preparation and to enhance its penetration into the skin. Although this can be a valuable technique in the short term, use of the occlusive dressing for an extensive period can increase the risk of local or systemic side effects from the use of topical corticosteroids. Make sure that you follow the product instructions and your doctor's recommendations, because topical corticosteroids can cause serious adverse side effects if you don't use them properly.

Oral antihistamines

As I explain in Chapter 16, oral antihistamines can often relieve the itching symptoms that frequently aggravate dermatitis conditions. Depending on the severity of your symptoms, your doctor may prescribe a less-sedating (Zyrtec) or a non-sedating second-generation antihistamine such as Allegra or Claritin. Or your doctor may prescribe an over-the-counter (OTC) sedating antihistamine if you can't sleep at night because of inflammation and intense itching. However, you should be aware that the sedative side effects of these products may still persist during the day.

Severe cases

If you suffer from a particularly acute and extensive allergic reaction, your doctor may prescribe a short course of oral corticosteroids, such as prednisone.

In cases where bacterial infection occurs — usually from scratching itchy rashes and lesions — I recommend using only oral antibiotics to clear the infection. Topical antihistamine and antibiotic products should not be applied because these drugs can actually aggravate the condition by provoking an allergic reaction if a patient is already sensitized to the substances in these products.

For the Love of Ivy

Poison ivy, poison oak, and poison sumac are native to many parts of North America and are widespread throughout the continent. The leaves of these poison plants contain *urushiol,* an *oleoresin* (oily resin). Making contact with the leaves of these plants, in most people who are sensitized to this oleoresin, can cause blisters and a characteristic, streaky red rash with linear lesions on skin areas of the skin brushed by the plant. (Because poison ivy is the most prevalent of these plants, I refer to it alone in the rest of this section.)

Resin reactions

The first exposure to urushiol is what sensitizes most people, but that exposure is usually not enough to trigger a reaction. It usually takes significant subsequent contact for the symptoms to appear. Most people will break out after a second major exposure to poison ivy or after several minor contacts, with symptoms usually occurring within two days.

Toxic transfers

Skin eruptions from poison ivy contact commonly result from the direct exposure of your bare skin to the plants while camping or hiking in the woods. However, other sources of exposure can include

- **Animals:** Pets or other animals (who usually don't break out) that roam outdoors and carry the resin in their fur.

- **Clothing:** Resin can stick to clothes and then transfer to people who touch the garments.

- **Firewood:** If poison ivy grows around your woodpile, or if you gather firewood in areas with poison ivy, the resin may stick on the logs and transfer onto your hands or clothes.

- **Gardening:** Performing yard work in areas with prevalent poison ivy can cause major resin exposure. For example, cleaning out lawn mower clippings can involve contact with urushiol if poison ivy grows in the grass that you mow. Poison ivy resin can also stick to garden tools, such as clippers, hedge trimmers, and rakes.

- **Smoke:** If you burn any of these poison plants, the smoke can trigger reactions if you're especially sensitive to the allergens. Tiny droplets of the oleoresin in the smoke can potentially come in contact with your body and trigger a reaction that may include symptoms affecting your eyes and skin.

Don't scratch that itch

Poison ivy skin conditions themselves aren't really contagious. Frequently the condition appears to spread to new areas of your body for several days after the initial outbreak. Contrary to popular belief, the fluid in blisters, rashes, and lesions does not contain the triggering allergen. Instead, the reason you may continue to experience outbreaks of poison ivy dermatitis is due to the different rates of absorption of the oleoresin by different parts of your body and the degree to which those areas were initially exposed.

However, in some cases, if you don't thoroughly clean and remove all the oleoresin from your hands — and especially from under your fingernails — then you may in fact spread the allergen with your fingers. This can occur by scratching unaffected areas around your existing blisters, thus triggering new eruptions. You could even potentially spread the oleoresin to other individuals (perhaps giving new meaning to the term "nailing them," don't you think?) In addition, scratching your own lesions, blisters, or rashes can also result in skin infections from any bacteria that may reside on your hands.

Avoiding poison problems

Avoiding all contact with poison plants is the easiest way to prevent exposure to the allergens that they contain. If you know that poison ivy grows on your property, you may want to consider killing it, as long as you can avoid exposure to its resin while doing so. Consider hiring a person who isn't sensitive to poison ivy to clean out the plants or do your yardwork. In addition, although poison ivy may be dormant in the winter, the dried vines still contain active oleoresin that can potentially trigger allergic contact dermatitis.

Some people with sensitivity to urushiol may also experience *cross-reactivity* (see Chapter 6) to the peel of mango fruit and the oil from the shell of cashew nuts. The appearance of a topical reaction after peeling mangos is the most common reaction, but more serious systemic symptoms, including nausea, vomiting, and diarrhea, can result if peelings contaminate the meat of the mango. However, mango that has not been contaminated by the peelings can be eaten without difficulty (Let someone else peel it!)

Leaves of three, let them be

One of the best ways of avoiding contact with poison ivy and other related plants is to recognize their appearance. The easiest way to recognize these plants is to look for the characteristic three-leaf cluster, hence the old saying quoted in the heading for this section. However, in winter, poison ivy loses its leaves and is less recognizable, so making yourself aware of the plants' possible locations can also help you avoid their resin's wrath.

Protecting yourself

You can lessen your chances of poison ivy contact by making sure that you expose your skin as little as possible when you're outside in areas where poison plants may grow. You can minimize exposure by following these suggestions:

- Wear clothing that covers as much of your skin as possible. In warmer weather, wear looser-fitting garments and fabrics that breathe. Following these guidelines can help you stay comfortable and avoid the temptation to take off your clothing articles to keep cool.

- Barrier creams such as Stokogard, Ivy Block, and Ivy Shield can provide some protection for exposed areas of your skin. However, check with your doctor before relying on these products because they can lose their effectiveness from perspiration, scratching, and abrasion. These products may not work for you if you plan to play or work extensively in areas where poison ivy exposure is a possibility.

Poison Pointers: Making It Better

If you think you've come into contact with poison ivy or other related poison plants, use these tips to help stop the spread of infection:

- Wash off any part of your skin that you may have exposed. If you wash off your skin within 5 to 30 minutes after contact — depending on your exposure and sensitivity levels to the plant — you may avoid developing a reaction. Soap and water work best to wash off the allergens, but sometimes even water alone can remove much of the plant resin that triggers your allergic contact reaction. If water isn't immediately available, wash as soon as you can to minimize the extent of your reaction.

- Carefully remove and wash (or dry clean as indicated) your clothes, including gloves and shoes, as soon as possible to minimize spreading the resin to other parts of your body or to other people around you.

- If you camp, wash any gear — blankets, towels, sleeping bags, tents — that may have contacted the poison plants.

- To relieve reaction symptoms, apply cold, wet compresses — using a clean, soft, uncontaminated cloth — to the inflamed areas of your skin. Calamine lotion, Burow's solution, and cool showers can also help relieve itching.

- If your face or genital areas are affected, or if your rash is widespread, see a doctor as soon as possible. In severe cases, usually when 20 percent or more of the body is affected, your doctor may prescribe a short course of oral prednisone.

In addition to the tips that I list at the beginning of this section, poison ivy treatment involves using the same medications that you use for other types of allergic contact dermatitis. See the "Treating Contact Dermatitis" section earlier in this chapter for more information.

Chapter 18

Hives and Angioedema

*H*ere's the rub on hives and angioedema: All that itches and erupts isn't allergic. Allergists see many patients with hives and *angioedema* (deep swellings) because almost a third of the U.S. population suffers at some point from these skin conditions and because most people assume that these itchy eruptions result from allergies.

For the most part, however, that assumption is a myth. Allergic reactions trigger only some cases of hives and angioedema, whereas a variety of other causes (which I describe in this chapter) trigger the majority of eruptions. Hives and angioedema are the subject of many myths and mistaken assumptions, as illustrated in the following list:

✔ **I'm breaking out because of my nerves.** If this myth were true, we'd all break out during rush hour, school exams, or when trying to figure out how to pay our children's college tuition. Anxiety and other psychological factors may aggravate hives, but many other illnesses can also worsen when you're under a lot of stress.

✔ **Hives are a minor problem, and they only bother me temporarily.** Hives may bother some people only temporarily, but hives can also develop into a chronic condition that lasts several months or years. A persistent hives outbreak can also signal a serious underlying medical disorder, such as an infectious or rheumatoid disease, which may worsen if you and your doctor don't diagnose, treat, and manage it appropriately.

- ✔ **Only prescription drugs like penicillin cause hives or angioedema.** This statement is simply untrue. In fact, plain old everyday, nonprescription aspirin is one of the most common causes of hives. Contrary to what you may expect — because hives and angioedema are inflammatory conditions and aspirin is an anti-inflammatory drug — you should not, under any circumstances, take aspirin or related anti-inflammatory medications to relieve hives or angioedema. This rule also applies to non-steroidal anti-inflammatory drugs (NSAIDs), most of which contain ibuprofen (Advil, Motrin), ketoprofen (Actron, Orudis), or naproxen (Aleve) as active ingredients. Also, avoid combination pain relievers that include any of these active ingredients.

- ✔ **My hives and angioedema are isolated disorders.** Doctors increasingly consider these conditions as possible symptoms of larger and potentially more serious underlying problems. As a result, more physicians are taking a global approach to the diagnosis and treatment of hives and angioedema. If your doctor can't precisely determine the cause of your eruptions, you should seek appropriate consultation with a specialist (an allergist or dermatologist) to help diagnose and manage your condition more effectively, as well as to make sure that you're not at risk for a more serious disorder.

In the past, medical texts referred to hives and angioedema as "vexing problems." Today, however, both patients and doctors call these related skin conditions *frustrating*. Indeed, for some patients, the search for a cure can seem like an endless journey from one clinic or treatment to another, with little resolution to the problem.

Although allergic triggers play important roles in some *acute* (rapid onset) forms of hives and angioedema, in many instances — particularly with chronic (long-term) hives — the causes of outbreaks aren't clear and appear to be unrelated to allergies. The vast majority of chronic hives and angioedema cases go undiagnosed. Your doctor may refer to undiagnosed types of disorders as *idiopathic* — which means "of unknown cause." (It doesn't mean that your doctor feels like an idiot for not identifying the source of your ailment.)

In most cases, you and your doctor can manage your outbreaks of hives and angioedema so that they don't adversely affect your quality of life. Even though no actual cure exists for many hives and angioedema, your doctor can recommend effective avoidance measures that lessen your exposure to potential causes of your eruptions. You can also use medications to prevent or provide relief from these eruptions. I explain treatment options in the "I Can't Go Out Like This: Managing Hives" section later in this chapter.

Hives: Nettlesome Conditions

The medical term for hives is *urticaria,* from the Latin word *urtica,* which means *nettles.* Indeed, the hallmark of hives is an outbreak of stinging, itchy welts, often resembling inflamed mosquito bites or the result of a close encounter between a thorny bush and your skin. These welts can worsen if you scratch them, and they may develop into *lesions* (a localized area of affected skin). The lesions can grow and run together into large areas, especially if you keep scratching them.

Classifying hives

Doctors classify most cases of hives either as acute urticaria or chronic urticaria. In cases of *acute urticaria,* hives erupt quickly after exposure to triggering allergens or irritants. The outbreaks often subside within two hours and rarely last longer than 24 hours in one area. The disorder usually disappears within six to ten weeks.

Chronic urticaria involves persistently recurring eruptions of hives that last longer than two months. Allergens rarely seem to trigger chronic urticaria, and in most cases, the causes are difficult, if not impossible, to determine.

Hives highlights

Here are other important aspects to consider about acute and chronic forms of hives:

- Children and young adults generally experience most of the acute urticaria cases.

- Upper respiratory viral infections, such as the common cold, are the most common infectious trigger of acute urticaria in children.

- Food allergies cause a larger number of acute urticaria cases in children than in adults.

- Chronic urticaria is more frequent among the middle-aged, especially women.

- Over one-third of patients who experience chronic urticaria for more than six months suffer recurring outbreaks of hives for at least ten years.

- Hive eruptions that persist in the same place on your skin for more than 24 hours may suggest symptoms of a more serious underlying condition, *urticarial vasculitis.* (See "Urticarial vasculitis and other systemic conditions," later in this chapter.)

Angioedema: Getting under Your Skin

In the previous section, I gave you some Latin to help explain urticaria. At the risk of turning this book into *Ancient Languages For Dummies*, here's some Greek for you: *angeion* means "vessel" and *edema* translates to "swelling." Hence *angioedema,* the medical term that refers to a skin condition similar to hives. The main difference between hives and angioedema is that the inflammation from angioedema extends into deeper tissues, resulting in a characteristic swelling of the skin.

Here are more key points that you need to keep in mind about angioedema:

- ✔ Angioedema occurs in deeper skin layers, where fewer mast cells and sensory nerve endings reside. Therefore, the lesions cause little or no itching, and the swelling more often produces painful or burning sensations.

- ✔ Angioedema may involve any part of the body. However, it affects the lips, eyelids, tongue, and genitalia more frequently. (These parts of your body have thinner skin and more blood circulation closer to the surface — that's why you bleed so much when you cut your lip.) In some cases, inflammation from angioedema can cause discomfort and temporary facial swelling.

- ✔ In rare cases, angioedema can cause life-threatening swelling of the tongue, throat, and airways.

- ✔ Angioedema often coexists with hives, but the two conditions can also occur independently. Among adults, angioedema develops in almost half of all hives cases in the U.S. In approximately 40 percent of adult cases of hives, angioedema isn't present. Angioedema that occurs alone (without hives) accounts for only 10 percent of adult cases. However, these types of cases often cause doctors special concern because angioedema that occurs alone can indicate a serious underlying disorder, such as hereditary angioedema (HAE), or it can indicate a severe drug reaction.

What Condition Is Your Skin Condition In?

Hives and angioedema can erupt as a result of different allergic and nonallergic mechanisms, including various irritants, allergens, underlying medical conditions, and other factors. These mechanisms provide the basis that doctors use to categorize hives and angioedema outbreaks, as I explain in the following sections.

Allergic mechanisms: Foods, drugs, and insects

Allergic mechanisms that trigger hives and angioedema are the result of systemic allergic reactions that involve IgE antibodies (see Chapter 2 for more information). The triggers usually include substances in certain foods, medications, and insect stings.

Use the following list to gather more information on the allergic substances that trigger hives and angioedema:

- **Foods:** Peanuts, shellfish, fish, tree nuts, eggs, milk, soy, wheat, and certain fruits are the most significant sources of allergens that can trigger hives as part of an allergic reaction in sensitized individuals. Food additives, including sodium benzoate and sulfites; food dyes, such as tartrazine; and substances in some vitamin products and dietary supplements can also trigger hive eruptions. (See Chapter 19 for more information on food hypersensitivites.)

- **Drugs:** Penicillin, sulfa drugs and other antibiotics, aspirin, NSAIDs, insulin, narcotic pain relievers, muscle relaxers, and tranquilizers can trigger hives and angioedema as part of a systemic reaction if you're sensitized to the allergens that these products contain. (See Chapter 20 for more information on drug reactions.)

- **Insects:** Yellow jackets, honeybees, wasps, hornets, and fire ants (all members of the *Hymenoptera* order) most commonly cause allergic reactions from their stings. Aside from the pain and discomfort of unfriendly encounters with these creatures, the reaction that most sensitized people experience is a variable degree of localized swelling at the site of the sting. However, in some rare cases, *anaphylaxis* (a life-threatening reaction that affects many organs simultaneously) can follow an insect sting or bite. Chapter 21 provides you with more information on diagnosing and treating insect stings, as well as dealing with cases of anaphylactic shock.

Physical mechanisms

Exposure to certain types of light, cold, heat, pressure, and exercise can also trigger reactions that cause hives and angioedema. Doctors refer to this type of skin condition, which accounts for nearly 20 percent of hives and angioedema cases, as *physical urticaria*. Under certain circumstances — depending on factors such as your occupation, activities, and sensitivity to triggering mechanisms — you can experience various manifestations of physical urticaria simultaneously, because different forms can coexist. The most common mechanisms of physical urticaria that have been identified include the following:

- ✔ **Dermatographism:** The name of this skin condition means "skin writing" in Greek (*derma* is "skin," *graphe* is "writing"). The ability to write letters or other symbols by stroking your skin (with your fingernails or a retracted ballpoint pen, for example), which results in *blanching* (whitening of your skin) that's followed by redness and swelling, is the most obvious sign of this often harmless form of hives (some doctors also refer to this condition as *urticaria factita*). Dermatographism affects approximately 5 percent of the U.S. population and can persist for years until the outbreaks disappear. Common triggers for dermatographism include rubbing, scratching, or stroking the skin. Tight clothing or pressure from leaning against hard surfaces (a chair or desk) can also cause this form of hives. A rarer, more severe form of dermato-graphism — known as *symptomatic dermatographism* — can occur following bacterial, fungal, or scabies infections, or after treating a bacterial infection with penicillin.

- ✔ **Cholinergic urticaria (CU):** This form of heat-induced hives (also known as *generalized heat urticaria*) causes at least 5 percent of chronic urticaria cases. In most cases, an increase in your body temperature triggers the eruption. Cholinergic urticaria is especially common among teenagers and young adults. Factors that can cause CU include hot baths or showers, exercise, perspiration, and strongly seasoned foods. The onset of CU symptoms is generally rapid, occurring within two minutes to half an hour of the triggering event. If you suffer from cholingeric urticaria, you may experience very itchy skin, tiny hives, tingling, an elevation of body temperature, or a burning sensation before a rash appears.

- ✔ **Cold urticaria:** In most cases of cold urticaria, symptoms develop at the site that comes into contact with a cold substance, and hives usually develop when the area reheats after removal of the cold substance. Ice cubes typically trigger this condition. Likewise, cold drinks may cause swelling of the lips and mouth. Cold urticaria can cause life-threatening reactions in cases of sudden, total-body immersion in cold water (if you fall into a half-frozen pond, for example). If you have a history of cold urticaria, your doctor may warn you to stay away from all water sports that may immerse you in cold water.

- ✔ **Delayed pressure urticaria (DPU):** As the name implies, this disorder takes time to develop; on average, from three to five hours after a triggering form of physical pressure occurs. Types of physical pressure that can trigger an attack include contact with hard surfaces, wearing tight clothes, or applauding (no, that doesn't mean you should boo — just clap more gently). Likewise, the pressure from shoulder straps of handbags, backpacks, shoulder bags, and other forms of baggage can also trigger DPU.

- ✔ **Papular urticaria:** The characteristic signs of this disorder include small groups of itchy pimples (*papules* in Latin) that often result from insect bites. This type of hives tends to affect the lower extremities more than other parts of the body. Papular urticaria symptoms often persist longer than other forms of hives, too. However, this condition doesn't involve the type of systemic reaction that can result from *Hymenoptera* insect stings. (See the preceding section for more information on the systemic reaction to *Hymenoptera* insect stings.)

✔ **Vibratory angioedema (VAE):** This rare skin condition manifests as an occupational disorder, with severe itching and swelling within minutes of vibratory exposure. Common triggers include vibrations from working in industries and professions such as metal grinding, carpentry, machine and tool making, and secretarial work. Rare cases can also occur from towel rubbing, riding on motorcycles, lawn mowing, bowling, applauding, and walking. Symptoms of VAE develop within minutes of vibratory activity and affect the body surface that experiences the vibrations most intensely.

✔ **Solar urticaria:** Ultra-violet (UV) light can trigger hives in some sunsensitive people within minutes of exposure, causing solar urticaria. Characteristic symptoms include itching, swelling, and hives at the site that receives direct exposure to UV rays. Symptoms may persist from 15 minutes to three hours. When large areas of the body are exposed, systemic reactions can occur, which include coughing, wheezing, shortness of breath, and even a drop in blood pressure.

✔ **Aquagenic urticaria:** The pinpoint hives characteristic of this condition usually result from skin contact with water (cold drinks, however, don't induce this condition — see "Cold urticaria"). The hives from this condition develop around the contact site, are often very itchy, and usually fade within 15 to 90 minutes. This diagnosis should only be made in cases where an individual has a rare positive response to a water-challenge test (hives appear within 2 to 30 minutes after water is applied to the skin) and after all other possible forms of physical urticaria have been eliminated.

Exercise-induced anaphylaxis (EIA)

As its name suggests, *exercised-induced anaphylaxis (EIA)* is an anaphylactic disorder. *Anaphylaxis* (a life-threatening reaction that affects many organs simultaneously) can result from severe allergic reactions, especially due to food, drug, and insect venom triggers. (For more anaphylaxis information, see Chapter 1.)

The trigger factor of EIA is physical activity. Symptoms of this rare syndrome can develop within two to 30 minutes of beginning exercise and usually progress in the following stages:

1. Rash, fatigue, and an increase in body temperature.

2. Eruption of hives and angioedema.

3. Wheezing and other respiratory difficulties, as well as nausea, diarrhea, or dizziness.

4. Severe headache, fatigue, and elevated body temperature. In most cases, all of these symptoms cease within three hours, although your headache can persist for one to two days after the onset of the condition.

As I explain in "Physical mechanisms," exercise can also trigger cholinergic urticaria (CU). However, unlike CU, a hot bath or shower or perspiration doesn't cause EIA in the absence of exercise. Hives associated with EIA are also usually larger than those that erupt as a result of CU. Exercising in hot, humid weather and a family history of allergies both increase the risk of EIA. Food allergies, from eating specific foods too soon before or after exercise, may also play a significant role in some EIA cases. (For more on food allergies and EIA, see Chapter 19.)

Contact mechanisms

Skin contact with certain irritants and allergens can also trigger hives. The two main categories of these types of hives include:

- **Allergic contact urticaria:** Hives may erupt after handling foods such as nuts, fish, shellfish, raw potatoes, and liver. Hives may also result after you contact allergens in antibiotics, epoxy, and treated woods. Contact with latex (in rubber gloves, for instance) may also induce this form of hives, as well as formaldehyde in clothing. (See Chapter 17 for more details on latex and other contact allergens.) Hive eruptions that occur from contact with latex, formaldehyde in new clothing, and handling certain foods result from the direct contact between your skin and allergens in these products. Hive eruptions from direct, topical contact with allergens are more limited than the systemic allergic reactions that you see after ingesting food and drugs, which are more characteristic of widespread hives, as I explain at the beginning of this section.

- **Nonallergic contact urticaria:** This disorder affects people who aren't sensitized to an allergen, but who react soon after skin contact with irritants such as insect and spider hairs (not stings or bites), alcohol, sodium benzoate, acetic acid, sorbic acid, balsam of Peru, and cobalt chloride.

Intolerance reactions

If you have an intolerance — rather than an allergy — to aspirin, NSAIDs, and other anti-inflammatory drugs, antibiotics, narcotic pain relievers, or any medications containing tartrazine (a substance in food dyes), using these products can lead to nonallergic reactions that can trigger eruptions of hives and angioedema. (I explain the difference between an allergic drug response and drug intolerance in Chapter 20.)

Urticarial vasculitis and other systemic conditions

Hereditary factors, such as a genetic predisposition to hives and angioedema, or other medical conditions, including serum sickness (potentially as a result of a delayed adverse reaction to medication — see Chapter 20) or pregnancy, can also cause eruptions. In other instances, hives can erupt as symptoms of a serious underlying disease, similar to the distinctive skin rashes that are characteristic of chicken pox and the measles.

The most significant forms of hives and/or angioedema related to systemic conditions include:

- ✔ **Pruritic urticarial papules and plaques of pregnancy (PUPPP):** This form of intensely itchy hives sometimes affects women in the third trimester of their first pregnancy. In many cases, PUPPP disappears after delivery and doesn't recur with subsequent pregnancies. For further information on medications that your doctor may advise for this condition, see Chapter 14.

- ✔ **Urticarial pigmentosa:** Pigmented lesions that swell when stroked into a cobblestone or leopard skin pattern of hives represent the characteristic sign of this rare disorder. The onset of this condition usually occurs before the age of 3 years. Because urticaria pigmentosa can serve as a warning symptom for *systemic mastocytosis* — a serious disease that can affect the bones, liver, lymph nodes, and spleen — you need to make sure that your doctor examines this type of outbreak. In addition, this form of hives can complicate symptoms of other allergies — especially those involving insect stings and bites — potentially causing severe or anaphylactic reactions.

- ✔ **Urticarial vasculitis:** The hives that erupt as a result of this syndrome — which affects women more than men — can resemble those that result from systemic reactions to food, drug, and insect allergies. Distinguishing symptoms of this disorder include burning sensations, itchy lesions, darkened skin coloring that remains even after lesions clear, and the persistence of individual outbreaks that last longer than 24 hours. These symptoms may indicate a more serious underlying condition such as hepatitis, mononucleosis, thyroid disorder, or rheumatoid infections. In "Diagnosing Hives and Angioedema," I explain the tests that your doctor may perform if you appear to have this form of hives.

- ✔ **Hereditary angioedema (HAE):** The hallmark of this disorder is angioedema episodes that can affect any part of your body and that are not associated with hives. Some cases of HAE can cause swelling of the gastrointestinal (GI) tract, leading to stomach cramps, nausea, vomiting, and intestinal and abdominal pain that may resemble appendicitis symptoms and last one to two days. The most severe complication is *laryngeal edema* (throat swelling), which can potentially be fatal. You should closely monitor this symptom because severe laryngeal obstruction can require a tracheotomy to prevent death by asphyxiation.

Diagnosing Hives and Angioedema

The first step in diagnosing your skin outbreak is to determine what specific condition is affecting you. As I explain in the preceding sections of this chapter, many different allergens, irritants, physical triggers, intolerance reactions, or underlying conditions can cause your hives and angioedema.

In order to narrow the range of possible causes of your hives and angioedema, your doctor should thoroughly evaluate your medical history and perform a complete physical exam.

Even if your doctor can't make a precise diagnosis, your medical history and physical exam enables your doctor to isolate the most likely causes of your eruptions, as well as to advise effective avoidance and treatment measures for your condition. Depending on the severity and extent of your outbreak, your doctor may also refer you to a dermatologist or allergist for further consultation.

Dealing with emergency situations

If you notice hoarseness, tongue swelling, and difficulty swallowing (symptoms typical of laryngeal edema) along with an outbreak of hives, seek immediate emergency treatment. These symptoms may represent a severe anaphylactic reaction such as EIA (exercise-induced anaphylaxis) or a severe form of HAE (hereditary angioedema). Don't waste time trying to figure out what may be causing your reaction — use your epinephrine (EpiPen or AnaKit — see Chapter 1) and get to the emergency room! After you're out of danger, you can proceed with any further needed investigation to try to get a diagnosis so you can possibly prevent similar occurences in the future.

Taking your hives seriously

When taking your medical history, your doctor should focus on the events and possible triggers in your life that might have been affecting you at the time of your outbreaks. Prepare to give your doctor as much information as possible about items and situations such as the following:

- ✔ Any medications (prescription or OTC products), supplements, or herbal products you take.

- ✔ Any exposure you may have to allergens — especially food, drug, and insect stings — in your occupation, school, home, or outdoors.

- ✔ Any exposure to physical urticaria triggers, including cold, heat, pressure, vibrations, sunlight, and other factors that I explain in "Physical mechanisms," earlier in this chapter.

- Viral or bacterial infections that you've recently experienced, including upper respiratory ailments, hepatitis, infectious mononucleosis, viral herpes, or other disorders.

- Any autoimmune disorder such as rheumatoid arthritis or lupus erythematous.

- Any contact you may have with allergens or irritants that trigger contact urticaria. (See "Contact mechanisms," earlier in this chapter.)

- If your outbreak isn't present at the time of your visit, prepare to tell your doctor where the condition typically appears on your body, how many eruptions occur, how long they persist, and how often they recur.

Examining eruptions

In addition to closely examining your skin, your physician should also perform a general physical examination to investigate other possible underlying disorders that may be contributing to your hives and angioedema.

Other disorders that may cause itching, inflammation, or lesions resembling hives and angioedema include

- Pregnancy; kidney, liver, thyroid, and lymph disorders; and diabetes can produce chronic itching, which you may mistake as a symptom of hives.

- Contact dermatitis (see Chapter 17), other skin disorders, skin infections (such as cellulitis), lymphedema, and injury can cause skin swelling that resembles angioedema.

- Stevens-Johnson syndrome, a potentially serious disorder, can cause lesions that resemble hives. Patients with this syndrome also often experience fever, burning sensations, sore throat, and general malaise.

- Viral herpes can trigger lesions that resemble outbreaks of papular and cholinergic urticaria. If your lesions appear in a symmetrical pattern, however, you may suffer from viral herpes.

- Serum sickness may trigger eruptions and other symptoms similar to the anaphylactic reactions of drug and insect allergies. With serum sickness, though, joint pain and fever also accompany the eruptions, and the reaction usually progresses more slowly than allergic cases.

If you're not sure whether your eruptions are hives, and if your outbreaks are infrequent and subside before you can see a physician, take color photographs (not black and white) of your eruptions while you can still see them. Showing these pictures to your doctor can help in making a diagnosis in some cases.

Keeping a diet diary

In cases of intermittent eruptions that may be due to food allergies, your doctor may advise you to keep track of what you consume. You usually need to record the foods and liquids that you ingest 24 hours before each episode of hives. Using this process can help you and your doctor possibly pinpoint potential food-related triggers of your condition.

Make sure that you consult with your doctor before assuming that you've identified a food allergen that triggers your hives and angioedema. Arbitrarily restricting your diet or the diet of a child who suffers from hives because of a suspected food allergy can cause nutritional deficiencies.

Testing for hives

Depending on what your doctor suspects as the trigger of your hives and angioedema, he or she may recommend certain medical tests to more precisely determine the causes and mechanisms of your condition. These tests may include the following types of procedures:

- **Challenge tests:** If a form of physical urticaria seems the likely cause of your condition, your doctor may perform procedures that provoke a small-scale reaction, similar to your outbreak. In most cases, these tests involve exposing your skin to a suspected physical mechanism such as heat, cold, UV light, pressure, water, or vibrations. Testing for exercise-induced anaphylaxis may involve eating and then exercising in a controlled setting to determine more precisely what combination of factors may trigger an anaphylactic reaction.

- **Allergy skin tests:** Your doctor may find skin testing for allergens useful when evaluating the cause of acute urticaria. In contrast with chronic urticaria, allergies more often cause eruptions in acute cases. (For more information on allergy skin testing, see Chapter 8.)

- **Blood tests:** If allergy skin testing is not advisable, your doctor may recommend a RAST blood test (see Chapter 8).

- **Skin punch biopsy:** This test involves extracting a small skin sample from your affected area for laboratory analysis. Doctors usually only perform a skin punch biopsy if they suspect that urticarial vasculitis causes your hives and if other lab tests show inconclusive results. A dermatologist usually performs the procedure, and a pathologist, who specializes in reading skin biopsies, evaluates the results.

I Can't Go Out Like This: Managing Hives

Avoidance measures and symptom relief are the keys to effective management of hives and angioedema. Some hives and angioedema cases resolve without major medical intervention and only require simple self-care and occasional medication to manage eruptions and associated symptoms (especially itching). Likewise, if you experience occasional outbreaks, you can improve your condition without treatment as long as you avoid exposure to the substances or mechanisms that trigger your symptoms.

If the cause of your eruptions is difficult to determine or if your outbreaks are more serious and persistent, your doctor may prescribe a preventive course of medication to help keep your condition from adversely affecting your quality of life. In the event of a widespread outbreak, seek immediate emergency medical attention.

Hives self-help

In addition to avoiding allergens, irritants, mechanisms, and intolerance reactions that may trigger your hives and angioedema, the most important concept to keep in mind when dealing with an outbreak is to not make your condition worse. If an outbreak occurs, follow these steps to relieve your symptoms and avoid making them worse:

✔ **Bathe and wash with lukewarm water.** Avoid hot baths and showers because they may intensify your symptoms and may also trigger conditions such as cholinergic urticaria. Likewise, avoid cold water and handling frozen items — such as ice cubes — because they can trigger cold urticaria outbreaks. (See "Physical mechanisms," earlier in this chapter.)

✔ **Don't use harsh soaps.** Using harsh soaps can damage your skin's natural protective layer and cause more itchiness. The less you itch, the less likely you are to infect your lesions through scratching.

✔ **Apply moisturizers immediately after bathing and avoid brisk drying.** Instead, gently use a soft towel to pat yourself dry.

✔ **Sport the loose look.** Wear comfortable, cotton, lightweight clothes and avoid tight, restrictive garments.

✔ **Stay out of hot environments as much as possible at work, home, or school.** Try to keep your home cool, especially your bedroom.

✔ **Avoid using any type of aspirin or NSAIDs, even after your outbreaks subside.** If you need medication for everyday aches and pains, your doctor may advise you to use acetaminophen products such as Tylenol. Likewise, avoid using alcohol or narcotic pain relievers.

Medication

Physicians mainly prescribe antihistamines from the H-1 class (see the nearby sidebar "Classifying antihistamines") to relieve and prevent the symptoms that accompany hives and angioedema. However, your doctor may prescribe more potent drugs if you suffer from more severe or persistent outbreaks.

Oral antihistamines

Antihistamines block the inflammatory effects of histamine to help reduce inflammation and can often relieve the itching associated with outbreaks of hives and angioedema (see Chapter 16 for more information on antihistamines and skin inflammations). Your doctor may prescribe a less-sedating (Zyrtec) or a non-sedating second-generation H-1 antihistamine (Allegra, Claritin). Or your doctor may prescribe an OTC sedating antihistamine such as Benadryl if you can't sleep at night because of discomfort from inflammation and itching. If these products don't provide you with sufficient relief, your doctor may prescribe a combination of an H-1 with an H-2 class antihistamine such as Tagamet or Zantac. (See the sidebar "Classifying antihistamines" for more information on H-1 and H-2 antihistamines.)

Other medications

If H-1 and H-2 antihistamine combinations fail to provide sufficient symptom relief, your doctor may consider prescribing more potent drugs. These drugs can include:

- **Prescription first-generation antihistamines:** These drugs can effectively treat cases of chronic hives that don't respond to prescription second-generation H-1 antihistamines. In some cases, your doctor may also prescribe a combination of prescription first-generation antihistamines with products from other antihistamine classes. For example, doctors often prescribe hydroxyzine (Atarax) to treat cases of cholinergic urticaria and as a preventive treatment for dermatographism. Cyproheptadine (Periactin) achieves good results in treating cold urticaria. However, because these products have sedating side effects that can significantly interfere with your daily life, your doctor may advise that you only use these drugs at night.

- **Antidepressants:** Doxepin (Sinequan) often provides a powerful antihistamine effect that your doctor may use to treat chronic hives. As with hydroxyzine and cyproheptadine, doxepin causes sedation, which may limit its use in some cases.

✔ **Corticosteroids:** If your hives or angioedema are particularly severe, extensive, and persistent, your doctor may prescribe a short course of oral corticosteroids, such as prednisone. If prednisone doesn't prove effective, your doctor may instead prescribe methylprednisolone (Medrol). Likewise, if your condition relapses after one or two short courses of these medications, your doctor may decide, as a last resort, to prescribe alternate-day single morning oral corticosteroid therapy for several weeks. If your doctor decides that you need this therapy, you must remain under close medical supervision for the duration of the medication course and make sure that you don't miss any of your scheduled appointments with your physician. You should also make sure that your doctor provides clearly written instructions for your dosage schedule before you leave the office.

✔ **Oral antibiotics and antihistamines:** In cases where bacterial infection develops — usually from scratching itchy rashes and lesions — I recommend using oral antihistamines to relieve itching and oral antibiotics to clear your infection. Using topical forms of these medications can result in allergic sensitization to these drugs, so you should clearly avoid topical forms when treating inflamed skin.

✔ **Emergency medication:** In the event that you suffer from a severe angioedema outbreak or an anaphylactic reaction that causes your tongue and mouth to swell and interfere with your breathing, you may need an emergency injection of epinephrine, the initial treatment for anaphylaxis, to keep your airway open. (See Chapter 1 for information on dealing with anaphylaxis.)

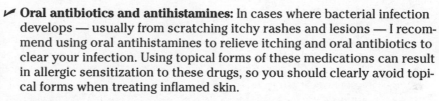

Classifying antihistamines

Antihistamines are classified by the types of histamine receptors, H-1 or H-2, that the drugs are designed to block. Your nasal cells have H-1 receptors, and your gastric (stomach) cells have H-2 receptors. Most people associate H-1 antihistamines with the treatment of allergies. However, your skin possesses both types of receptors, and your allergies may therefore require treatment with both H-1 and H-2 antihistamines.

Although the H-2 receptors in your stomach cells release histamine that secretes heartburn-causing acid, the release of histamine by H-2 receptors in your skin's blood vessels may also cause itching, swelling, and development of hives. Therefore, H-2 antihistamines such as Tagamet and Zantac (which are primarily marketed for relief of peptic ulcers and heartburn) can, in combination with H-1 antihistamines, provide a more comprehensive treatment of itching, swelling, and hives. Although these medications are generally safe, you should only use these products for the relief of hives and angioedema (or other medical conditions) on the advice of your doctor.

Part V

Food, Drug, and Insect Reactions: A Really Bad Trip

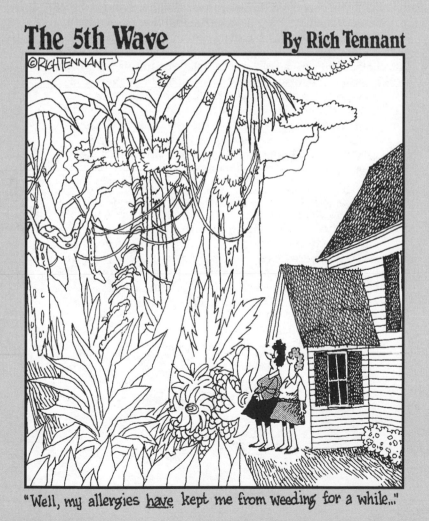

The 5th Wave — By Rich Tennant

"Well, my allergies <u>have</u> kept me from weeding for a while..."

In this part . . .

Are your allergies what you eat? Mostly, no, as I explain in Chapter 19. However, identifying the type of unfortunate food experiences that you may have, what specific food causes them, what to do about them, and how you can avoid those problems in the future is important, especially if you have a true food hypersensitivity, rather than a form of food intolerance.

I also deal with adverse drug reactions in this part. Drug reactions are also more often a result of nonallergic mechanisms rather than actual drug hypersensitivities. Understanding what may be affecting you so that you can take steps to avoid potentially serious reactions, especially to medications such as penicillin or aspirin and related nonsteroidal anti-inflammatory drugs (NSAIDs), is vital.

Insect stings may not seem like a big deal, unless you have a hypersensitivity to the venom of *Hymenoptera* insects (honeybees, yellow jackets, wasps, hornets, and fire ants). In extreme cases, life-threatening *anaphylaxis* (a sudden, severe reaction that affects multiple organs simultaneously) can result from insect stings, as I explain in Chapter 21. I also provide important and practical steps you can take to avoid painful encounters with these creatures.

Chapter 19

Managing Food Reactions

In This Chapter

▶ Understanding food allergies and food intolerance

▶ Evaluating causes of adverse food reactions

▶ Preventing food allergies in infants and children

▶ Avoiding allergenic foods

*I*f the food you eat bites you back with outbreaks of eczema, gastric distress, fits of wheezing, or other symptoms (perhaps even including life-threatening bouts of anaphylactic shock), you're not alone. Adverse food reactions affect at least one in four Americans at some point in their lives.

However, not all food ingredients that can cause adverse reactions are triggers of *food hypersensitivity* (the more precise term for *food allergy*). Even though 40 percent of Americans believe that their unfortunate gastronomical experiences result from allergies to certain foods, most cases involve various forms of food intolerance, food poisoning, and other nonallergic conditions that I explain throughout this chapter.

In fact, although allergic reactions to food can be severe (and should be appropriately diagnosed and managed), the actual number of adults in the United States who suffer from true food hypersensitivities is closer to 1 percent of the population. However, food sensitivities may affect as many as 6 percent of infants and children.

Because the range of adverse food reactions can include a constellation of nasal, respiratory, skin, gastrointestinal, and oral symptoms occurring separately or in combination, doctors usually classify these reactions according to the mechanisms that the reactions involve.

The following list provides a summary of the two main classifications of adverse food reactions:

- ✔ **Food hypersensitivity:** These reactions occur when your immune system responds to specific proteins in certain foods. The reactions can include allergic mechanisms involving IgE antibodies (see Chapter 1) as well as nonallergic mechanisms, which I explain in the next two sections of this chapter.

  - Allergic food hypersensitivities include gastrointestinal (GI) tract allergies, hives and other allergic skin reactions, and even anaphylaxis (a severe, abrupt reaction that affects many organs of the body simultaneously and can potentially be life-threatening).

  - Nonallergic food hypersensitivities (sometimes referred to as *non-IgE food reactions*) include syndromes such as food-induced enterocolitis, colitis, and malabsorption, as well as celiac disease, dermatitis herpetiformis, and pulmonary hypersensitivity. I discuss these medical conditions in greater detail in "Nonallergic (Non-IgE) Food Hypersensitivities," later in this chapter.

- ✔ **Food intolerance:** These types of reactions result from nonallergic, non-immunologic responses to offending substances in various foods. Forms of food intolerance include

  - Lactose intolerance

  - Pharmacologic food reactions

  - Metabolic food reactions

  - Food additive reactions

  - Food poisoning

  - Toxic reactions

Allergic Food Hypersensitivities

In the case of an *IgE-mediated food hypersensitivity,* commonly known as a *food allergy,* your immune system cooks up specific IgE antibodies (see Chapter 1) against specific allergens. The level of exposure required for your immune system to be sensitized to a particular food varies, depending on the allergens involved. The major food allergens that have been identified are mostly proteins, often found in the following foods:

✔ Peanuts (the leading cause of severe allergic food reactions), soybeans, peas, lentils, beans and other legumes, and foods containing these products as ingredients. Because a wide variety of foods include peanuts and soybean products as ingredients, these legumes often act as hidden triggers of food allergies. In "Anaphylaxis and allergic food reactions," later in this chapter, I provide more information on peanut issues. Likewise, you can find details on uncovering hidden allergenic ingredients in many common foods in "Avoiding Adverse Food Reactions" later in this chapter.

✔ Shellfish, such as shrimp, lobster, crab, clams, and oysters.

✔ Fish — both freshwater and saltwater.

✔ Tree nuts, including almonds, Brazil nuts, cashews, hazelnuts, and walnuts.

✔ Eggs, especially egg whites, which contain the predominant allergenic proteins, ovalbumin, and ovomucoid. The yolk is considered less allergenic than the egg white.

✔ Cow's milk and products that contain milk protein fractions, such as casein (80 percent of the protein in cow's milk) and whey, which includes lactalbumin and lactoglobulin.

✔ Wheat, an important ingredient in bran, malt, wheat flour, graham flour, wheat germ, and wheat starch. Corn, rice, barley, oats, and other grains and cereals are less common food allergy triggers.

Of these common ingested culprits, the products that trigger allergic food reactions in children most frequently are milk, eggs, peanuts, tree nuts, fish, soy, and wheat. In adults, the likeliest causes of allergic food reactions include fish, shellfish, peanuts, and tree nuts.

Although most children lose their sensitivity to milk and eggs by age 3, food allergies involving peanuts, fish, shellfish, and tree nuts can last a lifetime.

Other, less-obvious sources of food allergens may possibly cause adverse reactions in a smaller number of susceptible individuals. These much less frequently problematic food allergens (listed in family groupings to keep it all in the family) include the following:

✔ **Lily family:** Onions, leeks, garlic, asparagus.

✔ **Mustard family:** Broccoli, cabbage, cauliflower, horseradish, turnip, radish, mustard.

✔ **Plum family:** Apricots, cherries, peaches, almonds, plums.

✔ **Gourd family:** Watermelon, honeydew, cantaloupe, other melons, pumpkins, squash.

✔ **Nightshade family:** Tomatoes, potatoes, eggplant, bell pepper, red pepper.

✔ **Goosefoot family:** Spinach, beets, Swiss chard, pigweed.

Additives and allergies

Allergic mechanisms may or may not play a part in some adverse food reactions commonly associated with food additives. When additives are in the picture, identifying a suspected food allergen can get complicated, because finding out whether the food itself or the additive causes the problem is often difficult.

Additives, such as sulfites, are often used as antioxidants to preserve wine, dried fruit, shrimp, and potatoes. These additives have been implicated in cases of allergic food hypersensitivities, including potentially life-threatening *bronchospasm* (constriction of the airways) and asthma symptoms, especially in severe asthmatics who require long-term treatment with oral corticosteroids (see Chapter 12 for information on asthma medications).

Exposure to sulfites, when used in salad bars and in the guacamole served in some restaurants, can trigger asthma symptoms in susceptible asthmatics when they inhale the sulfite fumes from treated foods. These antioxidant additives are sometimes used to prevent discoloration and to keep greens looking perky. That's why some

salad bar lettuce — which may sit out for hours during the day — doesn't seem to wilt, unlike the salads most of us prepare at home.

The U.S. Food and Drug Administration (FDA) prohibits using sulfites on fresh fruits and vegetables meant to be eaten raw (as with a salad bar) and requires manufacturers to label products that contain sulfites. However, pre-cut or peeled potato products used in some restaurants to make common side dishes (such as french fries and hash browns) may still contain sulfites. Therefore, if you have asthma, I advise always asking questions about the food served in restaurants.

Doctors often need to be detectives to determine the causes of adverse food reactions. For example, if you experience an adverse food reaction to a hot dog, your doctor must determine whether your reaction is because of allergens in the meat, or whether you're suffering from hot dog headache due to nitrites used to retard meat spoilage, or even whether you're reacting to an added food dye that creates the pink coloring.

How allergic food hypersensitivities develop

Atopy, the genetic predisposition to develop allergies, is a significant factor in the development of food hypersensitivity. An infant's immune system can begin responding to food allergens soon after birth.

As I explain in Chapter 1, your inherited tendency to develop allergies can express itself in other allergic conditions also, such as allergic rhinitis (hay fever) and atopic dermatitis (eczema). The predisposition toward allergies passes between generations, but the specific allergies themselves may not. Therefore, Mom may be allergic to lobster, Junior may break out in hives after eating peanuts, and baby Betty may get congested after drinking cow's milk formula.

The severity of your symptoms may also depend on the level of your sensitivity to particular food allergens and the quantities of these foods you consume. In some cases, ingesting small amounts of these foods may not trigger adverse reactions. The following section provides more detail on the various forms of allergic food hypersensitivities.

Gastrointestinal tract allergies

Allergic reactions involving the digestive system can develop within a few minutes to several hours after ingesting food allergens, and they frequently result in abdominal pain, vomiting, and diarrhea. The most significant classifications of gastrointestinal (GI) allergies include

- **Gastrointestinal food hypersensitivity reaction:** This reaction generally occurs with other atopic conditions, such as allergic rhinitis and atopic dermatitis, and can cause nausea, stomach pain, vomiting, and, in some cases, diarrhea. In rare cases, a widespread systemic reaction such as anaphylaxis can also result. (See "Anaphylaxis and allergic food reactions" later in this chapter.)

- **Cow's milk allergy:** More than 2 percent of infants develop allergies to the proteins casein and whey (including lactalbumin and lactoglobulin) in cow's milk, resulting in adverse reactions (such as colic, vomiting, and diarrhea) even to minute amounts of these proteins. This reaction isn't the same as the more familiar syndrome known as *lactose intolerance,* as I explain in "Food Intolerance" later in this chapter.

- **Allergic eosinophilic gastroenteropathy:** This rare condition can cause nausea and vomiting following meals, abdominal pain, and diarrhea. If not managed effectively, this type of allergy can result in malabsorption and malnutrition, leading potentially to stunted or slowed growth in infants and weight loss in adults.

- **Oral allergy syndrome:** If you have allergic rhinitis (hay fever), you may also experience oral allergy symptoms after consuming certain fresh fruits and raw vegetables.

   This cross-reactivity syndrome can occur if you are sensitive to ragweed pollen (with bananas and melons such as cantaloupe, honeydew, and watermelon), birch pollen (with apples, carrots, potatoes, hazelnuts, and members of the plum family), and mugwort pollen (with celery, apple, and kiwi fruit). Your symptoms may include severe itching and swelling of the lips, tongue, and palate, as well as blistering of the throat and mucus lining of the mouth. You may be able to consume these fruits and vegetables in cooked or frozen forms; they seem to trigger reactions only in their raw state. However, make sure that you check with your doctor before you cook up that vegetable stir-fry or cool off with a melon sorbet. (See the nearby sidebar, "What's ragweed got to do with it?")

Hives and other food-related skin reactions

Allergic food hypersensitivities involving the IgE antibodies that I discuss earlier in this chapter can also trigger skin reactions in people whose atopic predisposition shows up through skin conditions. These conditions include

- **Atopic dermatitis (eczema):** In more than one-third of children affected by this skin condition, eggs, milk, peanuts, tree nuts, soybean, and wheat can contribute to outbreaks. (See Chapter 16 for more details on atopic dermatitis.)

- **Urticaria (hives):** These itchy welts can erupt from various types of reactions to many foods including peanuts, tree nuts, milk, eggs, fish, shellfish, soybeans, and fruits, as well as food additives such as sodium benzoates, sulfites, and food dyes. Skin contact with raw meats, fish, vegetables, and fruit can also trigger eruptions of acute contact urticaria. Allergic-food hypersensitivities are more likely to act as triggers of *rapid onset urticaria* (a particularly quick and severe eruption of hives) in children than in adults. (See Chapter 18 for more information on hives.) Food-related exercise-induced anaphylaxis (EIA), which I discuss later in this chapter, can also trigger hives and angioedema.

- **Angioedema:** Also known as *deep swellings,* this condition results in deeper tissue inflammation, causing swelling of the skin, and is more likely to produce painful and burning sensations rather than itching. Angioedema can erupt as a reaction to the same food allergens that trigger hives. (Chapter 18 provides more details on angioedema.)

What's ragweed got to do with it?

Symptoms of oral allergy syndrome can result from the cross-reactions that exist between particular pollens and foods. Your immune system expertly recognizes related allergens in seemingly unrelated sources. If you've been sensitized to allergenic cousins and are exposed to them at the same time, allergic symptoms can occur. This syndrome is called *cross-reactivity*.

For example, during ragweed season, in addition to typical allergic rhinitis (hay fever) symptoms, you may also experience itchy and swollen mouth and lips when eating melons such as cantaloupe, honeydew, and watermelon. Cross-reactivity can also affect you if you're allergic to latex (used in a host of everyday items such as gloves, rubber bands, erasers, sports gear, and condoms) when you consume fruits and nuts such as bananas, avocados, kiwi, papaya, and chestnuts.

In severe cases of hives and angioedema, symptoms can also include swelling of the tongue, throat, airway, and difficulty swallowing, as well as fainting. If angioedema affects your face, the swelling may potentially lead to breathing difficulties. If you experience swelling of your airway, get emergency care immediately.

Anaphylaxis and allergic food reactions

The most extreme of all allergic food symptoms is *anaphylaxis.* This abrupt, systemic allergic reaction, often caused by the same foods that trigger hives and angioedema eruptions, affects several organs simultaneously and can quickly turn life-threatening.

Generalized urticaria (Total body hives)

Generalized urticaria (widespread hives ocurring simultaneously over much of your body surface area) can often be the initial symptom of impending anaphylaxis and can result in a sudden swelling *(angioedema)* of the lips, eyelids, tonguc, and windpipe (laryngeal edema), as well as wheezing and dizziness. This particularly dangerous reaction can quickly progress to anaphylaxis, leading to shock, hypotension, *arrhythmia* (irregular heartbeat), and even cardiorespiratory arrest. In rare cases, this type of reaction can be fatal.

Common triggers of total body hives include foods such as peanuts and shellfish (in people who have extreme hypersensitivities to these foods), severe allergic reactions to medications such as penicillin and related compounds (or pseudoallergic reactions to aspirin and/or related NSAIDs; see Chapter 20), generalized hypersensitivity to latex (see Chapter 17), and/or extreme sensitivities to stings from insects of the *Hymenoptera* class, which includes honeybees, yellow jackets, wasps, hornets, and fire ants (see Chapter 21).

Food-dependent exercise-induced anaphylaxis

Food-dependent exercise-induced anaphylaxis, a variant of exercise-induced anaphylaxis (EIA) — which I explain in Chapter 18, — can occur when you exercise within three to four hours after eating a particular food. Two forms of this condition exist:

✔ In most instances, anaphylaxis results only if you ingest particular foods, especially celery, shellfish, wheat, fruit, milk, or fish prior to exercise. If you experience this type of reaction and you can identify the specific foods that trigger your episodes, your doctor may advise allergy skin testing (see Chapter 8) to confirm your sensitivity to the suspected foods.

✔ In rare cases, you may develop anaphylaxis while exercising, regardless of the type of food you've consumed.

Managing and preventing anaphylaxis

Food hypersensitivity is a leading cause of anaphylaxis. Current estimates are that as many as 125 people in the U.S. die each year from food-induced anaphylactic reactions. The most effective long-term method for preventing food-induced anaphylactic reactions is to avoid eating foods that trigger the reaction. I provide more details on avoiding food allergens and establishing a safe diet in "Avoiding Adverse Food Reactions," later in this chapter.

If your child suffers from food-induced anaphylaxis, notify baby-sitters, relatives, parents of other children, day care workers, teachers, and other school personnel of your child's sensitivities.

Avoiding peanut problems in children

As a parent of a peanut-allergic child, you need to pay close attention to products that might contain peanuts, because they can potentially cause life-threatening anaphylactic reactions in children (as well as adults) who are extremely allergic to this food.

Here are some important points to keep in mind about peanuts and children:

✔ Many foods contain peanuts as a not-so-obvious added ingredient. Therefore, you should examine all food labels for peanut ingredients and carefully select menu items when dining out with a child who is allergic to peanuts. (See "Avoiding Adverse Food Reactions," later in this chapter, for more information on foods that contain peanuts.) You may want to pack your child's lunch to reduce the risk of your child unknowingly consuming foods with minute traces of peanuts in school lunches.

✔ Because so many foods include peanuts as ingredients, you should teach your young child not only to avoid peanuts but also never to accept foods — particularly snacks and candy bars — from others, especially playmates and young siblings.

✔ Because the peanut hypersensitivity issue has received widespread media attention, some airlines are introducing peanut-free flights. If you suffer from food hypersensitivities of any kind, however, I advise asking a lot of questions about the food on your flight, even if the airline claims that no peanuts or peanut ingredients are in the snacks or meals.

✔ A child who has a peanut hypersensitivity should wear a MedicAlert bracelet, especially at school. Also, ask your family doctor about supplying your child's school with an emergency epinephrine kit. Make sure school personnel know how and when to administer this medication.

Emergency treatment for anaphylaxis

If you are prone to anaphylaxis, you should carry injectable epinephrine with you at all times and receive emergency care as soon as possible after an attack occurs. I also advise having an emergency plan in place that includes the following items:

✔ Medications your doctor has prescribed for you in the event of an anaphylactic reaction

✔ A list of your symptoms

✔ A written treatment plan prepared by your physician

✔ Your physician's name and contact information

Ask your doctor whether an emergency epinephrine kit, such as an EpiPen (or EpiPen Jr. for children under 66 pounds) or AnaKit, with an injectable dose of epinephrine, is advisable for you or your child. Parents and caregivers of children under 30 pounds (about 14 kilograms), who are too small for the dose of a pre-loaded EpiPen Jr., should be taught how to properly administer the correct dose of epinephrine by syringe to their infant or young child. I also strongly advise you to wear a MedicAlert bracelet or necklace in case you're unable to speak during a reaction. The appendix at the back of this book provides more information on how to obtain these items.

Nonallergic (Non-IgE) Food Hypersensitivities

Food hypersensitivity can also result from immune system reactions that don't involve the production of IgE antibodies. The most significant nonallergic food reactions include the following:

✔ **Food-induced enterocolitis syndrome:** This condition primarily occurs in infants between one and three months of age. Characteristic symptoms include prolonged vomiting and diarrhea, often resulting in dehydration. Triggers are usually the proteins in formulas that contain cow's milk or soy substitutes. Occasionally, breast-fed infants may also suffer from this syndrome, presumably as the result of a protein ingested by the mother and transferred to the infant in maternal milk. Similar symptoms can occur in older children and adults in response to eggs, rice, wheat, and peanuts. However, most children outgrow this type of hypersensitivity by their third birthday.

✔ **Food-induced colitis:** Cow's milk and soy protein hypersensitivity have been implicated in this disorder, which can occur in the first few months of life and is usually diagnosed through the presence of blood in the stools, either seen by the naked eye or hidden *(occult),* of children who otherwise appear healthy. This condition often diminishes after six months to two years if children avoid the implicated food allergens.

Feeding a hypoallergenic formula to your baby may help overcome food-induced colitis.

✔ **Malabsorption syndrome:** This condition involves hypersensitivities to proteins in foods such as cow's milk, soy, wheat and other cereal grains, and eggs. Symptoms include diarrhea, vomiting, and weight loss or failure to gain weight.

✔ **Celiac disease:** This condition is a more serious form of malabsorption syndrome, and it can cause intestinal inflammation. Symptoms range from diarrhea and abdominal cramping to anemia and osteoporosis. Celiac disease only seems to occur in people who inherit an atopic predisposition. Affected individuals develop a hypersensitivity to a component of gluten called *gliadin,* which you find in wheat, oats, rye, and barley. If you suffer from this syndrome, however, you're not necessarily doomed to a life without pasta and pancakes: Resourceful sufferers of celiac disease have come up with many gluten-free products, ranging from beer to pretzels.

✔ **Dermatitis herpetiformis:** This condition is a non-IgE-mediated food hypersensitivity to gluten that produces skin eruptions in addition to causing intestinal inflammation. Typical symptoms include a chronic, itchy rash that appears primarily on the elbows, knees, and buttocks, although the disease can affect other areas as well.

✔ **Pulmonary hypersensitivity.** This rare condition, induced by cow's milk, primarily affects young children. Characteristic symptoms include a chronic cough, wheezing, and severe anemia. Removing the offending dairy products from the diet can substantially alleviate symptoms.

Food Intolerance

As I explain at the beginning of this chapter, many adverse food reactions don't involve an immune system response. These types of direct, non-immunologic reactions are considered signs and symptoms of food intolerance and include the conditions that I explain in the following sections.

Lactose intolerance

If you are lactose intolerant, odds are your body doesn't produce sufficient amounts of the lactase enzyme in order for you to properly digest cow's milk. If you drink milk or consume foods with high milk content, you may experience stomach cramps, bloating, nausea, gas, and diarrhea.

Avoiding cow's milk and cow's milk products or adding the lactase enzyme to those foods are the standard ways of managing lactose intolerance. In contrast with the cow's-milk allergy (which I mention earlier in "Allergic Food Hypersensitivities"), you may be able to consume small quantities of cow's milk without suffering an adverse reaction.

Metabolic food reactions

In some cases, eating average or normal amounts of particular foods (especially fatty foods) may disrupt your digestive system because of various factors. These disruptions, called *metabolic food reactions,* may be caused by

✔ Medications (for example, antibiotics) you're taking for illnesses

✔ A disease or condition (such as a gastrointestinal virus) that may affect your digestive system

✔ Malnutrition (for example, due to vitamin or enzyme deficiency)

 Consult your doctor if everyday foods disrupt your digestive system frequently, especially if a prescribed medication seems to contribute to the condition.

Pharmacologic food reactions

 More serious forms of metabolic food reactions can result if you combine certain foods and drugs that don't mix well. Beware of the following potentially dangerous combinations:

✔ Grapefruit juice, which is usually harmless, sometimes causes harmful interactions when consumed by patients taking calcium channel blockers, such as Procardia.

 If you have a heart condition, ask your doctor about possible interactions between grapefruit juice and any over-the-counter (OTC) or prescription antihistamines you may take.

✔ If you take blood-thinning drugs such as Coumadin, check with your doctor before eating foods rich in vitamin K such as broccoli, spinach, and turnip greens, because these foods can reduce the medications' effectiveness.

 ✔ A harmful potassium buildup can occur if you overindulge on bananas while taking ACE inhibitors, such as Capoten and Vasotec.

✔ Avoid foods high in tyramine, such as cheese and sausage, if you take MAO inhibitors, because the combination can cause a potentially fatal rise in blood pressure. Tyramine may also aggravate or trigger migraine headaches.

✔ The caffeine in coffee, tea, and colas can interact badly with ulcer medications such as Tagamet, Zantac, and Pepcid AC. If your doctor prescribes theophylline for your asthma, you should reduce your caffeine intake, because caffeine can worsen side effects of the medication such as GI irritation, headache, jitteriness, and sleeplessness.

Food additive reactions

Doctors associate many types of food additives with adverse food reactions. The most frequently implicated food additives are

- **Monosodium glutamate (MSG):** When consumed in large quantities, this flavor enhancer reportedly causes burning sensations, facial pressure, chest pain, headache, and, in rare cases, severe asthma symptoms. Although many sufferers associate these types of reactions with eating Chinese or other types of Asian foods, no conclusive studies have determined a clear link between consuming MSG and adverse food reactions. In any event, with the recent increase of MSG-free restaurants in many parts of the U.S., you should have no trouble finding a place to chow down on chow mein without suffering ill effects.

- **Tartrazine (yellow dye #5):** This and other food dyes can aggravate chronic hives and may actually be an ingredient in the very same children's syrups used to treat allergic symptoms such as hives — another good reason to always check medication labels.

- **Sulfites:** Commonly found in processed foods and almost always in wines, sulfites can produce respiratory difficulties. In some cases, sulfites can also trigger potentially life-threatening bronchospasm (constriction of the airways) and asthma symptoms in some individuals (see the sidebar "Additives and allergies," earlier in this chapter).

Food poisoning

Food poisoning can result from bacterial contamination of improperly prepared or handled foods, especially meats or salads. You've probably heard of bacterial bad guys such as salmonella, e. coli, listeria, and staphylococcus enterotoxin. These bacteria are the usual suspects in outbreaks of food poisoning. Symptoms of food poisoning typically include nausea, vomiting, and diarrhea and can often mimic the flu. In rare cases, food-poisoning reactions can be fatal if not treated in time.

Researchers believe that many cases of illness mistakenly diagnosed as the 24-hour flu bug are actually the result of ingesting tainted foods.

If many people develop similar symptoms after eating the same meal (the potato salad with especially rich mayonnaise that sat in the sun all afternoon at the family picnic, for example), food poisoning is the likely cause of all those urgent trips to the restroom.

If you experience severe gastric distress that seems related to food poisoning, make sure you drink enough liquid to avoid dehydration, which is one of the most serious adverse effects of this reaction. If your condition doesn't improve within 24 hours, seek medical attention.

Toxic food reactions

Some foods are intrinsically poisonous to all humans, regardless of allergies or other conditions. Poisonous mushrooms, such as the Amanita variety, for example, are among the most dangerous foods you can consume. Other potent sources of toxic food reactions include shellfish caught in a red tide and exotic fish such as puffers, which can cause fatal reactions when consumed unless you prepare them properly.

 Use caution when picking those pretty toadstools during your hike through the forest. In some cases, the prettier the food, the more toxic it can be. Make sure your children (and you, for that matter) don't eat toxic garden plants such as azaleas, mistletoe, rhododendrons, jimsonweed, and daffodils.

Toxic food reactions can affect both the central nervous system and digestive system, causing symptoms such as

- Delirium, dizziness, unconsciousness, and convulsions.
- Breathing difficulties.
- Stomach cramps, nausea, vomiting, and diarrhea.
- Burning or severe pain in the mouth, throat, and stomach. (These symptoms characterize poisoning that occurs when you ingest poisonous products such as household or garden chemicals.)

 If you suspect that you or someone around you is experiencing a toxic reaction, call your local Poison Control Center, listed in the front pages of your community telephone directory. Toxic reactions very often require immediate emergency medical care.

Diagnosing Adverse Food Reactions

 In order to diagnose your adverse food reactions, your physician should take a detailed medical history and conduct a physical examination. Your doctor may also ask you about the specific details of your reaction to narrow the range of suspected food triggers that may cause your reactions.

Keeping a food diary

 A detailed food diary, in which you record everything you consume (even those midnight snacks) and describe your reactions, can help your doctor diagnose your condition.

A well-kept food diary can assist you in telling your doctor about the following items:

- ✔ The timing of your reactions. For example, do they occur immediately after you've consumed a food or liquid, and if not, how long afterwards?
- ✔ The amount of food that seems to trigger a reaction.
- ✔ The duration and severity of your symptoms.
- ✔ Any activities, especially exercise, associated with your reactions.

Considering atopic causes

As part of the physical examination, your doctor should also look for signs of atopic diseases, including

- ✔ Dry, scaly skin, which can indicate atopic dermatitis
- ✔ Dark circles under your eyes, which may indicate allergic rhinitis
- ✔ Wheezing and coughing, which can signal asthma symptoms

Eliminating possible food culprits

In some cases, your doctor may advise an elimination diet for you as a way of confirming what triggers your adverse reactions. This process involves eliminating suspected foods from your diet, one at a time, under your doctor's supervision. If your symptoms significantly improve, your doctor may then gradually reintroduce the likeliest food suspect to determine whether it's the source of your woes.

Only undertake an elimination diet under the direction of a physician. You don't want to deprive yourself of foods that may not cause your symptoms and are vital for your well-being. Your doctor may also advise an elimination diet in order to prepare you for an oral food challenge, which I describe later in this chapter.

Testing for food allergens

If your doctor can't readily identify the cause of your reactions, he or she may also recommend confirming a suspected food allergen with the allergy tests that I describe in the following sections.

Skin testing

Skin testing involves using specific food extracts to evaluate your sensitivity to suspected allergens. Only a qualified specialist, such as an allergist, should perform skin testing. Skin testing for food allergens is not always recommended.

In some cases, your doctor may not advise skin testing because a positive reaction may involve unacceptable risks of inducing anaphylactic shock, particularly if you're highly sensitized to certain foods, such as peanuts.

In general, prick-puncture tests are the only skin tests that your doctor needs to administer when attempting to identify suspected food allergens. *Intracutaneous tests* (small injections of weakened allergen extract just under the surface of the skin on the patient's arm) are rarely advisable in these cases. (See Chapter 8 if you're on pins and needles about prick-puncture tests.)

Oral food challenges

Oral food challenges involve actually ingesting — under medical supervision — minute quantities of food that contain suspected allergens.

To ensure the most accurate diagnosis, your doctor should administer an oral food challenge while you're symptom-free, usually as a result of a food elimination diet. Depending on the severity of your adverse food reactions and the type of food allergen that your physician suspects as the cause, your doctor may choose to administer one or more of the following types of oral food challenges:

✔ **Open challenge:** In this type of test, your doctor informs you of what type of food you're ingesting.

✔ **Single-blind challenge:** With this test, you aren't told what you're fed. However, your doctor or the clinician administering the test knows the ingredients.

✔ **Double-blind, placebo-controlled oral food challenge (DBPCOFC):** This elaborate procedure is the gold standard for identifying food allergens. Neither you nor your doctor (nor the clinician who administers the test) knows the contents of the test. In most cases, your doctor schedules a DBPCOFC so you can fast for a prescribed amount of time beforehand. You also need to stop taking antihistamines (based on your doctor's advice) prior to the challenge, because these drugs can interfere with the accuracy of a DBPCOFC. The initial dose of the suspected food in this type of challenge is usually half of the minimum quantity that your doctor estimates as the trigger for your reaction.

Take this challenge only in a facility equipped to treat potentially severe reactions. If your history of adverse food reactions is life-threatening, your doctor will most likely advise you that an oral food challenge is too risky.

Radioallergensorbent testing (RAST)

Your doctor may recommend *radioallergensorbent testing,* a type of blood test that measures levels of food-specific IgE antibodies (see Chapter 1) in your blood, if skin testing or oral food challenges seem too risky.

Most allergists rarely use RAST because it isn't as accurate as skin testing and may result in an incomplete profile of your allergies. For more information on this test, see Chapter 8.

Avoiding Adverse Food Reactions

After your doctor determines the source of your adverse food reactions, the most effective long-term approach to managing your condition and preventing further reactions is strict avoidance of the implicated food. That may seem like an obvious solution. However, you may need to become an expert at reading ingredient listings when you buy groceries. In some cases, food allergens and other types of precipitants may hide under arcane names in food labels. For updates and information on food allergens and related issues and to find out how to decipher ingredients listed on food labels, contact the Food Allergy Network at 800-929-4040.

You should make sure that your family, friends, and colleagues all understand what causes your adverse food reactions. You can then minimize the chances of erupting in hives at the Thanksgiving meal or during that crucial dinner with your boss and the company's new clients.

If you have a life-threatening food hypersensitivity, you may need to avoid certain restaurants. In many cases, food servers don't have enough information about the ingredients in the establishment's menu to guarantee you an allergen-free meal, although some restaurants actually do offer dishes without common food allergens. However, I strongly advise double-checking all the ingredients in the menu item with the chef or restaurant manager. In particular, you need to inquire whether the restaurant prepares allergen-free meals using surfaces, cookware, and utensils that are separated from the other items in the kitchen.

If effective management of your adverse food reactions involves excluding common food groups from your diet for long periods, consider professional dietary advice in order to prevent nutritional deficiency or malnutrition.

Chapter 20

Treating Drug Reactions

In This Chapter

▶ Defining adverse drug reactions

▶ Diagnosing drug hypersensitivities

▶ Avoiding medications that cause problems

*T*he term *wonder drug* is a very apt description of the benefits that many modern-day medications bring to us. These products — such as antibiotics, insulin, anti-inflammatories, and other drugs — enable doctors to treat or cure conditions that once seemed beyond remedy. When prescribed and used properly, most of these medications — such as the ones I discuss for treating nasal allergies (see Part II) and asthma (see Part III) — cause few if any serious side effects.

However, adverse drug reactions are a concern for some people. Although these reactions occur much less frequently than the known potential side effects you may hear about at the end of a medication's television commercial, adverse drug reactions account for as many as 75,000 deaths in the United States each year, according to recent estimates.

Any unexpected adverse consequence of taking medication, other than for the purpose it is intended, is considered to be an adverse drug reaction. This definition does not include intentional or accidental poisoning, drug abuse, overdose, or treatment failures.

Patients most at risk for adverse drug reactions include those who have

✔ Serious illnesses that require high doses and/or many types of medications.

✔ Impaired liver and kidney functions, especially patients who consume large quantities of alcohol.

✔ Compromised immune systems, especially those with AIDS. In these cases, the drugs most likely to cause adverse reactions are sulfadiazine, acyclovir, and zidovudine.

Even though adverse drug reactions may affect as many as one-third of all people taking medications, of these reactions, less than 10 percent are due to actual hypersensitivities (allergies) to substances in the drugs themselves. In fact, most adverse drug reactions result from other types of mechanisms, as I explain in this chapter.

Understanding Adverse Drug Reactions

Adverse drug reactions can be classified as those that are predictable and those that are unpredictable. (I discuss unpredictable reactions in "Drug Intolerance and Idiosyncrasy," later in this chapter.) Predictable adverse drug reactions include the following:

- **Known side effects:** The product information package inserts that accompany all types of medications list these types of reactions. For example, a typical side effect of aspirin in some people is stomach irritation, and a frequent side effect of many over-the-counter (OTC) antihistamines is drowsiness.

- **Drug interactions:** As I explain in Chapters 7 and 12, you should always make sure that any physician who treats you knows about any and all products you take for other medical conditions. This list includes any OTC drugs you may take, even for minor aches and pains, as well as any vitamins and nutritional supplements. Some of these drugs don't work well together, as I explain in these two examples:

  - If you have asthma and are also taking oral beta-blockers such as Inderal, Lopressor, and Corgard (for migraine headaches, high blood pressure, angina, or hyperthyroidism) or beta-blocker eyedrops such as Timoptic (for glaucoma), these medications might block the effect of your inhaled short-acting adrenergic bronchodilator, thus depriving you of quick relief when you need it for your respiratory symptoms. Occasionally, taking beta-blockers can trigger asthma episodes in susceptible individuals who have not previously experienced any respiratory symptoms.

  - Drug combinations may also result in other serious consequences. For example, if you take theophylline (which doctors use to treat some cases of asthma) and then also take prescribed erythromycin (an antibiotic) for a bacterial infection, the combined effects of these two drugs may impair your liver's ability to metabolize and clear theophylline from your system. This could result in overly high levels of theophylline in your bloodstream and a possible toxic reaction.

- **Accidental or intentional overdose:** Remember, too much of anything can be bad for you. Use only products and preparations — whether prescription or OTC — that are clearly labeled to treat the symptoms you are experiencing. Also, always carefully read the product information package insert and take the medication only as the label or your doctor instructs.

You can also define adverse drug reactions according to the mechanisms that cause them, although doctors don't yet fully understand what makes some of us react to certain drugs in certain ways. The following three sections summarize these mechanisms.

Drug hypersensitivities

Also known as drug allergies, *drug hypersensitivities* involve specific immunologic responses (see Chapter 2) to certain drugs in people who have developed allergic sensitivities to allergenic substances in these drugs. The most frequent type of adverse allergic reactions to medications occur with penicillin and its related compounds. Other drugs that can cause allergic reactions include cephalosporins, sulfanomides, insulin, and anti-sera (horse serum for anti-venom treatment of snake bite).

Aspirin, OTC nonsteroidal anti-inflammatory drugs (NSAIDs) such as ibuprofen (Advil, Motrin), ketoprofen (Actron, Orudis), naproxen (Aleve), and newer prescription NSAIDs, known as COX-2 inhibitors — including celecoxib (Celebrex) and rofecoxib (Vioxx) — and other drugs can also trigger adverse reactions. However, these reactions are not truly considered "allergic" because in most cases, immunologic mechanisms are not involved.

Non-immunologic drug reactions

Most adverse drug reactions are *non-immunologic* — not involving any of the four types of immunolgic processes that I explain in Chapter 2. Aspirin and nonsteroidal anti-inflammatory drugs (NSAIDs) are the main culprits in these types of reactions, which include the following categories:

- **Drug idiosyncrasy:** An unexpected and unpredictable effect that doesn't relate to the intended action of the drug (for example, severe anemia occuring, in certain groups of people, after taking medications such as anti-malarials, sulfanomides, and pain relievers).

- **Drug intolerance:** An undesirable effect that occurs at lower than normal doses of a drug, for which no scientific explanation has yet been discovered. For example, *tinnitus* (ringing in the ears) can occur in some individuals after taking just a single aspirin tablet.

Pseudoallergic drug reactions

Pseudoallergic drug reactions often mimic drug hypersensitivity reactions and can result in anaphylaxis. These reactions aren't truly the result of an immunolgic mechanism involving IgE antibodies (agents that cause the release of inflammatory chemicals such as histamine from the mast cells that line tissues in many parts of our bodies, thus inducing allergy symptoms), but a response similar to drug hypersensitivity occurs nonetheless.

If you're susceptible to a pseudoallergic reaction from a particular drug, you may have an immediate and severe reaction the very first time you use the substance instead of after more than one exposure to allergenic substances in the drug, as is the case with true hypersensitivities or allergies.

Aspirin and NSAIDs are also often implicated in pseudoallergic cases. Other medications that can produce pseudoallergic reactions include

- Radio-contrast media (RCM), containing organic iodine, used in some diagnostic tests, such as intravenous pyelogram (IVP) to check for kidney and urinary tract problems

- Colloid volume substitutes (used for severe cases of shock) such as dextran, gelatin, hydroxyethel starch, and human serum albumin

- Opiates such as codeine, meperidine, and morphine prescribed for pain management

Forms of Drug Hypersensitivities

Contrary to popular belief, only a small number of adverse drug reactions occur as a result of *drug hypersensitivities* (also known as drug allergies).

Drug allergies can develop if you've been sensitized to one of the otherwise harmless components of a drug. As a result, your immune system produces agents (known as IgE antibodies) as a response to these allergens. The more exposure you receive to a drug that may trigger an allergic response, the greater chance you have for developing a hypersensitivity to that substance (see Chapter 2 for an extensive explanation of this process).

Factors that determine your risk of developing a drug hypersensitivity can include

- The dosage level of your medication

- How the drug is administered — orally, topically, via injection, or intravenously (IV)

- How long you take the drug

- How many courses of the drug you've taken before

- Other concurrent illnesses you may have, such as asthma, cystic fibrosis, mononucleosis, human immunodeficiency virus (HIV), or full-blown AIDS, in addition to the ailment for which your doctor prescribes the drug

- Your age, gender, and family history

Skin sensitizing and drug allergies

While medicating your skin, you may also sensitize your body to substances that a topical product contains. This problem frequently occurs with ethylenediamine (EDA), a chemical that has been widely used as a stabilizer in topical anti-infective medications, such as Mycolog Cream and similar generic products. I discuss this topic in greater detail in Chapter 17, in the section on EDA.

I strongly advise against using topical forms — whether in prescription or OTC strengths — of antibiotics (such as neomycin), local anesthetics (such as benzocaine), and antihistamines (such as Benadryl and Caladryl) without first asking your doctor. You could develop a sensitivity to the substances in these topical preparations, which can subsequently result in a potentially serious systemic reaction if you take the drug in an oral or injected form.

Signs of drug hypersensitivities

Certain drugs have a tendency to produce reactions in specific tissues and organs. Although drug hypersensitivity reactions most frequently target the skin, the reaction can affect any organ system in your body, including mucous membranes, lymph nodes, kidneys, liver, lungs, and joints.

Common signs of allergic reactions that affect various organs and functions include the following symptoms:

- ✔ **Skin rashes:** Allergic drug rashes, which often take the form of red, itchy bumps, may appear all over your body. If a topical drug causes the reaction, the rash usually appears at the site where you applied the product. However, you may also have a reaction on your hands or any other part of your body that came into contact with the product. (See Chapter 17 for more information on topical drugs and contact dermatitis.)

- ✔ **Urticaria (hives) and angioedema (deep swelling):** These red, itchy welts and swollen lesions can appear anywhere on your body as a systemic allergic reaction to certain drugs. The most frequent allergic triggers of urticaria and angioedema for sensitized people include penicillin, sulfanomides, cephalosporins, insulin, and anti-sera (such as horse serum). Pseudoallergic reactions, frequently caused by aspirin, NSAIDs, and narcotic pain relievers, also commonly trigger hives and angioedema.

- ✔ **Other skin reactions:** In rare cases, more serious skin conditions can result from adverse allergic drug reactions. These more serious conditions can include

  - • **Exfoliative dermatitis:** This potentially life-threatening reaction may cause the top skin layer of your skin to shed over much of your body, with the remaining layer becoming red and scaly.

TECHNICAL STUFF

> ## What's acetyl got to do with hives?
>
> Aspirin (acetylsalicylic acid) is one of the most common triggers of hives. Although hives and angioedema are inflammatory conditions, you generally should not take acetylated forms of aspirin or other related anti-inflammatory medications to relieve these conditions without first consulting your physician. This advice also applies to OTC nonsteroidal anti-inflammatory drugs (NSAIDs), most of which contain ibuprofen (Advil, Motrin), ketoprofen (Actron, Orudis), or naproxen (Aleve) as active ingredients, and
>
> newer prescription NSAIDs, known as COX-2 inhibitors — including celecoxib (Celebrex) and rofecoxib (Vioxx). Likewise, avoid combination pain relievers that include any of these active ingredients.
>
> In many cases, you can use acetaminophen (Tylenol) or salicylsalicylic acid (Disalcid, Salflex), a non-acetylated form of aspirin known as *salsalate*, as substitutes for acetylated aspirin and NSAIDs.

- **Erythema multiforme:** This widespread reaction can produce itchy rashes on many parts of your body, most characteristically on the backs of your hands and feet. Very often, the hallmark pattern of this eruption resembles a bull's-eye, or in medicalese, a *target* or *iris lesion*. In many cases, you may also have a headache and fever.

- **Stevens-Johnson syndrome:** This extremely rare but serious condition can produce substantial tissue damage, often involving mucous membranes, such as your mouth, throat, and eyes. The reaction can also target internal organs such as your liver, kidney, and lungs. This syndrome can also result from a nonallergic, viral-precipitating factor, especially a herpes simplex infection.

✔ **Internal organs and functions:** Adverse drug reactions can also affect the lungs, liver, kidneys, gastrointestinal tract, and mucus membranes. Reactions involving your lungs may trigger asthma symptoms, such as wheezing, or can lead to pneumonia.

✔ **Fever:** In some patients, an allergic drug reaction may also cause a *drug fever*, occasionally accompanied by shaking chills and a skin rash.

✔ **Blood:** In some cases, adverse drug reactions can destroy and impair your body's ability to produce red blood cells, leading to low blood pressure and/or anemia.

✔ **Anaphylaxis:** In less frequent, but more serious cases, an immunologic adverse drug reaction can result in *anaphylaxis*, a severe, potentially life-threatening response that affects many organs simultaneously. According to recent estimates, anaphylaxis from penicillin hypersensitivity is the leading cause of drug-related anaphylactic deaths in the U.S., usually due to injections of penicillin. Fortunately, the use of penicillin shots has significantly decreased in recent years.

Mechanisms of drug hypersensitivity

Your immune system can respond to different types of allergens in a variety of ways. Although drug hypersensitivities can involve all four types of immune system mechanisms (see Chapter 1), in most allergic drug reactions, one mechanism usually predominates.

The following section explains various mechanisms of drug hypersensitivities:

- ✔ **IgE-mediated reactions (Type I):** This category of hypersensitivity results in immediate reactions such as anaphylaxis and includes symptoms of hives, swelling of the throat, wheezing, and cardiorespiratory collapse. The most common culprits for this extreme drug reaction are penicillin and its relatives. If you've had a prior allergic reaction to penicillin, you are six times more likely than the general population to experience another severe allergic reaction if you take this antibiotic again.

- ✔ **Cytotoxic reactions (Type II):** These reactions are serious and potentially life-threatening. They involve cell destruction, possibly resulting in the breakdown of your red blood cells, leading to anemia and decreased numbers of platelets in your blood (needed to make your blood clot). Drugs known to cause these reactions include penicillin, sulfonamides (Bactrim, Septra), and quinidine (Apo-Quinidine, Quinalan).

- ✔ **Immune complex reactions (Type III):** Manifestations of this reaction include fever, rash, hives, and symptoms that affect the lymph nodes and joints. This reaction, which physicians refer to as *serum sickness,* typically appears one to three weeks after taking the final doses of drugs such as penicillin, sulfonamides, thiouracil, and phenytoin.

- ✔ **Cell-mediated reactions (Type IV):** Contact dermatitis is the primary sign of this localized, non-systemic reaction (see Chapter 17). In cell-mediated reactions, symptoms appear on your skin after using topical drug preparations to which you're sensitized. The most frequent medication causes of this reaction are topical antibiotic preparations such as neomycin (Neosporin), topical anesthetics such as benzocaine and other -caines (Lanacane, Solarcaine), and antihistamines such as diphenhydramine (Benadryl).

Drug Intolerance and Idiosyncrasy

Unlike drug hypersensitivities, the production and interaction of IgE antibodies by your immune system are not factors in drug idiosyncrasy (medicalese for "we don't know") and drug intolerance reactions. For this reason, these types of reactions are far less predictable than those that result from drug hypersensitivities. Although the mechanisms involved in these kinds of reactions are less well documented, most adverse drug reactions fall into this category.

The drugs most often associated with drug idiosyncrasy and drug intolerance include

✔ **Quinidine:** Even a small dose of this medication, prescribed for arrhythmia (irregular heartbeat), can lead to *tinnitus* (ringing in the ears) in some heart patients.

✔ **Aspirin and NSAIDs (including newer prescription NSAIDs, known as COX-2 inhibitors):** If you're an asthma patient with nasal polyps and an aspirin sensitivity, using these pain relievers or related anti-inflammatories can lead to the potentially serious and even life-threatening symptoms of severe bronchoconstriction (constricted airways). This syndrome is known as the *aspirin triad* — asthma, nasal polyps, aspirin sensitivity, and a history of sinusitis — which I explain more extensively in Chapter 11.

✔ **Angiotensin-converting enzyme (ACE) inhibitors:** These inhibitors can produce coughing and angioedema. The coughing usually disappears within several weeks of discontinuing ACE medications. However, angioedema resulting from use of these medications can cause life-threatening complications, sometimes requiring hospitalization.

Other symptoms of non-immunologic aspirin and NSAID drug reactions can include *generalized urticaria* (total body hives), *rhinoconjunctivitis* (inflammation of nasal passages and eyes), and *airway edema* (swelling of the airways).

Diagnosing Adverse Drug Reactions

As you may suspect from reading previous sections of this chapter, diagnosing adverse drug reactions — such as a suspicious rash, fever, swollen and tender lymph nodes, or lung, kidney, or gastrointestinal disturbances — soon after starting a new drug can present a challenge. In fact, the testing options for determining whether an allergic mechanism causes your reactions are limited. In most cases, your medical history is the most important factor in making an accurate diagnosis.

Taking your drug reaction history

To evaluate the likelihood of an adverse drug reaction as the cause of the types of symptoms I discuss previously in this chapter, your doctor needs to take a thorough medical history. Be prepared to provide your doctor with detailed information about your medication use, because your physician probably needs to ask questions such as

✔ What drugs are you currently using and what drugs have you taken in the past?

✔ How long did you take a particular drug before symptoms started?

✔ Have you had similar episodes in the past?

✔ Has anyone in your family experienced adverse drug reactions?

Keeping track of your drugs

Determining the source of your adverse drug reaction can prove particularly tricky when you take more than one medication. Keeping a symptom diary can enable you to help your doctor narrow down the likeliest causes of your adverse reactions. (In Chapter 10, I discuss this topic in greater detail.)

In addition to a symptom diary, I also recommend establishing a drug record that lists all the medications — prescription and/or OTC — you take over your lifetime. Think of this diary as similar to recording your checks in your check register.

Your drug record should include information such as

✔ The brand and generic names of all the drugs you've used and are currently taking

✔ The conditions you're treating or have treated with particular drugs

✔ The effectiveness and/or results of taking these drugs

✔ For prescription products, the names of the doctors who prescribed those drugs and the dates when you received the prescription

✔ Any side effects and/or adverse reactions you may have experienced while taking the drugs

Skin testing for drug hypersensitivities

Allergy skin testing can prove helpful for diagnosing allergies to a few drugs, such as penicillin and related antibiotics, insulin, local anesthetics, and vaccines. However, I advise skin testing for these drugs only if your doctor considers these products essential for treating a medical condition that severely affects you and if your medical history indicates a likelihood of hypersensitivity to these medications.

Also keep in mind that skin testing isn't advisable if penicillin and related antibiotics are implicated in a previous, severe, non-immunologic systemic reaction, such as exfoliative dermatitis, erythema multiforme, or Stevens-Johnson syndrome (see "Signs of drug hypersensitivities," earlier in this chapter). For an in-depth discussion of allergy skin testing, see Chapter 8.

Patch testing for drug reactions

For cases involving cell-mediated reactions, such as localized, non-systemic reactions to topical preparations (characteristic of contact dermatitis), patch testing is the gold standard for diagnosing drug hypersensitivities.

Patch testing involves applying patches that contain small amounts of suspected allergens directly to your skin. A positive reaction usually appears as a small area of allergic contact dermatitis within one to four days (see Chapter 17 for more information on contact dermatitis).

If you have a severe or widespread outbreak of contact dermatitis, I don't advise using a patch test. Your doctor should also instruct you to immediately remove any patch that causes severe irritation.

General clinical testing for drug reactions

For cases involving potential late-phase drug-hypersensitivity reactions that appear days or weeks after you take a particular medication, your doctor may advise other types of testing. These tests can include the following:

- In the event that lung and/or heart complications develop days or weeks after starting a drug, your doctor may advise a chest X-ray and/or electrocardiogram (EKG).

- If your doctor suspects that an adverse drug reaction may affect your liver or kidneys, he or she may advise tests for those organ functions.

- If your doctor suspects a cytotoxic reaction, he or she may advise complete blood and platelet counts.

- If a suspected adverse drug reaction involves symptoms such as drug fever (see "Signs of drug hypersensitivities" earlier in this chapter), eosinophilic pneumonia (a form of pneumonia that features nonproductive coughing as the main symptom and is characterized by elevated levels of eosinophils; see Chapter 2), or an immune system disorder, your doctor may advise further tests to confirm the diagnosis.

Reducing Adverse Drug Reaction Risks

Your best bet for managing adverse drug reactions, as with other kinds of allergies, consists of avoiding the problematic substances. Using medications — particularly topical drugs — only when you really need them, instead of resorting to products and preparations for every ache and pain, can reduce your risks of developing drug sensitivities.

In addition, the overuse of antibiotics, especially for inappropriate treatment of viral infections such as the common cold and flu (for which antibiotics are ineffective), contributes to an increased incidence of drug sensitivity throughout the world.

Treating your reactions

For mild reactions, simply stopping the drug in question is the best remedy. When you experience more severe symptoms, your doctor may institute drug therapy to counteract your adverse reaction.

Drug therapy usually involves using one or more antihistamines, such as hydroxyzine (Atarax) and/or diphenhydramine (Benadryl), as well as a short course of oral corticosteroids (especially for symptoms such as persistent joint inflammation and discomfort) if needed. For pain, I often recommend acetaminophen (Tylenol) as the first choice, or a nonacetylated form of aspirin, known as *salsalate,* such as salicylsalicylic acid (Disalcid, Salflex).

Managing severe adverse drug reactions

If an adverse reaction causes severe skin problems, such as rashes, hives, or angioedema, or if you experience drug-induced anemia or platelet problems, your doctor may advise a short course of oral corticosteroids.

A life-threatening reaction such as anaphylaxis usually requires immediate administration of epinephrine (adrenaline), oxygen, antihistamines, and corticosteroids.

If you experience a non-immunologic adverse reaction to a drug that is essential for treating another medical condition from which you suffer, your doctor may treat you preventively with a short course of oral corticosteroids and antihistamines. This preventative treatment can often enable you to use the potentially problematic drug in the short term with a much-reduced risk of an adverse reaction.

If your doctor determines that you may experience a serious adverse drug reaction to particular drugs, wear a MedicAlert tag or bracelet. In the event that you're unable to communicate during a medical emergency, the information on the tag can prevent you from receiving an accidental dose of a drug that can trigger an adverse reaction.

Preventing penicillin problems

Simply staying away from a specific drug may not sufficiently eliminate your adverse drug reaction. If you're allergic to penicillin, you also need to avoid other antibiotic relatives of this drug, including frequently prescribed antibiotics such as ampicillin and amoxicillin. In addition, some patients with penicillin sensitivities may cross-react with certain cephalosporin antibiotics.

If you experience an allergic reaction, such as a rash, to an antibiotic, I suggest that you stop taking the medication (with your doctor's consent) and wait until your reaction resolves before starting another antibiotic as an immediate substitute. Many experts believe you're in a hypersensitive state during the period of time that an allergic reaction takes place, and you risk developing a sensitivity to another antibiotic if you begin taking it while your allergic symptoms are still present.

For example, if you develop a mild rash while taking an antibiotic such as amoxicillin/potassium clavulanate (Augmentin) for your sinusitis, your doctor may advise you to wait a few days or more (depending on the severity of your response) until the reaction resolves before you switch to an alternative, unrelated antibiotic, such as clarithromycin (Biaxin). Doing so may reduce the risk of sensitizing your immune system to other families of antibiotics.

Desensitizing your drug hypersensitivities

If you have a hypersensitivity to a medication that your doctor considers essential to your treatment, he or she may suggest skin testing, followed by rapid desensitization. The desensitization process requires rapidly administering incremental doses (starting with very small amounts) of the allergenic drug. The steady increase in the dose desensitizes your immune system so that it doesn't trigger an allergic response when you get a therapeutic dose of the drug in question.

Desensitization should only be performed under the supervision of an experienced physician and in a medical facility equipped to handle emergency situations.

Chapter 21

Preventing Insect Sting Reactions

●●●

In This Chapter

▶ Knowing what's stinging you

▶ Diagnosing insect sting hypersensitivities

▶ Treating serious insect sting reactions

▶ Preventing insect stings

●●●

*I*nsect stings are part of life. These creepy, crawly, and flying creatures have been around at least 400 million years (much longer than our own species), and they show no signs of going away. Although some insects spread diseases or harm crops, many of these creatures are essential and beneficial participants in the complex workings of this planet's ecosystems — for example, insects pollinate many crops, especially fruit.

Insect stings usually produce only local nonallergic reactions (as I explain in the next section) — such as redness, itching, swelling, and pain — due to the potent chemicals contained in their venom. However, according to recent estimates, 3 percent of adults and 1 percent of children in the United States may be at risk for serious allergic reactions to certain insect stings, potentially resulting in the following types of systemic symptoms:

✔ Hives (on your skin — not where bees live), itching, and skin swellings on parts of your body other than the sting site — for example, more than just a large local reaction

✔ Bronchospasm (airway constriction), tightness of the chest, and difficulty breathing

✔ Hoarseness and swelling of the tongue, throat, and upper airway (laryngeal edema — see Chapter 18)

✔ Dizziness

✔ Hypotensive shock (sudden drop in blood pressure)

✔ Anaphylaxis (a potentially life-threatening reaction affecting many organs simultaneously)

The good news is that although many insects bite or sting, only a very small percentage of stinging insects produce venom that can actually trigger allergic reactions. In fact, in terms of insect venom hypersensitivity, in the vast majority of cases, you only need to watch out for five groups of the estimated three million insect species, as shown in Figure 21-1:

- Honeybees (bumblebees, which are solitary bees, are rare causes of insect sting reactions).

- Yellow jackets.

- Wasps (specifically the social wasps, more commonly known as *paper wasps*).

- Hornets (white-faced and yellow hornets).

- Fire ants (both the red and black species). (See "Fire ants," later in this chapter, for more information.)

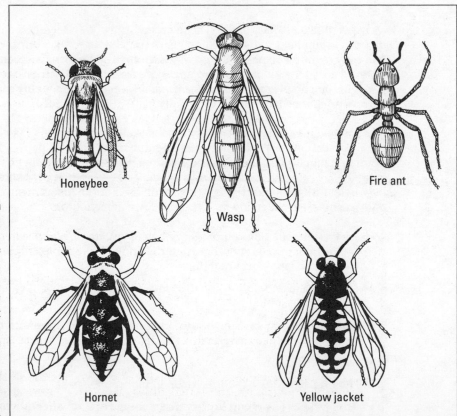

Figure 21-1:
These five groups of insects are the ones whose venom most often triggers allergic insect sting reactions in humans.

The stinging insects that can cause hypersensitivity reactions all belong to the *Hymenoptera* order — the third largest insect order — which encompasses more than 100,000 species. This insect order gets its name from Hymeno, the Greek god of marriage (whose name derives from the Greek word "hymen," which means *membranous*), because the flying species of this order have two pairs of membranous front and back wings ("optera" in Greek), held together by tiny hooks so that they function as one unit (the way married couples are supposed to work).

Mosquitoes and most other biting insects can cause painful and/or irritating bites and may also spread diseases, but they rarely cause severe allergic reactions. However, bites from genus *triatoma* (kissing bug or cone-nose bug, found primarily in rural areas of the southwestern U.S.), which are usually painless and almost always occur at night, have been associated with severe allergic reactions, including cases of anaphylaxis, due to the allergen contained in the insect's saliva.

Reacting to Insect Stings

Insect sting hypersensitivities are equal-opportunity allergies. Even if you have other allergic conditions — such as allergic rhinitis (hay fever), asthma, atopic dermatitis (eczema), or food allergies — or have a family history of atopy (a genetic susceptibility to developing allergic disease), you are not at any greater risk than anyone else for having an allergic reaction to *Hymenoptera* insects.

However, if you have a chronic heart or lung condition (such as coronary artery disease or asthma) and also have a stinging insect hypersensitivity, you may be at greater risk for developing more serious reactions if one of those creatures stings you.

Insect sting reactions are classified according to the type and severity of symptoms they produce. Here's what you should know about these reactions:

- ✔ **Small, local reactions:** Most insect stings cause localized reactions that pose few serious medical consequences and that don't require special treatment. However, you may experience redness, itching, swelling, and pain for several days at the sting site. Irritating enzymes and chemicals in insect venom, rather than an allergic mechanism, create these kinds of reactions.

- ✔ **Large, local reactions:** These responses involve extreme swelling that extends from the sting site, sometimes affecting an entire arm or leg. However, the swelling usually disappears in two to three days. As with small, local reactions, these large, local reactions result from the enzymes and chemicals in the insect's venom. You're at no greater risk than the general population of developing a serious, systemic reaction to an insect sting if you've ever experienced a large local reaction.

- **Systemic reactions:** *Cutaneous* (skin-related) eruptions, such as *urticaria* (hives) and *angiodema* (deep swellings), over a large area of the body often are a feature of these more serious reactions. A systemic reaction results from an allergic mechanism. Unlike small or large local reactions, symptoms of a systemic reaction appear on areas of your body other than the sting site. After you've had one systemic reaction to a sting, you're likely to have the same or worse reaction if the same type of insect stings you again. However, treating the discomfort associated with these skin reactions is usually the only treatment necessary, because these symptoms are rarely life-threatening.

- **Life-threatening reactions:** Anaphylactic symptoms, such as swelling of the tongue and/or throat (laryngeal edema), breathing difficulty, and dizziness or fainting (due to a fall in blood pressure) are signs of this type of systemic reaction to insect venom. Approximately 40 people die each year in the U.S. from anaphylaxis resulting from severe allergic reactions to insect stings. If you experience a life-threatening reaction, you need immediate emergency treatment (see "Treating urgent insect sting cases," later in this chapter). In addition, because these potentially life-threatening reactions result from allergic triggers in the insect venom, your doctor may recommend skin testing and a course of venom immunotherapy (VIT) to prevent future reactions. (Read "Long-term treatment: Venom immunotherapy," later in this chapter, for more information on VIT.)

What's bugging you?

The *Hymenoptera* insects responsible for producing allergic reactions belong to these three separate families:

- **Apidae:** Honeybees are members of this family. Flowers and bright colors usually attract these busy bees. The bees in this family generally aren't aggressive, except for Africanized honeybees (so-called killer bees), as I explain in the next section.

- **Vespidae:** This family includes yellow jackets, hornets, and wasps. These insects generally feed on human food, which is why you may see them hovering or crawling over garbage cans, leftover food on the picnic table, or at any outdoor event that includes food and sugary beverages such as soft drinks.

- **Formicidae:** These ant families include the two types of fire ants — red and black — that plague the southeastern U.S. and Puerto Rico and that are spreading throughout the rest of the southern states. These ants get their name from the painful, burning pustules that result from their (often) multiple stings. You certainly don't want these ants in your pants, or anywhere else in your vicinity, for that matter.

Venom varieties

The stinging insect species in the three families that I list in the preceding section produce different venoms, as distinct from each other as ragweed and dust-mite allergens. However, cross-reactivity to these stinging insects' venoms does exist *within* families. For example, if you have a sensitivity to yellow jacket venom, you may also have an allergic reaction if you're stung by a hornet.

On the other hand, you'll be happy to know that cross-reactivity is far more limited between the stinging insect families. For example, multiple sensitivity to both honeybees (Apids) and yellow jackets (Vespids) is much less common than multiple sensitivity to hornets and yellow jackets (both members of the Vespid family).

The following sections provide more details on the stinging *Hymenoptera* insects and how they can affect you.

Honeybees

Bees are the most important pollinators in the insect world, and they also make honey, one of the oldest crops harvested by humans. Honeybees are either domestic — raised in hives for commercial purposes — or wild. Wild honeybees usually build their hives, which may contain thousands of bees, in tree hollows or old logs. Here's more important information about these hard-working insects:

- **Appearance:** Honeybees have hairy bodies with yellow and black markings.

- **Habitat:** These insects are widespread throughout most of the U.S. However, because honeybees prefer warmer climates, they tend to cause more problems in areas such as southern California, where they're one of the leading causes of insect sting reactions.

- **Behavior:** Honeybees aren't usually aggressive away from their hives. Female workers are the only honeybees that sting. They give their lives to protect their hives when they leave their large stingers in their victims — the only stinging insect that does this.

Yellow jackets

These ground-dwelling insects are the most frequent causes of stings in most of the U.S., particularly the northern states. Like paper wasps (see "Wasps," later in this chapter), yellow jackets build paper nests, but they enclose them. Other important characteristics of yellow jackets are

- **Appearance:** Similar to hornets, these insects have bright yellow and black markings. Unlike hornets, however, they don't have a dark band under their eyes.

- ✔ **Habitat:** Yellow jackets usually build their nests in the ground, wall tunnels, crevices, and hollow logs. Therefore, you may encounter them more often while working in your yard, gardening, or farming.

- ✔ **Behavior:** Yellow jackets can be very aggressive and may sting — sometimes repeatedly — with minimum provocation, especially if food is around. They like the taste of soft drinks and may dive right into the container. In fact, many people get stung while drinking a beverage. Because female yellow jackets require protein in their diets, they may also go after meat (for example, hamburger at your cookout) as a food of choice.

Wasps

Watch for the so-called *paper wasps,* which get their name from the papier-mâché honeycomb nests that they build. These nests can be several inches in diameter, and the wasps often locate them in shrubs, under the eaves of houses and barns, and sometimes in pipes on playgrounds or under patio furniture. Here are other important points to keep in mind about wasps:

- ✔ **Appearance:** Wasps have hairless bodies with narrow waists and black or brown markings.

- ✔ **Habitat:** Wasps are primarily a problem in the southern half of the United States.

- ✔ **Behavior:** Wasps are easy to provoke and can sting repeatedly and in large numbers when disturbed.

Most solitary wasps — except for velvet ants (also wasps, in spite of their name) — are much less aggressive and usually sting humans only if handled. In spite of their bad reputation, farmers often consider wasps useful, because many of them feed on other insects that harm crops and trees.

Hornets

Related to yellow jackets and wasps, hornets build large papier-mâché nests several feet in diameter, which are often hard for humans to see, because hornets frequently nest in tree hollows or high in tree branches. In North America, the two varieties of this insect that concern people the most are white-faced hornets (also known as *bald-faced hornet*) and yellow hornets.

- ✔ **Appearance:** Hornets are usually larger than other *Hymenoptera,* with short waists, compact black bodies, sparse hair, multiple yellow or white stripes, and a dark band under the eyes.

- ✔ **Habitat:** Hornets often build their oval or pear-shaped nests in trees and shrubs. They're especially prevalent in the southern United States.

- ✔ **Behavior:** Hornets are extremely aggressive, especially when close to their nests (hence the term *hornet's nest*) and, like wasps, can sting repeatedly.

The buzz on killer bees

Killer bees, the infamous result of breeding between wild South American bees and African honeybees that were accidentally released in Brazil in 1956, have been grabbing a lot of headlines. More properly called *Africanized honeybees,* these hybrid bees have gradually migrated northward from South America, establishing themselves in many parts of Central America and entering southern Texas in 1990.

At the time this book was written, Africanized honeybees were present in parts of Texas, Arizona, and California and were gradually spreading through other southern parts of the United States. They don't survive in colder climates, but occasionally forage into northern parts of the United States during the summer months. These bees are less selective in their hive sites than native honey bees — the descendants of European honeybees brought to the Americas from the Old World by colonists and immigrants over the last three centuries — and may nest in holes in outside walls, old tires, in the ground, around fence posts, and even in water meter vaults in front yards of some homes.

The venom of so-called killer bees isn't any different or more dangerous than most other wild or domestic native bees. Killer bees have a bad reputation primarily because of their aggressive behavior. When provoked, killer bees tend to attack in swarms, inflicting many more stings on their unfortunate targets than other types of bees do. If a swarm of killer bees (or any other stinging insect) attacks you, drop facedown on the ground, curl up, and protect your head as much as possible.

Scientists hope that, as they slowly migrate northwards, these belligerent bees will breed with less aggressive homegrown honeybees, thus resulting in mellower and better-behaved subsequent generations, although this has yet to occur. The main damage that killer bees actually cause is economic, because they often interfere with the pollination of crops by domestic honeybees.

Fire ants

Although you may think it's odd that these insects are included with buzzing, stinging insects, fossil evidence indicates that ants probably evolved from wasps. Count your blessings that out of the estimated one quadrillion ants living on this planet (even more numerous than *...For Dummies* books), you only need to contend with four species of stinging fire ants in the United States, depending on where you live.

Of the fire ant species, two are native and two were inadvertently introduced from South America in the early decades of the 20th century. Here's what you need to know when dealing with these fierce insects:

- **Appearance:** Fire ants are red or black and resemble typical, non-stinging ants, except they have a well-developed rear stinger. (If they've ever stung you, you know how well-developed that stinger is!)

- **Habitat:** These ants are well established in the Gulf Coast states of the U.S. and Puerto Rico and are spreading to other southern states. They build large, hardened mounds several inches high and one to two feet wide, which are very common along sidewalks and roadways in the southeastern U.S. Because fire ants' nests are underground, getting rid of these creatures is extremely difficult.

✔ **Behavior:** These insects are very aggressive, especially if you disturb their mounds. They've developed a particularly effective way of inflicting damage: They anchor themselves to their victims with their powerful jaws and then pivot themselves (they're also quite limber) to deliver multiple stings, in a semi-circular pattern, from their rear stinger. Fire ant stings usually produce pustules, sometimes within 24 hours. The most aggressive fire ants are the red imported fire ant, *Solenopsis invicta*. This species stings livestock, injures crops, and can cause short circuits by building mounds around electrical equipment.

Diagnosing Your Stings

In addition to physically examining your sting reaction, taking a thorough medical history is the first step in properly diagnosing and effectively managing insect hypersensitivity (as with any other allergic condition). Your doctor needs to know whether you've been stung in the past and the symptoms you've experienced. Providing your doctor with as much possible information about your current sting is also very important.

Know your stinger

Figuring out which bug is bugging you may be a little easier if your doctor knows all the circumstances about your sting. For example:

✔ If you're clipping the hedges when you get stung, yellow jackets or hornets are likely suspects.

✔ A hornet may sting you while you're sitting under a tree or near a bush without obvious provocation.

✔ Insects that sting your feet while you're walking outside barefoot or in sandals are most likely yellow jackets — just like you and me, they don't like getting stepped on!

✔ Getting stung while lounging on a patio chair may indicate that your chair harbors a wasp nest.

> ✔ Stinging that occurs while you stop to smell the roses is usually a result of honeybees, which like to feed among flowers.
>
> ✔ If you're stung while changing your tire on a rainy night in Georgia, you may be on top of a fire ant mound.

To further identify the insect responsible for your reaction, try to provide your doctor with the following information:

> ✔ Your activities at the time you were stung.
>
> ✔ Where you were when you were stung.
>
> ✔ Where the insect stung you on your body.
>
> ✔ The types of insects that seem active in the area where you were stung.

If you're able to capture the creature that stung you, bring it with you to your doctor's office. Knowing exactly what stung you greatly helps your doctor determine how to treat your reaction and hopefully may help you prevent future reactions. As I mention earlier in this chapter, if a honeybee stings you, you'll probably have a stinger and a dead bee as evidence of a "close encounter of the unkind."

Allergy skin testing

If you've had a serious, systemic reaction to an insect sting, your doctor will usually recommend allergy skin testing (see Chapter 8). This procedure can determine whether your reaction is the result of an allergic response. If it is, allergy testing can determine the specific cause of your reaction — you may be sensitive to more than one insect — and the extent of your sensitivity.

Because you may be at a higher risk of having a similar reaction in the future (due to increased sensitization from your previous insect sting), and considering that such reactions can be potentially dangerous, allergy skin testing for insect sting hypersensitivity will help your doctor to determine appropriate and effective prevention measures.

To determine whether you have one or more sensitivities to the various *Hymenoptera* insects, your doctor will need to perform skin tests by using venom extracts from each of the stinging insects. The results can help your doctor determine the advisability of initiating venom immunotherapy (VIT), which I explain in the final section of this chapter. Allergen extracts for skin testing and immunotherapy for the diagnosis and treatment of bites of *triatoma* and other biting insects are not currently commercially available.

Preventing and Managing Insect Reactions

Effectively managing your sensitivity to insect stings can mean the difference between enjoying the great outdoors relatively worry-free or risking recurrences of serious allergic reactions.

The first step you can take to effectively manage your sensitivity to insect stings (and this should come as no great surprise!) is to avoid getting stung. When it comes to insect stings, an ounce of avoidance is worth a pound of medication.

If you have an insect sting hypersensitivity, I advise consulting your doctor about taking preventive measures, such as the following:

- Avoid bugging insects, and they usually won't bug you. If stinging insects are in your vicinity, don't provoke them, but move as quickly and calmly out of the area as possible. If you run, flap your arms, or otherwise get agitated, the insect may sting in self-defense. In general, avoid jerky, fast movements, because these can startle and provoke stinging insects.

- Make sure that your children don't poke, prod, hit, or otherwise play with insect hives, nests, or mounds.

- Hire a trained extermination professional to check your home and its surroundings for insect nests. (I don't advise doing this home improvement project yourself.)

- Stay away from strongly scented lotions, perfumes, colognes, and hair products. Likewise, don't wear brightly colored or flower-print clothing. Try khaki and other light-colored apparel. Also, avoid loose clothing that may trap insects.

- Don't use electric hedge clippers and power mowers. For some reason, electricity really excites *Hymenoptera* insects, and you don't want to be part of their excitement. In general, I advise against doing yard work yourself if you have a stinging insect hypersensitivity.

- If you work outdoors, cover up from head to toe with long pants, a long-sleeved shirt, socks, closed shoes, a hat, and work gloves. Wear closed shoes (not sandals) or sneakers when you're outdoors and don't go out in your stocking feet or barefoot.

- Practice caution near flowery plants, blooming orchards (they're in bloom because something's busy pollinating them), bushes, clover fields, eaves, attics, garbage containers, and picnic areas.

- Have insecticides at hand to zap stinging insects before they zap you (insect repellents don't work on stinging insects). Bear in mind that if these products kill insects, then they're also not too good for you either.

Therefore, make sure that you use insecticides properly as per the manufacturer's instructions, to limit your exposure to the toxins in these products.

✔ Be careful when eating or drinking outdoors or when you're near areas where food and beverages are served. Also, cover the opening to your beverage in between sips, and never drink from an open container that's been left outdoors.

✔ Check to see whether the insect left a stinger, which usually looks like a black thorn or splinter, in your skin. Carefully remove the stinger, using a tweezer to pry or a credit card to flick or scrape the stinger from your skin (certainly the least expensive way to use a credit card!). Never squeeze the stinger with your fingers in an effort to remove it from your skin. Doing so only pumps more venom into your body, making your reaction worse.

✔ After a sting, walk slowly, don't run. Running may increase your body's absorption of the venom. (See "Treating local reactions" for more important tips on treating stings.)

Treating local reactions

You can manage the symptoms of local reactions (itching, swelling, and pain) until they pass with simple remedies, such as:

✔ **Cold compresses,** which can help reduce local pain and swelling.

✔ **Local anesthetic cream, oral antihistamines, and oral analgesics,** which may help relieve the pain and itching of skin reactions.

Treating systemic reactions

Hives and angiodema (deep swellings) can sometimes be the first signs of an impending anaphylactic insect sting reaction. Because it's impossible to predict whether these systemic symptoms will or will not progress to anaphylaxis, it's therefore safer to immediately administer epinephrine (see the next section) than to wait until the reaction potentially becomes life-threatening.

If the systemic reaction is limited to hives and angioedema, then your best strategy is to avoid further aggravating your skin while soothing it as much as possible. Advisable steps include

✔ Bathing and washing with lukewarm water and using gentle soaps instead of harsh ones to reduce itching. Hot baths and showers may intensify your symptoms. Likewise, avoid hot environments and keep your home — especially your bedroom — cool.

✔ Patting yourself dry with a soft towel after bathing and applying moisturizers immediately afterward to seal in moisture.

✔ Wearing comfortable, loose, cotton clothing instead of tight-fitting garments.

✔ Taking oral antihistamines may also be advisable to help relieve your symptoms.

Treating urgent insect sting cases

If you're prone to serious systemic insect sting reactions and you get stung despite taking protective measures, you should be prepared to prevent a life-threatening reaction (anaphylaxis). Consult with your doctor about getting a prescription for an injectable epinephrine kit (such as an EpiPen, EpiPen Jr. for children under 66 pounds, or AnaKit), which contains an injectable dose of epinephrine.

Make sure that your doctor shows you how to use the epinephrine kit. Learning the proper technique for administering epinephrine in your physician's office is much better than to trying to figure it out for the first time when you're having a reaction.

Keep these important points about using an epinephrine kit in mind:

✔ Having more than one injectable epinephrine kit is a good idea. That way, you can keep one at home and have one with you when you may be exposed to stinging insects, for example during a picnic, while hiking, or other outdoor activities. You may want to keep more than one kit with you when traveling or going on an extended outing, because the initial injection wears off in 30 minutes and you may need another injection before you can get emergency care.

✔ Store any kits you're not keeping with you at room temperature, and protect them from sunlight.

✔ If your child is at risk for anaphylactic reactions to insect stings, you should keep a kit at home and consider keeping one at his or her school or day care (in consultation with the personnel at these places). Make sure personnel at those locations know how and when to administer this medication.

✔ Many people also keep an antihistamine such as diphenhydramine (Benadryl) with them in the event of a serious insect sting reaction. However, I strongly advise you not to rely solely on an antihistamine, which can take up to 30 minutes to start becoming effective. In addition, this medication will not prevent anaphylaxis. Clearly, injectable epinephrine should be the intial treatment for anaphylaxis prior to the use of any antihistamine.

- ✔ Remember that you need to get emergency treatment immediately after using your epinephrine kit, because the drug's effect usually doesn't last more than 30 minutes.

- ✔ If you're at risk for anaphylaxis, I strongly advise you to wear a MedicAlert bracelet or necklace in case you're unable to speak during a reaction.

Long-term treatment: Venom immunotherapy

If you've had a serious systemic reaction to an insect sting, your doctor will probably advise you to consider *venom immunotherapy* (VIT). This form of immunotherapy (allergy shots) is effective in about 98 percent of cases.

VIT injections are usually initially administered on a weekly basis, beginning with an extremely small dose of venom from the insect to which you react. Very often, doctors will initiate a rapid *desensitization* process so that you reach a maintenance dose as soon and as safely as possible. After you've worked up to a *maintenance dose,* shots are usually given every four weeks during your first year of immunotherapy and every six to eight weeks in subsequent years.

After three to five years of VIT, depending on the degree of your sensitivity and the level of your initial allergic episode, your doctor may recommend that you discontinue immunotherapy if skin tests are negative or the venom-specific IgE antibodies in your system have dropped to an insignificant level. Most experts agree that at the end of five years, VIT can usually be safely discontinued. For the vast majority of patients who have completed a course of VIT, the threat of another life-threatening reaction to an insect sting is remote.

Part VI
The Part of Tens

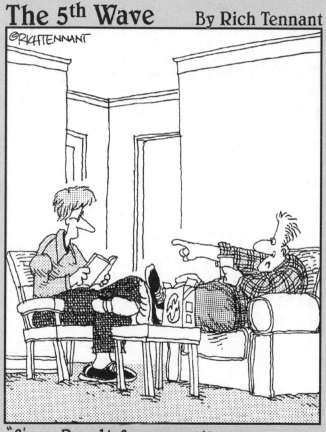

The 5th Wave   By Rich Tennant

"C'mon, Darrel! Someone with asthma shouldn't be lying around all day. Whereas someone with no life, like myself, has a very good reason."

In this part . . .

The Part of Tens is a tradition in *...For Dummies* books. In Chapter 22, I discuss what you should take with you — and what you should take into account — when traveling with allergies and asthma.

In Chapter 23, I provide you with examples of significant people from ancient times to today who have excelled in many impressive ways in spite of their asthma. I hope this chapter inspires you to further seek out the care that you deserve, which can give you the freedom to pursue your own personal goals and aspirations.

Chapter 22

Ten Tips for Traveling with Allergies and Asthma

*1*f only airlines could lose your allergies or asthma the way they sometimes lose your baggage. Imagine if you could leave your allergic rhinitis (hay fever) instead of your heart in San Francisco. And wouldn't it be nice to wake up in the city that never sleeps because the Big Apple stirs you to the very core — instead of an asthma episode interrupting a good night's rest?

Of course, getting away from allergies and asthma isn't that easy. Extensive studies over the past 15 years show that these ailments are ongoing conditions that you usually don't outgrow, although they can certainly vary in character and severity throughout your lifetime.

Think of asthma and allergies as constant companions. Wherever you may roam, these types of conditions probably accompany you to some degree. Knowing how to control the symptoms of these ailments is vital to ensuring that no matter what else may go wrong during your vacation or business travel, your allergies or asthma won't complicate or ruin your plans.

Planning a Safe, Healthy Trip

A key element in proper travel planning is avoiding places where you know pollens, dander, tobacco smoke, or other allergens and irritants may be prevalent and could, depending on your specific sensitivities, trigger your allergy and/or asthma symptoms.

The following points are general guidelines for preventing problems frequently associated with these triggers:

✔ **Ragweed:** Avoiding travel to the eastern half of the United States and Canada from mid-August through October is probably advisable (if you don't already live there) if you're sensitized to ragweed pollen. If you must travel to those areas during ragweed season, ask your physician about preventive medications you can take to keep your symptoms under control (see Chapter 6). Also, the National Allergy Bureau (NAB) of the American Academy of Allergy, Asthma, and Immunology (AAAAI) has a "United States Pollen Calendar" that charts the prevalence of allergenic pollens from certain trees, grasses, and weeds, as well as several other allergens, around the country throughout the year. Check out the NAB Web site at www.aaaai.org/nab/ or call 1-800-9-POLLEN (1-800-976-5536). (See Chapter 5 for more information on pollens.)

✔ **Dander:** Beware of visiting or staying in the homes of people who live with cats, dogs, and other animals, including rabbits, birds, and gerbils and other pet rodents. Even if the animal is removed from the area during your stay, you could still suffer an adverse reaction because of the residual dander and/or hair in the room. Horseback riding also may not be advisable. Before you saddle up for a dude ranch out west, make sure you can control any symptoms that Trigger's horsehair might just trigger. Consult your doctor about preventive medications (and see Chapters 6 and 11).

✔ **Food allergens:** The foods that trigger allergic reactions most frequently in adults with food hypersensitivities include peanuts, fish, shellfish, and tree nuts; for children, the most common triggers are milk, eggs, peanuts, tree nuts, soy, and wheat (see Chapter 19). Because of the swiftness and severity with which a food allergy reaction can strike (especially with peanuts), be especially vigilant in avoiding these triggers when traveling. In particular, if you or your child is sensitive to peanuts and you're planning to travel where these seemingly harmless legumes are a regular part of local cuisine (many parts of East Asia, for example), ask your doctor about additional precautions you can take. Not only is it possible that peanuts will be a clearly identifiable ingredient added to numerous dishes, but they also may be a hidden part of the cooking process itself in many cases. When in doubt, you should probably avoid local fare in these parts of the world, rather than risk reactions such as an asthma attack, hives (see Chapter 18), or worse yet, a potentially life-threatening case of anaphylaxis.

✔ **Insect stings:** If you're sensitized to the venom of *Hymenoptera* insects (honeybees, wasps, yellow jackets, hornets, and fire ants), a sting from one of these creatures can mean discomfort, swelling, itching, hives, or, in rare cases, potentially life-threatening adverse reactions. When traveling to Puerto Rico and the southeastern U.S. (particularly the Gulf Coast), be especially careful: In addition to wasps, fire ants are prevalent there and have been spreading to other southern parts of the country as well (see Chapter 21).

✔ **Poison ivy:** Walking in the woods can be one of life's great pleasures, unless you're sensitized to plants in the *Toxicodendron* family (such as poison ivy) and have a close encounter of the contact dermatitis kind with the resin of these plants. The resulting skin irritation can turn the rest of your vacation into a very uncomfortable experience. The simplest advice is to avoid areas where poison ivy and related plants grow and to remember the old scout saying: "Leaves of three, let them be." For more tips and information on poison ivy and other contact dermatitis sensitivities, see Chapter 17.

Adjusting Treatment for Travel

Prevention is the key to a safe and trouble-free trip, which usually means consulting your physician ahead of time to evaluate your asthma management plan or your course of allergy treatment and to make any advisable adjustments, based on where and when you're going and what you'll be doing while traveling. You may need to adjust your medication because of increased exposures to triggers. In addition, remember that changes in time zones may affect the dosage schedule of some medications you're taking (for any ailment, not just asthma or allergies).

After you've established the best way to manage and control your condition while away, you need to make sure that you'll be able to stick with the program that your physician advises. If possible, get a letter from your doctor summarizing your medical history, as well as the treatments and medications you're currently taking. If you're at risk of acute allergic or asthma attacks, ask your physician about wearing a MedicAlert pendant on your wrist or around your neck. (See the appendix for information on this and other valuable asthma and allergy products.)

Taking Medications and Other Essentials

Make sure you have all your necessary medical supplies, devices, and prescriptions with you when traveling. If flying (or riding on a train or bus), keep these items in your carry-on bag. After you arrive at your destination, keep your essentials with you instead of leaving them in your hotel room (or other accommodation) when you're out and about. If you need to leave your medications in the room (for example, while using hotel recreational facilities), make sure you store these products in a safe and secure location such as the room safe or in a locked suitcase, instead of leaving them out on the bathroom countertop.

Keep medications in their original containers and never mix pills of different types into one receptacle. By keeping them in their original containers, you'll have the proper dosage information readily available, which could be especially important if someone else needs to administer your medication to you. Also, if you're traveling internationally, customs officials are generally less suspicious of pills and capsules in their original containers.

If you or your child uses a nebulizer at home, ask your doctor about taking one with you on your trip. If you're traveling overseas, don't forget to bring whatever adapters and converters (available in most luggage, electronics, and travel stores) you may need in order to use your domestic devices in different countries. The electric current in many other parts of the world is 220 volts rather than the 110 voltage that is standard in the U.S. and Canada. If you have a portable nebulizer, remember also to bring extra batteries.

Getting Medications and Medical Help Abroad

Ask your doctor about special medical considerations for specific countries and areas. Some countries require that you take certain vaccine shots before your visit. As for medications, don't assume that every place you visit has pharmacies stocked with the supplies you need. Write down both the brand names of your medications and their generic names. In a pinch, having both names available may allow a local pharmacist to find what you need.

When planning your trip, you may want to obtain a booklet that lists qualified, English-speaking physicians in just about every country of the world. The International Association for Medical Assistance to Travelers (IAMAT), a voluntary organization based in Canada, offers this booklet. You can contact them at 716-754-4883 or via their Web site at `www.sentex.net/~iamat` for further information.

Also, if you're a U.S. citizen, the U.S. State Department's American Citizens Services can provide help in case of an emergency. Call 202-647-5226 before your departure to receive information on contacting U.S. embassies and consulates for assistance in dealing with medical matters in the areas where you plan to travel.

Flying with Allergens and Irritants

Your fellow airplane passengers may make you sick. Studies show that airplane passenger cabins are some of the worst indoor dust mite and dander sites. Because airliners are tightly sealed environments that often lack adequate air filtering or cleaning, they often concentrate sky-high quantities of allergens and irritants that hundreds, even thousands of passengers constantly track in with them. So be advised: Your seat may already be occupied by frequent flier allergens.

Many airplane seats house thriving colonies of dust mites and their allergenic waste products. In addition, while all U.S., Canadian, and many European flights ban smoking anywhere on the aircraft (and in most parts of airport terminals), some international flights still allow smoking.

If exposure to tobacco smoke triggers your allergy or asthma symptoms, find out as much as possible about an air carrier's smoking policies. If your travel includes flying an airline that permits smoking, try to get seating as far away from the smoking section as possible.

Here's my general advice to patients who are planning air travel:

✔ Pack your medications in a carry-on bag so they're immediately available in the event of a serious allergic reaction and in case the airline loses your luggage. (You want to avoid finding yourself in strange territory without your medications.)

✔ Stay hydrated during your flight. Avoid alcohol and drink plenty of water. Not only does drinking water help minimize your problems with allergies and asthma, but it'll also probably put a dent in whatever jet lag you may otherwise develop.

✔ If you have the opportunity, consider upgrading to first or business class. If available, the leather seats might be less likely to harbor allergy triggers, and at the very least, you'll give yourself more breathing room.

Considering Allergy Shots and Travel

When you're traveling, I usually recommend transferring your immunotherapy (allergy shots) program to another location only if you'll be gone at least a month or more (if you're a snowbird from the North wintering in southern California or southern Florida, for example). If, in fact, you'll be gone for a month or more, ask your physician for a referral to a doctor in the area where you'll be staying and have that physician administer your shots in a medical facility.

Although practices vary in different areas of the U.S. and the world, I strongly advise not giving yourself allergy shots. The risk, although low, of a bad reaction or even anaphylactic shock means you need qualified medical personnel around you, just in case (see Chapter 8). When visiting the physician in the new location, bring your allergy serum (vaccine) vials in a refrigerated or ice-insulated pack, and make sure you have clear written instructions from your doctor back home regarding your dose.

Reducing Trigger Exposures in Hotels and Motels

Tobacco smoke and its lingering traces can cause problems, especially outside the U.S. or Canada, where hotels and other accommodations are less likely to restrict smoking on their premises. Wherever you happen to stay, I advise reserving a room on a smoke-free floor. Likewise, if feathers pose a potential allergy problem for you, bring your own pillow and pillowcase (see Chapter 6).

Inspect the room before you occupy it, looking for signs of animal hair, dirty air vents, dust, or mold. If you find evidence suggesting that staying in the room will lead to breathing problems, ask for another room that appears safer and more comfortable. In some cases, your doctor may advise bringing along a portable HEPA air filter system (see Chapter 11).

Avoiding Food Allergies during Your Trip

As you travel from city to city and country to country throughout the world, you may come into contact with foods to which you have an allergy (not just an intolerance — see Chapter 19 for the difference between the two conditions). In some cases, the menu in a given restaurant, hotel, or café reveals all you need to know regarding potentially problematic ingredients. But more often than not, you need to ask a lot of questions about the cuisine, its component parts, and how it's prepared. Don't be rude, but definitely don't be shy.

As I explain in Chapter 19, you may need to do more than simply determine that a particular dish doesn't contain foods to which you're allergic. For example, in many restaurants, various dishes are all prepared on the same grill. In this case, if you're allergic to shellfish, for example, make sure that the cooking surface and utensils used to prepare your chicken, steak, or other food haven't also been previously used to prepare shellfish. If they have, allergens from the shellfish may end up in your meal, potentially causing a distressful dining experience.

If your food hypersensitivities put you at risk for anaphylaxis, you should wear a Medic Alert pendant or bracelet. I also advise asking your doctor about prescribing an epinephrine kit such as an EpiPen or AnaKit (see Chapter 19), and be sure to carry the kit with you.

Finding Help in Case of Emergencies

Although the local hospital probably isn't at the top of your sightseeing list when you travel, I strongly advise finding out the location of the nearest medical facility equipped to treat you in case of a serious adverse allergic reaction or severe asthma episode. Knowing where the closest help is available can help ensure that you get effective treatment if you experience a life-threatening reaction.

Depending on your destination, you can easily obtain local hospital locations from the organizations that I list earlier in this chapter, the organizations that I list in the appendix, your doctor, or your travel agent. In some cases, you may need to do more homework; however, your health and safety are worth the effort.

Traveling with Your Allergic or Asthmatic Child

When traveling with a child who has allergies or asthma, many of the same considerations that adults must contend with also apply. These points include the following:

- ✔ Pack two containers of all medications, and make sure that you've labeled them properly. Keep one container as a carry-on with you, and keep the other in a purse, backpack, or briefcase.

- ✔ Obtain a MedicAlert bracelet or necklace for your child.

- ✔ Teach your child how to pack his or her asthma and/or allergy medications properly. In addition to preparing your child for trips that he or she may take without you, this lesson can also help your youngster learn more about managing his or her condition appropriately.

- ✔ Take at least two epinephrine kits (such as an EpiPen, EpiPen Jr. for children under 66 pounds, or AnaKit) if your child is at risk for anaphylaxis to ensure that you'll always have one at hand. Make sure that you and/or your child (depending on the youngster's age) know how to use the kit. Knowing how to use the kit means you should receive instructions on the proper use of the injector in your doctor's office, rather than waiting for a potential emergency to figure it out.

✔ Ask questions about meals. If your child has peanut allergies, be especially vigilant on airplanes (particularly with the contents of those appealingly packaged snack bags), where peanuts can be as common as delayed flights (see Chapter 14).

Asthma camps

Children with asthma can benefit from a special type of vacation experience. A number of organizations, including the American Lung Association (ALA), sponsor children's asthma camps. If your child has asthma, you may want to consider sending him or her to one of these camps for a healthy, safe, educational, and fun nature-oriented vacation. Asthma camps generally offer one- to two-week programs that teach children how to recognize the signs of asthma and allergy triggers, use medications and inhaler devices properly, and the basics of asthma management. Call the ALA at 800-586-4872 for a list of asthma camps throughout the U.S. and Canada.

Chapter 23

Ten Famous Folks with Asthma

Rarely do you think of famous figures such as Augustus Caesar, Ludwig van Beethoven, and Charles Dickens in the same breath — unless you're considering the many great achievers throughout human history who had asthma.

The modern world also abounds with asthmatics who have had a significant impact on human events, including John F. Kennedy, Jackie Joyner-Kersee, Kenny G, and Liza Minnelli, to name only a few. Living with asthma doesn't mean you're sentenced to life's sidelines.

Renowned leaders, writers, musicians, doctors, and athletes have overcome their asthma to achieve greatness in their field of endeavor — in some cases, long before the development of the medications and therapies that help today's asthmatics.

Imagine Dickens, coughing deeply and incessantly while trying to finish *David Copperfield,* or Beethoven suffering from attacks of *dyspnea* (shortness of breath) and wondering whether he was fated to die of a respiratory disease, as his mother did. These brilliant creative spirits persevered, fighting past the restrictions of asthma, and created transcendent literature and music that still speaks to us today.

Perhaps you're a budding Beethoven, a youthful Jackie Joyner-Kersee, or an up-and-coming Teddy Roosevelt. You can accomplish your dreams and hopes for the future, despite having asthma — especially if you and your doctor ensure that you receive the necessary treatment to appropriately and effectively manage your condition. As I explain throughout Part III of this book, you can control your asthma — don't let your asthma control you.

Augustus Caesar

The grand-nephew of Julius Caesar, Gaius Octavius (63 B.C.- A.D. 14) began his life with a slight advantage over his future rivals. However, when his powerful great-uncle was assassinated on the Ides of March (March 15) in 44 B.C., 18-year-old Octavius could hardly have known that he would someday become the first, and ultimately most famous, ruler of the ancient Roman Empire. Octavius fought battles, both political and military, for 17 years before consolidating his power, eliminating his foes (most notably Mark Antony, who was distracted by Cleopatra, the exotic Egyptian queen), and creating the position of Roman Emperor for himself. When he became emperor, Octavius also took on a new name: Augustus, which means "the Exalted."

Augustus acquired his empire while also fighting asthma, according to ancient writings on his life. However, instead of using respiratory difficulties as an excuse — no accounts of Augustus saying, "I came, I saw, I coughed" have come to light — he forged an empire that encompassed everything from England to Egypt.

Peter the Great

The youngest son of Czar Alexis, Peter (1672-1725) wasn't expected to become head of state, but when his older half-siblings died early, he became co-ruler at the age of 10 and sole czar at age 24. While his lungs fought asthma, Peter battled the Turks and later the Swedes, eventually winning access to the Baltic Sea and founding Russia's "window on the West," Saint Petersburg.

Peter the Great's early experiences of learning from foreigners, especially Dutch traders and merchants, helped fuel his desire to open Russia to Western trade, inventions, and ideas, setting in motion a process that continues (with considerable challenges) to the present day.

Ludwig van Beethoven

Most people know that Beethoven (1770-1827) contended with the worst affliction any musician could face: deafness. And yet, even as his hearing began to deteriorate at age 29 and continued until he became completely deaf at age 46, Beethoven managed to compose some of the most dramatic and beautiful works ever written in the Western classical music tradition.

Beethoven's hearing wasn't his only challenge: The first recorded account of illness in Beethoven's life was an asthma attack he experienced at age 16. He subsequently suffered "numerous colds and bronchitis" for most of his adult life. However, Beethoven pushed the *Pathetique* side of his existence away and aimed for the *Eroica,* becoming one of the world's greatest composers. (No one knows whether a coughing fit inspired the famous opening motif of Beethoven's Fifth Symphony.)

The great German master may have taken some solace from the fact that the Italian composer Antonio Vivaldi (1678-1741) was also asthmatic. Short of breath or not, Vivaldi composed many wonderful works that music lovers continue to enjoy — most notably, *The Four Seasons.*

Charles Dickens

"Please, sir, I want some more." Although Oliver Twist, hero of one of Dickens' best-loved novels, speaks that famous line, it's not hard to imagine the author himself pleading for a bit more oxygen to reach his lungs — without a coughing fit to go with it. Although Dickens (1812-1870) grew up in London, where the air was dank with the smoke and fog (hence, smog) of the Industrial Revolution, the great writer apparently didn't experience real respiratory trouble until he was 37. A vacation retreat to the seaside town of Bonchurch left him allergy-ridden, coughing, and sick to his stomach. Dickens felt relief only after he departed for the inland country surroundings of Broadstairs in Kent.

Over the next few years, asthmatic characters filled Dickens' novels, from Mr. Omer in *David Copperfield* to Mr. Sleary in *Hard Times*. In his correspondence with friends and relations, the author cited nights in which he couldn't sleep because of constant coughing. Dickens also reported that only opiates, which were popular asthma remedies of the time, helped his symptoms. As I explain in Chapter 12, more effective medications (with far fewer side effects) now exist for treating asthma. Despite his condition, Dickens wrote dozens of terrific books and stories, becoming (along with Shakespeare) one of the two most popular writers of all time in the English language.

Dickens was not the only writer and social commentator who rose above asthma. Other significant literary figures with asthma include French author Marcel Proust (1871-1922), Welsh poet Dylan Thomas (1914-1953), and American author John Updike (born 1932).

Teddy Roosevelt

Theodore (Teddy) Roosevelt (1858-1919) lived with asthma from infancy but overcame the disease in a big way, becoming a prolific author, military hero, and, at age 42, the 26th president of the United States. Perhaps more important for children, he also provided the namesake for the teddy bear.

Roosevelt did everything in a big way: Throughout his childhood, he dealt with numerous diseases, bad eyesight, and unsuccessful asthma remedies. But a course of vigorous exercise, which "TR" — as he was also known — began at age 12, eventually helped lessen his attacks. (See Chapter 14 for more information on how exercise can help youngsters with asthma.)

Roosevelt's positive outlook on life, in spite of the many challenges facing him, also kept him from turning his asthma into an excuse for self-pity or losing his wry sense of humor. Referring to one asthma episode, the 15-year-old Teddy wrote, "Except for the fact that I cannot speak, without blowing like an abridged edition of a hippopotamus, it does not inconvenience me much."

In 1884, a terrible pair of tragedies struck Roosevelt: His first wife and his mother died on the same day. Beset by grief, which may have contributed to the serious asthma episodes that plagued him in the wake of his loss, Roosevelt's doctor advised leaving the cooler, humid weather of upstate New York for the drier climate of the West. Horseback riding and a change in surroundings seemed to help TR's recovery.

As I explain in Chapter 5, however, relocating to a drier climate rarely works these days because of the abundance of non-native plants that so many settlers and developers introduced to the western parts of North America during the last century. (Take a look under *allergists* in the yellow pages of the Phoenix telephone directory, and you'll see what I mean.)

Roosevelt, who was quite the fun-loving, rough-housing parent, sometimes suffered asthma episodes after pillow-fights with his children. Therefore, some medical scholars suggest that Teddy was allergic to feathers. However, old "Rough and Ready" fought his asthma well enough to lead his volunteer troops up San Juan Hill during the Spanish-American War and subsequently become a successful two-term president, with his face carved into Mount Rushmore.

Years after he left office, TR ran for president again, this time as an independent candidate. Although he survived an assassination attempt during that campaign, he eventually lost the election to Woodrow Wilson (1856-1924), himself an asthmatic.

John F. Kennedy

So much has been written about John F. Kennedy's tragic and untimely death at the age of 46 that it's easy to overlook the many health problems he faced throughout his life. From his early childhood, Kennedy (1917-1963) was prone to disease, including asthma. His medical history also included childhood scarlet fever and diphtheria; adolescent afflictions such as bronchitis, sinusitis (see Chapter 9), and an irritable colon; hepatitis in college; malaria during World War II; and struggles with hypothyroidism, ulcers, and urinary tract infections later in life.

In 1954, complications from back surgery led to a staph infection that nearly killed the future president. In addition to these ailments, *atopy* (a genetic predisposition to developing allergic conditions), which ran in the Kennedy family, showed up throughout John's life in the form of food allergies and (most significantly) allergic reactions to animal dander, particularly dog and horsehair. These reactions often triggered asthma episodes, which plagued Kennedy throughout his life.

As a result, during Kennedy's teenage years, his family kept their beloved dogs outdoors — a less than adequate attempt at avoidance and allergy-proofing (see Chapters 6 and 11). The Kennedys loved dogs: Think of all those images of the clan roughhousing with furry friends in Hyannisport. Therefore, JFK (as Kennedy was also known) was often exposed to these potent asthma triggers (see Chapter 11), either through direct contact with canines or from dander that invariably collected on the clothes of friends and family members and which then permeated indoor environments.

But JFK was remarkably resilient, fighting through his many obstacles to become a U.S. senator from Massachusetts and, in 1960, the youngest elected president in U.S. history. Kennedy contended with his allergies, the related asthma attacks, and the laryngitis that occasionally followed during his years in public office. Not until his years in the White House was Kennedy able to appreciably reduce his sensitivities to animal dander — thanks to a long course of allergy shots (see Chapter 8) that his allergist, Paul F. de Gara (1903-1991), administered.

Because he also suffered from Addison's disease, a condition marked by insufficient adrenal function, Kennedy required cortisone to boost his adrenal levels. This cortisone therapy may have helped control his asthma, reducing the underlying airway inflammation (see Chapter 10).

Ultimately, Kennedy led an extraordinarily productive and successful life despite his physical ailments, championing anti-discrimination policies, supporting the arts and culture, and facing down Soviet missiles in Cuba, all in inspiring fashion. Although a standoff with Khrushchev or Castro might have flustered others, JFK didn't flinch. (And neither did Castro's fellow Latin American revolutionary Ché Guevara [1928-1967], also a longtime asthma sufferer.)

Leonard Bernstein

Arguably the most famous American-born conductor of classical music, and certainly one of the most influential figures in American culture, Leonard Bernstein (1918-1990) made his mark on the world despite living with asthma from infancy. In fact, Bernstein had numerous childhood asthma episodes, sometimes turning blue from lack of oxygen.

Lenny had an incredible will to learn and succeed, however, insisting on taking piano lessons even though his father was willing to pay only the tiniest of fees in an ultimately unsuccessful attempt at dissuading his son from a career in music. In his early 20s, Bernstein graduated from Harvard with honors and became the assistant conductor of the New York Philharmonic. Lenny's first big break came in 1943 when he replaced ailing music director Bruno Walter on the podium at the last minute, leading a performance that wowed the Big Apple's classical music establishment.

Bernstein had an immeasurable impact on the arts in his native land and around the world. He showcased his talent as the composer of dynamic, innovative Broadway musicals such as *West Side Story* and *Kaddish,* a dramatic, semi-liturgical piece. Likewise, Bernstein flamboyantly conducted symphony orchestras and incisively taught TV audiences about the wonders of great music.

Bernstein's asthma was a constant presence throughout his success, largely because he aggravated the condition by chain-smoking from early adulthood until the end of his life. Lenny's wheezing was often so severe that audiences heard it over the sound of the orchestra during performances.

Because of his incessant smoking, Bernstein developed emphysema, which, unlike asthma, often leads to irreversible, destructive lung damage. (See Chapter 11 for more reasons why smoking is a bad idea, especially if you have a respiratory condition such as asthma.) When he finally succumbed to a heart attack in 1990, Bernstein was suffering from asthma complicated by emphysema, a lung tumor, and progressive heart failure.

Liza Minnelli

"What good is sitting alone in your room? Come hear the music play," sang Liza Minnelli (born 1946) in her Academy Award-winning performance from the 1972 film *Cabaret*. Throughout her life, Minnelli has followed that advice and then some, as one of the few performers in history to win the triple-stakes of an Oscar, an Emmy, and a Tony, in addition to building a worldwide following of devoted fans.

Beginning in early childhood, Minnelli performed in films and on stage, first as a guest of her legendary mother, Judy Garland, and on her own in her late teens. Considering the extraordinary vocal power that Minnelli displays night after night in concert, you may not suspect that she has asthma or other lung problems.

Although she has dealt with bouts of bronchitis in recent years and several physical mishaps have sidelined her at times, Minnelli continues to make the music "play," as a committed singer, actress, and humanitarian who inspires others rather than "sitting alone in her room."

Kenny G

Despite his asthma, inhaling enough oxygen to make his instrument sing doesn't seem to be a problem for the soprano saxophonist Kenny Gorelick (born 1956), better known as Kenny G. Likewise, asthma hasn't stopped this tuneful reed player from becoming the most commercially successful instrumental artist in the history of recorded music.

In fact, the biggest-selling album of all time by an instrumentalist is Kenny G's ironically titled *Breathless*. More than 15 years into his solo career, Kenny G continues his string of chart-topping releases and has recently dedicated efforts to raise money for school music programs, helping students learn about the power of music.

On the other side of the musical coin, veteran shock-rocker Alice Cooper (born 1947) has also carved out a long career despite having asthma.

Jackie Joyner-Kersee

Growing up in a rough East St. Louis neighborhood, Jackie Joyner (born 1962) had plenty to overcome as a child. She avoided drugs and violence, and she struggled to find money to support her athletic training. Joyner persevered and concentrated her considerable abilities on several sporting pursuits at once, becoming a high-school basketball star, excelling in various track and field events, and playing volleyball. She graduated in the top 10 percent of her class and won a basketball scholarship to UCLA, where she met her track-and-field coach and future husband, Bob Kersee.

In 1983, a year before she competed in her first Olympics, Joyner-Kersee was diagnosed with asthma. Although she began taking medication for her condition soon afterwards, she often used her prescribed products only when she thought she needed them rather than following her doctor's instructions for regular use. A serious asthma episode during Olympic training in 1988 — triggered by breathing cold air — made her realize the vital importance of using her medication as prescribed, on a consistent basis, to keep her condition under control. (See Chapter 11 for more information on exercise-induced asthma, or EIA.)

Neither her respiratory condition nor her related allergies have kept Joyner-Kersee from reaching the pinnacle of her sport. She won three gold medals in track and field and still holds the world record for the heptathlon, a demanding seven-part grouping of events. She is the only woman to have received the *Sporting News Man of the Year* award. Many sports analysts consider Joyner-Kersee the greatest woman athlete in the world, perhaps of all time.

Likewise, other famous athletes have also overcome asthma to reach the top of their fields. Some of these stellar achievers include

- ✔ Dennis Rodman, a leading rebounder in the NBA and a key member of several championship teams (also part-time actor and fashion trendsetter)
- ✔ Art Monk, one of the most successful wide receivers in NFL history
- ✔ Jerome Bettis, a top NFL running back who has rushed over 1,000 yards per season for several years
- ✔ Greg Louganis, Olympic diving gold medalist
- ✔ Amy Van Dyken, Olympic swimming gold medalist
- ✔ Nancy Hogshead, Olympic swimming gold medalist

Appendix

Resources for Additional Information

● ●

*T*his appendix lists organizations, publications (books and periodicals), other forms of media (such as videotapes), and Web sites related to the subjects that I discuss throughout this book.

Organizations

The organizations in this section, which I list in alphabetical order (to make these listings easier to use), can provide you with valuable information about many aspects of dealing with allergies and asthma.

Allergy and Asthma Network
Mothers of Asthmatics, Inc.
2751 Prosperity Ave.
Suite 150
Fairfax, VA 22031
800-878-4403 703-641-9595
www.aanma.org

Allergy Foundation of Canada
Box 194
Saskatoon, Saskatchewan S7K 355
306-652-1608

American Academy of Allergy,
Asthma, and Immunology
611 East Wells St.
Milwaukee, WI 53202
800-822-2762 414-272-6071
www.aaaai.org

American College of Allergy,
Asthma, and Immunology
85 W. Algonquin Road, Suite 550
Arlington Heights, IL 60005
847-427-1200
www.acaai.org

American College of
Chest Physicians
3300 Dundee Road
Northbrook, IL 60062-2348
847-498-1400 800-842-7777
www.chestnet.org

American Dietetic Association
216 W. Jackson Blvd., Suite 800
Chicago, IL 60606-6995
800-366-1655 312-899-0040
www.eatright.org

American Lung Association
1740 Broadway
New York, NY 10019
800-LUNGUSA (586-4872)
212-315-8700
www.lungusa.org

American Thoracic Society
1740 Broadway
New York, NY 10019
212-315-8700
www.thoracic.org

Asthma and Allergy
Foundation of America
1233 20th St. N.W., #402
Washington, DC 20036
800-727-8462 202-466-7643
www.aafa.org
*Contact the AAFA for information on
the regional chapter nearest you.*

Asthma Society of Canada
425-130 Bridgeland Ave.
Toronto, Ontario M6A1Z4
416-787-4050 416-787-5807
www.asthma.ca

Canadian Society of Allergy
and Clinical Immunology
774 Echo Drive
Ottawa, Ontario K1S 5N8
613-730-6272 800-668-3740
http://csaci.medical.org
E-mail: csaci@rcpsc.edu

Environmental Protection
Agency Indoor Air Quality
Information Clearinghouse
401 M St. SW
Washington, D.C. 20460
800-438-4318 703-356-4020
www.epa.gov
E-mail: iaqinfo@aol.com
*Contact this EPA office for
information on indoor air quality.*

Food Allergy Network
10400 Eaton Place, Suite 107
Fairfax, VA 22030-2208
800-929-4040 703-691-3179
www.foodallergy.org

Food and Drug Administration
FDA, HFI-40
Rockville, MD 20857
310-827-6250 888-463-6332
(INFOFDA)
www.fda.gov

Healthy Kids
79 Elmore St.
Newton, MA 02459-1137
617-965-9637
E-mail: erg_hk@juno.com

Immune Deficiency Foundation
25 W. Chesapeake Ave., Suite 206
Towson, MD 21204
800-296-4433 410-321-9165
www.primaryimmune.org

International Food
Information Council
1100 Connecticut Ave. NW,
Suite 430
Washington, D.C. 20036
202-296-6540
ificinfo.health.org

Joint Council of Allergy, Asthma,
and Immunology
50 N. Brockway, Suite 3-3
Palatine, IL 60067
847-934-1918
www.jcaai.org
*Guidelines for allergy and asthma
treatment are located at this
Web site.*

Journal of American
Medical Association
JAMA Asthma Information Center
American Medical Association
515 N. State St.
Chicago, IL 60610
800-262-2350
www.ama-assn.org/asthma

Latex Allergy Information Service
176 Roosevelt Ave.
Torrington, CT 06790
860-482-6869
www.latexallergyhelp.com

The Lung Association
1900 City Park Drive, Suite 508
Blair Business Park
Gloucester, Ontario K1J 1A3
613-747-6776
www.lung.ca/ca/

National Allergy Bureau
611 E. Wells St.
Milwaukee, WI 53202-3889
414-272-6071
Year-round indoor allergy report
877-9-ACHOOO
Pollen and mold report
800-9-POLLEN (976-5536)
www.aaaai.org
*Contact the NAB for information on
its bureaus throughout the U.S. and
Canada and in many other countries, which report on local pollen
and mold conditions.*

National Asthma Education
and Prevention
NHLBI Information Center
P.O. Box 30105
Bethseda, MD 20824-0105
301-592-8573
www.nhlbi.nih.gov

National Eczema Association
for Science and Education
1220 SW Morrison
Suite 433
Portland, OR 97205
503-228-4430
www.eczema-assn.org

National Heart, Lung,
and Blood Institute
NHLBI Information Center
P.O. Box 30105
Bethseda, MD 20824-0105
301-592-8573
www.nhlbi.nih.gov

National Institute for
Occupational Safety and Health
U.S. Dept. of Health
and Human Services
4676 Columbia Parkway
(Mail Drop R2)
Cincinnati, OH 45226
513-533-8236
800-35-NIOSH (356-4674)
www.cdc.gov/niosh

National Institute of Allergy
and Infectious Diseases
Building 31, Room 7A-50
31 Center Dr.
Bethseda, MD 20892-2520
301-496-5717
www.niaid.nih.gov

National Jewish Medical and
Research Center
1400 Jackson St.
Denver, CO 80206
303-388-4461
800-222-LUNG (5864)
www.njc.org

Asthma Camps

The American Lung Association (ALA) and other organizations sponsor children's asthma camps to educate youngsters about their conditions, while also providing them with safe and healthy experiences in natural settings.

Contact the ALA, the Asthma and Allergy Foundation of America, or Allergy and Asthma Network•Mothers of Asthmatics, Inc. (find their numbers in "Organizations," earlier in this appendix), for information regarding a camp in your area.

Asthma and Allergy Environmental-Control Products

This section provides contact information for manufacturers and suppliers of the items that I mention throughout the book, especially for controlling exposure to allergens (see Chapters 6 and 11), devices for inhaling asthma medications (Chapter 12), and devices that you can use to test your lung function at home (Chapter 13).

Suppliers

The following companies distribute allergy and asthma control products, including allergen barrier encasings for mattresses, box springs, comforters, and pillows; allergenic blankets and linens; HEPA and ULPA air filters, filters, and vacuum cleaners; humidifiers and inhaled medication delivery systems; nebulizers and spacers; and numerous mold, dust mite, and dander control products.

Allerguard, Inc.
40 Cindy Lane
Ocean, NJ 07712
800-234-0816 732-988-6868

Allergy Asthma
Technology, Ltd.
8224 Lehigh Ave.
Morton Grove, IL 60053
847-966-2952 800-621-5545

Allergy Clean Environments
PO Box 9067
San Rafael, CA 94912
800-882-4110 415-459-4003

Allergy Control Products, Inc.
96 Danbury Rd.
Ridgefield, CT 06877
203-438-9580 800-422-3878
www.allergycontrol.com

American Allergy Supply
PO Box 722022
Houston, TX 77272
800-321-1096 713-995-6110
www.americanallergy.com

Enviro Remedies Allergy
Relief Products
693 West Reading Ave.
Reading, PA 19611
610-371-0123 800-315-3461
www.enviro-remedies.com

National Allergy Supply, Inc.
1620-D Satellite Blvd.
Duluth, GA 30097
760-623-3237 800-522-1448
www.nationalallergy
supply.com

Manufacturers of asthma and allergy products

The following list provides contact information for manufacturers that sell specific allergy and asthma products, which I describe throughout this book, directly to consumers.

Ferraris Medical, Inc.
(Manufacturers of Pocket Peak Flow Meters and distributors of Mini-Wright Peak Flow Meters.)
9681 Wagner Rd.
PO Box 344
Holland, NY 14080
716-537-2391
419-535-7490 (order department in Toledo, OH)
800-205-7187
www.ferrarismedicalusa.com

Honeywell
(Manufacturers of HEPA and ULPA air filtration systems.)
101 Columbia Road
Morristown, NJ 07962
973-455-2000
www.honeywell.com

MedicAlert Foundation
(Manufacturers of emergency medical information necklaces and bracelets. Ask your doctor about wearing a medical tag if you're at risk of anaphylaxis from a life-threatening allergic reaction.)
2323 Colorado Ave.
Turlock, CA 95382
209-668-3333 800-432-5378
www.medicalert.org

Respironics Health Scan Asthma Allergy Products
(Manufacturers of Assess Peak Flow Meters.)
908 Thompton Ave.
Cedar Grove, NJ 07009
973-857-3414 800-962-1266
www.respironics.com

Vitaire Corporation
(Manufacturers of Vitaire HEPA air purifiers and allergen barrier encasings for
mattresses, box springs, and pillows.)
141 Lanza Ave.
Garfield, NJ 07026
973-473-2244
800-552-5533

In Other Words: Other Writings and Media about Asthma and Allergies

The books, periodicals, and videos in this section cover a wide range of
topics related to asthma and allergies. I highly recommend all the titles that I
list here as sources of valuable information.

Books

*A Parent's Guide to Asthma: How You Can Help Your Child Control Asthma at
Home, School, and Play*
Nancy Sander
Plume/Penguin, 1994. $10.95

Asthma & Exercise
Nancy Hogshead and Gerald Couzens
Henry Holt and Company, 1990. $19.95

Complete Book of Children's Allergies
B. Robert Feldman, M.D., with David Carroll
Times Books, 1986. $17.95

Dr. Tom Plaut's Asthma Guide for People of All Ages
Thomas F. Plaut M.D. with Teresa B. Jones, MA
Pedipress, Inc., 1999. $25.00
125 Red Gate Lane
Amherst, MA 01002
800-611-6081
www.pedipress.com

One Minute Asthma: What You Need to Know
(also available in Spanish as *El asma en un minuto: Lo que usted
necesita saber*)
Thomas F. Plaut, M.D.
Pedipress, Inc., 1998. $5.00

Taking Charge of Asthma
Betty B. Wray, M.D.
John Wiley & Sons, 1997. $14.95

Periodicals

Asthma Magazine
3 Bridge St.
Newton, MA 02458
800-527-3284
Six issues per year; $19.95

Allergy and Asthma Health
Allergy and Asthma Network ∑ Mothers of Asthmatics, Inc.
2751 Prosperity Ave., Suite 150
Fairfax, VA 22031
800-878-4403
Web site: www.aanma.org
E-mail: aanma@aol.com
Quarterly: Full-color magazine provides in-depth coverage of allergy and asthma issues from leading medical and consumer experts. Includes mini-magazine just for kids. $12.95 per year.

The Reporter and Breathing Matters
Asthma and Allergy Foundation of America (AAFA) newsletters
1233 20th St. NW, Suite 402
Washington, D.C. 20036
800-7-ASTHMA (727-8462)
www.aafa.org

Videotapes

Breathe Easy: Getting the Most From Your Asthma Medication
Gary Rachclefsky, M.D., and Colleen Lum Lung, R.N., M.S.N., C.P.N.P.
Key Pharmaceuticals, Inc.
Videotape: 30 minutes

It Only Takes One Bite
Food Allergy Network
800-929-4040
Videotape: 18 minutes; $20.00

Food Allergies: Fact or Fiction
Food Allergy Network
800-929-4040
Videotape: $20.00

The Elephant Who Couldn't Eat Peanuts
Food Allergy Network
800-929-4040
Videotape: $15.00

Internet Resources

This section provides Web site addresses for selected organizations and topics that provide helpful information online about products, services, topics concerning asthma and allergy, as well as news about developments in related medical research.

`healthwatch.medscape.com`: tune into the Asthma channel for the latest asthma features, news, and advice from experts on asthma.

`webmd.com`: serves all aspects of the healthcare industry, from consumers to medical professionals. Allows you to stay up to date with breaking health news, ask experts questions during live chat events, and share your feelings with others on message boards devoted to your interests.

`gazoontite.com`: Yes, it's meant to sound like *gesundheit,* but the company spells its name differently. Site provides allergy and asthma products and information.

`allergy.mcg.edu`: Allergy, asthma, and immunology online. An information and news service for patients, parents of patients, purchasers of group health care programs, and the news media.

`askdrbob.com`: Witty and informative Web site featuring Dr. Bob Lanier's *60-Second Housecall* segments, many on allergy and asthma topics.

`drkoop.com`: Web site affiliated with the former Surgeon General, containing library of allergy articles with information about the latest news, research, and treatment options.

Index

Notes